Problem-Based Behavioral Science and Psychiatry

Anthony Guerrero · Melissa Piasecki
Editors

Problem-Based Behavioral Science and Psychiatry

Foreword by Richard T. Kasuya

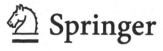 Springer

Editors
Anthony Guerrero
University of Hawai'i
John A. Burns School of Medicine
Honolulu, HI
USA
GuerreroA@dop.hawaii.edu

Melissa Piasecki
University of Nevada School of Medicine
Reno, NV
USA
mpiasecki@medicine.nevada.edu

ISBN: 978-1-4419-2653-1   e-ISBN: 978-0-387-78585-1

Printed on acid-free paper

9 8 7 6 5 4 3 2 1

springer.com

We dedicate this book to our parents, with love.
Celina and Reuben Guerrero
Joan and Leo Piasecki

Foreword

Learning behavioral science is an important part of becoming physicians. More and more, professional and accrediting organizations are explicitly endorsing the necessity of physicians being skilled and well trained in these areas.

Physicians themselves are increasingly aware of the importance of behavioral health and psychiatric issues in their practices. Whether one intends to practice in a primary care or subspecialty area, an appreciation of behavioral health issues and basic principles of psychiatry is critically necessary. In addition to topics that are more specific to the practice of psychiatry, the authors of this textbook have chosen to cover a range of topics important to all aspects of clinical medicine, including culture, violence, physician–patient relationships, adherence and substance abuse. Almost any practicing physician will admit that effectively addressing these types of behavioral issues is among the more challenging of the tasks they face.

Teaching and learning about psychiatry and behavioral sciences can be difficult. Basic textbooks do not easily connect their lessons with the complexity of clinical reality. Students cannot easily find the clinical importance from classroom lectures. Even clinical clerkships in psychiatry have difficulty exposing students to the breadth of clinical experiences they need to learn about.

This long overdue book holds the promise of becoming a solution to these challenges. The study of psychiatry and the behavioral sciences is perfectly matched with the problem-based learning methods utilized in this book. Problem-based learning (PBL) is a widely utilized approach to learning that involves the detailed study of patient cases, with a primary goal of identifying topics for self-study relevant to the cases. This approach helps students find meaning in learning a wide variety of topics and provides an opportunity to apply new knowledge to clinical situations. Through understanding the cases, they learn psychiatry.

For those familiar with the PBL process, this book offers a welcome resource in the area of behavioral sciences and psychiatry. Students are sometimes reluctant to vigorously pursue a study of behavioral issues. They often cite a difficulty in finding reliable, evidence-based resources for their independent learning. Unlike the biological and clinical sciences, where there are scores of readily available textbooks, review articles and web-based resources, students often report frustration with the relative dearth of medical student-friendly resources in the behavioral sciences. This book represents a significant addition to student learning resources in behavioral health and should become a familiar and well-worn companion to students in PBL environments.

For those new to the PBL process, this book will also serve as a useful guide to approaching clinical problems. By working through the case studies in this book, the reader will not only be able to learn important material related to psychiatry and the behavioral sciences but also develop a systematic approach to life-long learning that will serve them well in their clerkships and beyond.

In addition to providing opportunities to work through clinical vignettes in a problem-based learning format, the authors incorporate other useful and practical learning tools such as mechanistic case diagramming and the bio-psycho-social-cultural-spiritual formulation. In the long term, readers will benefit as much from these exercises as they will from learning the content within the pages of this book. The authors have also incorporated content areas for the United States Medical Licensing Examinations, making this textbook relevant for preparation and review for these examinations. So, in many ways, this book represents a learning tool as much as a content resource.

I am also particularly encouraged to see that a number of the contributors to this book are themselves graduates of PBL medical schools. Their experiences should provide them with a unique and valuable perspective in what they have chosen to offer in the pages that follow.

Readers will find the methodology and approaches offered in this book to be refreshing and educationally rewarding. I hope that this text will prove to be the first of a number of books that skillfully and thoughtfully blend authoritative content with effective problem-based learning exercises.

Director, Office of Medical Education   Richard T. Kasuya, M.D., M.S.Ed.
Professor of Medicine

School of Medicine   John A. Burns
University of Hawai'i at Mānoa

Contents

Part I   Introduction

1   **How to Use This Book** 3
Anthony P.S. Guerrero, Melissa Piasecki, and Nathanael W. Cardon

Part II   Human Behavior

2   **Childhood Development** 17
Maya Strange and Andrea Sorensen

3   **Effects of Experience on Brain Development** 31
Jeffrey Raskin, Whitney Waldroup, Nikhil Majumdar,
and Melissa Piasecki

4   **Learning Principles of Human Behavior** 49
David O. Antonuccio and Amber Hayes

5   **Sexuality Throughout the Life Cycle** 67
Kevin Allen Mack and Anthony P.S. Guerrero

6   **Adaptation and Coping in a Medical Setting** 77
Maria-Christina Stewart

7   **Violence and Abuse** 89
Jeanelle J. Sugimoto and Anthony P.S. Guerrero

Part III   Healthcare Principles

8   **The Physician–Patient Relationship** 107
My Kha and Melissa Piasecki

9 **Ethics and Professionalism** 121
Jacob Doris and Marin Gillis

10 **Adherence in Medicine** 133
Maxwell Takai Frank and Eriko Takai Frank

11 **Stress and Health** 141
Michael K. Daines and Nikhil Majumdar

12 **Health Care 101** 151
David C. Fiore and Jason P. Crawford

13 **Stigma and Medicine** 171
Barbara Kohlenberg, Melanie Watkins and Lindsay Fletcher

14 **Culture, Ethnicity, and Medicine** 183
Anthony P.S. Guerrero

15 **Quantitative Measures in Healthcare** 193
M. Anand Samtani, Earl S. Hishinuma, and Deborah A. Goebert

16 **Death, Dying, and End-of-Life Care** 215
Lori Murayama-Sung and Iqbal Ahmed

Part IV Behavioral Neuroscience and Clinical Psychiatry

17 **Basic Principles of Evaluation: Interviewing, Mental Status
Examination, Differential Diagnosis, and Treatment Planning** 231
Anthony P.S. Guerrero, Daniel A. Alicata, and Nathanael W. Cardon

18 **Disorders of Childhood** 253
Erika Ryst and Jeremy Matuszak

19 **Substance Use Disorders** 269
William F. Haning III and Anthony P.S. Guerrero

20 **Psychotic Disorders** 289
Steven J. Zuchowski and Ryan Ley

21 **Mood Disorders and Suicide** 309
Mireille Anawati

22 **Anxiety Disorders** 325
Mireille Anawati

23 Somatoform Disorders 339
Jonah Shull and Catherine McCarthy

24 Personality Disorders 353
Latha Pai, Melissa Piasecki, and M. Nathan Mason

25 Cognitive Disorders 367
Russ S. Muramatsu and Junji Takeshita

26 Sleep Disorders 381
Ole J. Thienhaus and Nathanael W. Cardon

27 Eating Disorders 393
Hy Gia Park and Cathy K. Bell

28 Sexual Disorders 409
Crissa R. Draper, Nikhil Majumdar, William T. O'Donohue,
and Melissa Piasecki

29 Other Disorders 423
Anthony P.S. Guerrero

Index 435

Contributors

Iqbal Ahmed, M.D., FRCPsych (UK)
Professor of Psychiatry, University of Hawai'i John A. Burns School of Medicine,
University of Hawai'i

Daniel A. Alicata, M.D., Ph.D.
Assistant Professor of Psychiatry, Psychiatry Clerkship Director, University of
Hawai'i John A. Burns School of Medicine

Mireille Anawati, B.A.
Fourth Year Medical Student, University of Hawai'i John A. Burns School of
Medicine

David O. Antonuccio, Ph.D.
Professor of Psychiatry, University of Nevada School of Medicine

Cathy K. Bell, M.D.
Assistant Professor of Psychiatry, Program Director Child and Adolescent
Psychiatry Residency Program, University of Hawai'i John A. Burns School of
Medicine

Nathanael W. Cardon, D.O.
Resident in Psychiatry, University of Nevada School of Medicine

Jason P. Crawford, M.D., M.P.H.
Assistant Professor, Family and Community Medicine, University of Nevada
School of Medicine

Michael K. Daines, M.D.
Assistant Professor of Psychiatry, University of Nevada School of Medicine

Jacob Doris, M.D.
Resident in Psychiatry, University of Nevada School of Medicine

Crissa R. Draper, M.S.
Graduate Student in Psychology, University of Nevada, Reno

David C. Fiore, M.D.
Associate Professor, Family and Community Medicine, University of Nevada
School of Medicine

Lindsay Fletcher, B.A.
Graduate Student, Psychology, University of Nevada, Reno

Marin Gillis, L.Ph., Ph.D.
Director of Medical Humanities and Ethics, University of Nevada School of
Medicine

Deborah A. Goebert, Dr.P.H.
Associate Professor of Psychiatry, Associate Director, Research Division,
Department of Psychiatry, University of Hawai'i John A. Burns School of Medicine

Anthony P.S. Guerrero, M.D.
Associate Professor of Psychiatry and Pediatrics, Associate Chair for Education
and Training, Department of Psychiatry, University of Hawai'i John A. Burns
School of Medicine

William F. Haning, III, M.D., FASAM, FAPA
Associate Professor of Psychiatry, Program Director, Addiction Psychia-
try/Addiction Medicine, Director, Graduate Affairs, University of Hawai'i John A.
Burns School of Medicine

Amber Hayes, M.D.
Resident in Family Medicine, University of Nevada School of Medicine

Earl S. Hishinuma, Ph.D.
Professor of Psychiatry, Associate Chair for Research, Department of Psychiatry,
University of Hawai'i John A. Burns School of Medicine

My Kha, M.D.
Resident in Psychiatry, University of Nevada School of Medicine

Barbara Kohlenberg, Ph.D.
Associate Professor of Psychiatry, University of Nevada School of Medicine

Ryan Ley, M.D.
Resident in Psychiatry, University of Nevada School of Medicine

Kevin Allen Mack, M.S., M.D.
Assistant Professor, University of California, Berkeley/San Francisco

Nikhil Majumdar, M.D.
Resident in Psychiatry, University of Nevada School of Medicine

M. Nathan Mason, M.D.
Resident in Psychiatry, University of Nevada School of Medicine

Jeremy Matuszak, M.D.
Fellow, Child Psychiatry, University of Nevada School of Medicine

Catherine McCarthy, M.D.
Assistant Professor, Family and Community Medicine, University of Nevada
School of Medicine

Russ S. Muramatsu, M.D.
Fellow in Geriatric Psychiatry, University of Hawai'i John A. Burns School of
Medicine

Lori Murayama-Sung, M.D.
Chief Resident, General Psychiatry Program, University of Hawai'i John A. Burns
School of Medicine

William O'Donahue, Ph.D.
Professor in Psychology, University of Nevada, Reno

Latha Pai, M.D.
Resident in Psychiatry, University of Nevada School of Medicine

Hy Gia Park, M.P.H., M.S.
Fourth Year Medical Student, University of Hawai'i John A. Burns School of
Medicine

Melissa Piasecki, M.D.
Associate Professor of Psychiatry, University of Nevada School of Medicine

Jeffrey Raskin
Medical Student, University of Nevada School of Medicine

Erika Ryst, M.D.
Assistant Professor of Psychiatry, University of Nevada School of Medicine

Mohan Anand Samtani, M.A.
Statistician, Department of Psychiatry, University of Hawai'i John A. Burns School
of Medicine

Jonah Shull, M.D.
Fellow, Child Psychiatry, University of Nevada School of Medicine

Andrea Sorensen, M.D.
Child and Adolescent Psychiatry Fellow, University of Nevada School of Medicine

Maria-Christina Stewart, M.A.
Department of Psychology, University of Hawai'i, Currently a Research Fellow at
the Center for Anxiety and Related, Disorders, Boston University

Maya Strange, M.D.
Assistant Professor of Psychiatry, University of Nevada School of Medicine

Jeanelle J. Sugimoto, B.S.
Program Manager, Asian/Pacific Islander Youth Violence Prevention Center,
Department of Psychiatry, University of Hawai'i John A. Burns School of Medicine

Eriko Takai Frank, M.S.W., M.P.H.
Staff Social Worker, Beth Israel Deaconess Medical Center

Maxwell Takai Frank, M.D.
Resident in Psychiatry, Boston University Medical Center

Junji Takeshita, M.D.
Associate Professor of Psychiatry, Program Director, Geriatric Psychiatry
Residency Program, Associate Chair for Clinical Services, Department of
Psychiatry, University of Hawai'i John A. Burns School of Medicine

Ole J. Thienhaus, M.D., M.B.A.
Professor and Chair of Psychiatry, University of Nevada School of Medicine

Whitney Waldroup, M.D., M.P.H.
University of Nevada School of Medicine

Melanie Watkins, M.D.
Resident in Psychiatry, University of Nevada School of Medicine

Steven J. Zuchowski, M.D.
Assistant Professor, University of Nevada School of Medicine

Part I
Introduction

Chapter 1
How to Use This Book

Anthony P.S. Guerrero, Melissa Piasecki, and Nathanael W. Cardon

Welcome to *Problem-Based Behavioral Science and Psychiatry*. In this chapter, our aims are to illustrate how the problem-based learning process works so that you can apply it to the other cases in this textbook.

The goals of this chapter are:

1. To provide the reader with a guided experience on "how to use this textbook"
2. To review basic principles of problem-based learning and the rationale for why this approach is used
3. To illustrate, with a sample case, the processes of

    (a) "Progressive disclosure"
    (b) Identifying facts/problems, hypotheses/differential diagnoses, additional clinical information needed, and learning issues
    (c) Thinking about underlying neurobiology and other physiological mechanisms to understand the signs and symptoms of a case

4. To review the more generic process of bio-psycho-social-cultural-spiritual formulation, in order to understand the various perspectives offered by patient cases

Because a textbook is not the same as a patient encounter or face-to-face small group discussion, we are not claiming to represent problem-based learning (PBL) in a pure or "authentic" form (Barrows, 1986,2000). However, we hope to integrate many of the principles and potential benefits of PBL into this textbook.

PBL, as described by Norman and Schmidt (1992), aims to endow learners with the skills of clinical reasoning, cooperative learning, and patient-based integration of knowledge. In its ideal form, it begins with an initial free-inquiry process, in which learners explicitly discuss hypotheses and additional lines of investigation. This is followed by a period of self-directed learning and a synthesis and application of information back to the case. The student then has an opportunity to critically evaluate the initial clinical reasoning process. Because PBL attempts to integrate information from multiple disciplines, all phases of the process emphasize attention

A.P.S. Guerrero
Associate Professor of Psychiatry and Pediatrics, Associate Chair for Education and Training, Department of Psychiatry, University of Hawai'i John A. Burns School of Medicine

A. Guerrero, M. Piasecki (eds.), *Problem-Based Behavioral Science and Psychiatry*,
© Springer Science+Business Media, LLC 2008

to the biological, behavioral, and populational aspects of the case. Certain articles (Guerrero, 2001; Guerrero et al., 2003) have discussed how certain learning tools can be used to ensure that beneficial PBL processes actually occur in the course of studying a case. We will illustrate these tools, including "mechanistic case diagramming," as part of this sample case.

When compared to traditional learning methods, PBL may enhance the application of concepts to clinical situations, long-term retention of knowledge, and lifelong interest in learning (Norman and Schmidt, 1992). It has been shown to improve student and faculty satisfaction and educational outcomes in numerous clinical disciplines, including family medicine, pediatrics, obstetrics, and psychiatry (Washington et al., 1999; McGrew et al., 1999; Kaufman and Mann, 1999; Curtis et al., 2001; Nalesnik et al., 2004; McParland et al., 2004). Furthermore, we believe that psychiatry and the behavioral sciences, because of the inherently integrative and holistic approaches of these subject areas, are particularly well suited for study in a PBL format (Frick, 2005; Zisook, 2005). Peters et al. (2000) reports on the longitudinal outcomes of a randomized controlled trial and concludes that the New Pathways Program at Harvard Medical School—of which PBL is one important component—improved students' interpersonal skills and humanistic approach to patient care, with no loss in medical knowledge.

We will illustrate the problem-based learning process as applied to cases in this textbook. Typically, each chapter will begin with an introductory paragraph for a case. An example has been provided below.

Case Vignette 1.1.1 Presenting Situation: Melanie Crystal

Melanie Crystal is a 39-year-old woman who is the single mother of a 17-year-old boy. She was referred for psychiatric assessment at the local emergency room because a police officer on foot patrol found her crying and confused in a nearby parking lot. She is tearful and hostile. She told the screening nurse that she would kill herself "at the first opportunity." On screening for substance use, she stated that she used "dope." Needle marks were visible on both arms.

At this point, the student will see the following sign, which is a prompt to "Proceed with the PBL process" before moving on to the remainder of the case.

 Please proceed with the problem-based approach!

Learning from these cases will be maximized if the student carefully digests all components of the case and engages in the clinical reasoning processes that a clinician uses to effectively evaluate and manage the case. For example, in the case above, it may be worthwhile to:

1. Highlight or underline the facts.
2. Specifically identify the clinical signs and symptoms that are present, as these are likely to be the relative "endpoints" of a mechanism that must be subsequently understood. Below we show a graphical way of identifying signs and symptoms through use of boxes.

   Melanie Crystal is a 39-year-old woman who is the single mother of a 17-year-old boy. She was referred for psychiatric assessment at the local emergency room because a police officer on foot patrol found her ⎡crying⎤ and ⎡confused⎤ in a nearby parking lot. She is ⎡tearful⎤ and ⎡hostile⎤. She told the screening nurse that she ⎡would kill herself⎤ "at the first opportunity." On screening for substance use, she stated that she used "dope." ⎡Needle marks⎤ were visible on both arms.
3. Organize these findings as shown in Table 1.1 (blank samples are provided for photocopying in Appendix).
4. Use this grid to guide the clinical reasoning process that will guide further evaluation and management of the case.

Obviously, there will be variations in the specific items one will choose to put under each of the columns. The main principles to follow are:

1. To develop specific hypotheses, ask the question "What are the possible *mechanisms* (biological or otherwise) behind the signs and symptoms present in the case?" In this text we emphasize the neurological and physiological mechanisms that are known to be associated with normal and pathological behavior.
2. Additional clinical information ("What do you want to know next?") reflects your hypotheses and should follow a logical clinical organization.

In this textbook, the use of the clinical reasoning process will prompt or answer many of the questions in the rightmost column. Each clinical case includes text coverage of the learning issues likely to be most relevant to medical student learners. Therefore, if this sample chapter were an actual textbook chapter, it might contain sections on:

- The mechanisms behind abnormal mood and confusion
- The mechanisms of action of common illicit drugs
- Definitions of child abuse and neglect

Some chapters offer high-density tables and figures to illustrate mechanisms of action. Examples include: the mechanism of psychotic symptoms (see Fig. 20.1) and the mechanism of action of common substances of abuse (see Table 19.1).

With an effective clinical reasoning process, the subsequent sections of the case will address items in the "what do you want to know next" column. A sample continuation of the case vignette is shown below.

Table 1.1 Grid to guide the clinical reasoning process that will guide further evaluation and management of the case

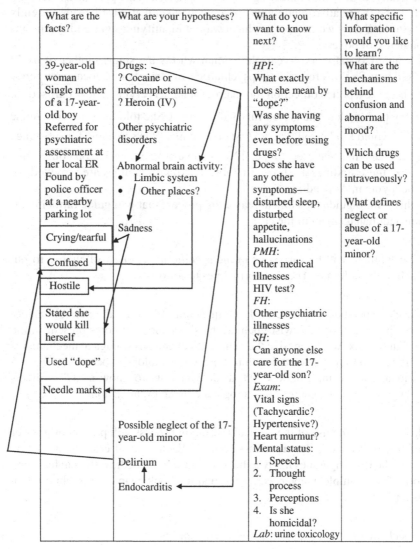

What are the facts?	What are your hypotheses?	What do you want to know next?	What specific information would you like to learn?
39-year-old woman Single mother of a 17-year-old boy Referred for psychiatric assessment at her local ER Found by police officer at a nearby parking lot	Drugs: ? Cocaine or methamphetamine ? Heroin (IV) Other psychiatric disorders Abnormal brain activity: • Limbic system • Other places? Sadness	*HPI*: What exactly does she mean by "dope?" Was she having any symptoms even before using drugs? Does she have any other symptoms— disturbed sleep, disturbed appetite, hallucinations	What are the mechanisms behind confusion and abnormal mood? Which drugs can be used intravenously? What defines neglect or abuse of a 17-year-old minor?
Crying/tearful		*PMH*:	
Confused		Other medical illnesses	
Hostile		HIV test?	
Stated she would kill herself		*FH*: Other psychiatric illnesses	
Used "dope"		*SH*: Can anyone else care for the 17-year-old son?	
Needle marks		*Exam*:	
	Possible neglect of the 17-year-old minor	Vital signs (Tachycardic? Hypertensive?) Heart murmur?	
	Delirium	Mental status: 1. Speech 2. Thought process	
	Endocarditis	3. Perceptions 4. Is she homicidal?	
		Lab: urine toxicology	

Case Vignette 1.1.2 Continuation

Ms. Crystal was uncooperative with further questioning. Attempts to reach collateral informants were unsuccessful. On examination, vital signs were as follows: temperature 100.3 °F, pulse 106 per minute, blood pressure 142/88, respiratory rate 22 per minute. The remainder of the physical examination was unremarkable except for: thin appearance, poor dentition, and needle marks on her skin. Mental status examination was remarkable for: poor cooperation and eye contact, mumbled rapid speech, labile and tearful affect, tangential thoughts, possible auditory hallucinations, and suicidal ideations.

Please proceed with the problem-based approach!

Once again, this is the prompt to analyze the case and complete the table as shown above.

Case Vignette 1.1.3 Conclusion

After admission to an inpatient unit, Ms. Crystal went to sleep and remained asleep for almost 14 hours. She was ravenously hungry and only marginally cooperative with measurements of vital signs or attempts at interview. She remained irritable and was verbally abusive to staff for the next day.

Three days later, Ms. Crystal became conversant with the staff. On the fourth day she was pleasant and social. She described her history of methamphetamine dependence beginning in her twenties, with 10 years of abstinence. She stated that she stopped going to meetings and "it only took one guy" who showed her the drug at his home. She reported that as soon as she saw and "smelled" methamphetamine, she began to have intense cravings and immediately relapsed. She has used daily for the last month or so and is not sure where her adolescent son is. She thinks he will be graduating from high school "one of these days."

The case and text discussion cover core curricular material relevant to the general subject matter. For example, if the goal of the chapter were to review methamphetamine abuse and dependence (please refer to Chap. 19), the following topics may be covered:

Epidemiology (including the recent epidemic, age groups affected, mortality statistics)
Differential diagnosis (including mood, psychotic, and other substance disorders)
Etiology and neurobiological mechanisms
Clinical findings (including cognitive changes, psychotic symptoms, motor symptoms, acute and secondary drug effects, and craving)
Treatment (psychosocial and pharmacological)
Social, cultural, and legal factors
Prognosis

Bio-psycho-social-cultural-spiritual Model

In all our teaching, we invite students to conceptualize patient problems by using a bio-psycho-social-cultural-spiritual formulation. This model is used throughout the psychiatric curriculum at the authors' institutions. The goal of these patient formulations is to consider the complexities of patient presentations and to drive treatment planning. Formulations help explain "how did this patient get to this psychiatric state at this time?"

What follows is a description of the components of the bio-psycho-social-cultural spiritual formulation (adapted from Kohlenberg and Piasecki, 2006). We have added prompts for the students to help them think about and organize clinical material. Students are encouraged to include each component in formulations.

This model generally includes the following:

Biological

Past:

  Genetics:

- Consider whether any blood relatives have had psychiatric problems, substance use problems or suicide attempts/suicides. Is there a history of close relatives who have been hospitalized for psychiatric reasons? What kind of treatments did they get, and how did they respond?

  History of pregnancy and birth:

- Consider pregnancy variables: Was there in utero exposure to nicotine, alcohol, medications, or illicit substances? Was there anything unusual about pregnancy?
- Note birth complications, such as prematurity, birth trauma, or extended periods of hospitalization.

  Relevant previous illnesses:

- Consider any history of head injury, endocrine disorders (e.g., thyroid, adrenal), seizures, malignancies, or neurological illnesses.
- Consider potential lasting effects of past substance use on brain functions such as cognition, affective regulation, etc.

Present:

  Current illnesses:

- Identify current illnesses and any direct impact they may have on psychiatric presentation.

  Medications:

- Assess current medication regimen. Consider whether these medications have psychoactive effects (e.g., steroids, beta blockers, pain medications, benzodiazepines, serotonin-selective reuptake inhibitors, antipsychotics). Consider possible side effects of current medications. Note any noncompliance with medications.

Substances:

- Consider the influence of nicotine, alcohol, and illicit drugs on current psychiatric symptoms.
- Consider the possible effects of substance withdrawal.

Endocrine/hormonal:

- Consider the impact of onset of adolescence.
- Consider the impact of the menstrual cycle, pregnancy, postpartum period, menopause.

Psychological

Past:

- Comment on any past history of trauma (child abuse, combat, rape, serious illness), as well as resiliency (how the patient coped with trauma, e.g., through friends, family, religion).
- Consider the sources of positive self-image and positive role models.
- Comment on the patient's experience with loss.
- Comment on the patient's quality of relationships with important figures, such as grandparents, friends, significant teachers, or significant employers.
- Comment on how past medical problems, substance use, or psychiatric problems impacted the patient's development and their relevance to the patient today.

Present:

- Describe the recent events and experiences that precipitated the admission or appointment.
- What are the current stressors? Do they have any symbolic meaning?
- Assess and comment on coping skills, defense mechanisms, presence or absence of cognitive distortions.
- Consider current developmental demands on the person, such as marriage, divorce, birth, children leaving home, loss, aging, etc. What stage of development is the patient at now? Is it appropriate to chronological age?
- What is the developmental impact of the patient's illness?

Social

- How adequate is the patient's current support system?
- What is the current status of relationships with important figures?
- What are the possible peer influences?
- Consider the patient's current housing arrangement.
- Comment on vocational/financial status.
- Comment on any relevant legal problems.
- Consider the role of agencies (e.g., Veteran's Administration, Child Protective Services, Criminal Justice System) on the patient.

Cultural

- Comment on cultural influences and acculturative pressures that may impact the current situation.
- Comment on cultural influences on understanding of illness and/or help-seeking behavior.

Spiritual

- Comment on the role of spirituality in the patient's life.
- Is the patient affiliated with a spiritual community of some sort?
- How does spirituality contribute to the patient's ability to hope, his/her position on suicide if relevant, or his/her contact with a supportive community?

A sample formulation for Ms. Crystal would be as follows:

This is a 39-year-old woman with acute psychiatric symptoms. Biological factors that contribute to her presentation include the acute effects of methamphetamine on her mood and behavior. Methamphetamine is likely also contributing to her abnormal vital signs. There is no history of current or previous medical problems, family history of substance use disorder/mental illness or current medication use.

Psychologically, this patient has recently experienced a relapse. Cues for drug use included the sight and smell of the drug. She apparently lacked coping skills for resisting relapse. There is no information about recent stressors, past trauma, or relationship history. Her role as the mother of a 17-year-old has been seriously compromised but there is little information about how she perceives this. Her relationship with a man appears to be superficial and based on mutual drug use.

Socially, we have little information about her employment status, housing, legal situation, or social supports. She appears to have benefited from meetings in the past and may have been lacking the social support she needed to remain abstinent prior to her relapse.

Spiritually, we have little information about her history and current beliefs.

In addition, we believe that both pre-clerkship behavioral science students and clerkship psychiatry students can benefit from seeing a "big-picture" graphic representation of the formulation. This graphic uses arrows to detail how one aspect of the case leads to another and ultimately results in her presenting concerns. It also shows how the biological, psychological, and social/spiritual/cultural aspects are ultimately related and suggests how all knowledge learned (including basic neurobiological mechanisms) can be used to benefit the patient in the form of specific treatments (shown as circled items, connected to the rest of the diagram using dotted arrows). An example is shown in Fig. 1.1.

While it is up to the readers to decide on the degree to which such an exercise suits their learning needs, the textbook chapters will provide such diagrams on some of the cases, in order to integrate knowledge learned in the chapter and to provide closure to the case vignettes, particularly those that cover major psychiatric illnesses and symptoms (e.g., substance use disorders, mood disorders, anxiety disorders, cognitive disorders, and eating disorders). It is our hope that this feature

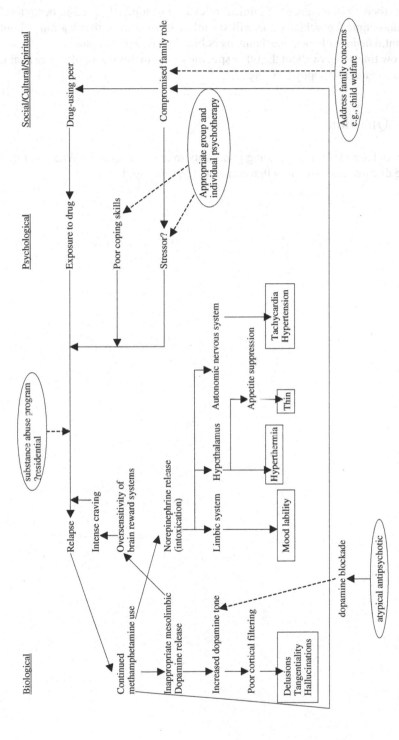

Fig. 1.1 Sample diagram to integrate knowledge and provide closure to case vignettes

of this textbook will enhance the clinical relevance of topics learned in behavioral science and clinical psychiatry and will stimulate interest in further learning about fundamental neurobiological mechanisms behind behavioral symptoms.

It is now time to learn about the other specific topics in this textbook. Once again, welcome aboard, and happy learning!

Review Question

1. Problem based learning is gaining popularity in medical schools. What are three of the documented outcomes that contribute to this popularity?

Appendix PBL Worksheet to Guide Case Studies

What are the facts?	What are your hypotheses?	What do you want to know next?	What specific information would you like to learn about?
		History of Present Illness:	
		Past Medical History:	
		Family History:	
		Social History:	
		Exam:	
		Labs:	

References

Barrows HS. A taxonomy of problem-based learning methods. Med Educ 1986;20:481–486.

Barrows HS. Authentic problem-based learning. In Teaching and Learning in Medical and Surgical Education: Lessons Learned for the 21st Century. Distlehorst LH, Dunnington GL, Folse JR, eds. Mahwah, NJ: Lawrence Erlbaum Associates, 2000.

Curtis JA, Indyk D, Taylor B. Successful use of problem-based learning in a third-year pediatric clerkship. Ambul Pediatr 2001;1:132–135.

Frick E. Teaching somatoform disorders in a "nervous system and behaviour" course: the opportunities and limitations of problem-based learning. Educ Health (Abingdon) 2005;18(2): 246–255.

Guerrero AP. Mechanistic case diagramming: a tool for problem-based learning. Acad Med 2001;76(4):385–389.

Guerrero AP, Hishinuma ES, Serrano AC, Ahmed I. Use of the mechanistic case diagramming technique to teach the biopsychosocial-cultural formulation to psychiatric clerks. Acad Psychiatry 2003;27(2):88–92.

Kaufman DM, Mann KV. Achievement of students in a conventional and problem-based learning (PBL) curriculum. Adv Health Sci Educ Theory Pract 1999;4(3):245–260.

Kohlenberg B, Piasecki M. Bio Psycho Social Spiritual Model, personal communication, 2006.

McGrew MC, Skipper B, Palley T, Kaufman A. Student and faculty perceptions of problem-based learning on a family medicine clerkship. Fam Med 1999;31:171–176.

McParland M, Noble LM, Livingston G. The effectiveness of problem-based learning compared to traditional teaching in undergraduate psychiatry. Med Educ 2004;38(8):859–867.

Nalesnik SW, Heaton JO, Olsen CH, Haffner WH, Zahn CM. Incorporating problem-based learning into an obstetrics/gynecology clerkship impact on student satisfaction and grades. Am J Obstet Gynecol 2004;190:1375–1381.

Norman GR, Schmidt HG. The psychological basis of problem-based learning: a review of the evidence. Acad Med 1992;67:557–565.

Peters AS, Greenberger-Rosovsky R, Crowder C, Block SD, Moore GT. Long-term outcomes of the New Pathway Program at Harvard Medical School: A randomized controlled trial. Acad Med 2000;75(5):470–479.

Washington ET, Tysinger JW, Snell LM, Palmer LR. Implementing problem-based learning in a family medicine clerkship. Fam Med 1999;31:306–307.

Zisook S, Benjamin S, Balon R, Glick I, Louie A, Moutier C, Moyer T, Santos C, Servis M. Alternate methods of teaching psychopharmacology. Acad Psychiatry 2005;29(2):141–154. Review.

Part II
Human Behavior

Chapter 2
Childhood Development

Maya Strange and Andrea Sorensen

In order to detect and diagnose pathology in children and adolescents, clinicians need to recognize the bounds of normal behaviors. Rapid changes in the developing child make "normal" behavior a moving target. These three cases illustrate some of the challenges to parents and professionals.

At the end of this chapter, the reader will be able to

1. Describe normal emotional development in a preschool age child, a middle-school age child and an adolescent.
2. Discuss protective factors for normal development and how parents can foster normal development in a child.
3. Identify ways in which stages of development, personality traits, family, culture and society influence adaptation and coping.
4. Describe some risk factors for developing psychopathology at various stages of development.
5. Relate how a child's developmental stage influences the physician–patient interview.

Case Vignette 2.1.1 Presenting Situation: Caleb

You are a third-year resident at a pediatric clinic where 34-month-old Caleb is brought in by his parents with the concern that he has emotional outbursts. With further discussion, Caleb's mother shares that she has a sister diagnosed with Bipolar Disorder and is concerned that he has a mood disorder or Attention-Deficit Hyperactivity Disorder "like his cousins." The parents describe that Caleb can "rage." They say that he lies on the floor and flails around while screaming or runs from them and slams doors. He sometimes stands with stiff arms and legs and cries inconsolably.

M. Strange
Assistant Professor of Psychiatry, University of Nevada School of Medicine

A. Guerrero, M. Piasecki (eds.), *Problem-Based Behavioral Science and Psychiatry*,
© Springer Science+Business Media, LLC 2008

Please proceed with the problem-based approach!

Case Vignette 2.1.2 Continuation

The parents note that the "rages" can last up to 10 minutes and may occur several times a day. They both agree that triggers for the outbursts may be when he doesn't get what he wants, when they may not understand him, and when it is around nap or bed time. The father says that he is able to speak sternly with Caleb or sit him in a chair for 1–2 minutes, after which he usually calms down. The mother says that she can become frustrated with him and usually ends up yelling at him to be quiet. When you ask, she gives an example from that morning: she gave Caleb crayons and paper but he only colored for a few minutes and then wanted to play with blocks. She redirected him to the coloring and he sat on the floor and "raged" for 5 minutes. She yelled "Stop it!" then felt guilty, so she gave him the blocks and walked away.

Caleb was the product of a full-term first pregnancy without exposures or complications. He was easy to feed and has always slept well at night. He responded appropriately socially, with babbling and peek-a-boo play in infancy, pointing at objects as a toddler, and enjoying being with other children as a toddler. He crawled at 10 months and walked at 15 months. Currently, he can eat with a fork, undress, ride a tricycle, color a circle and a line, and identify colors and much of the alphabet. He speaks in three-word sentences and demonstrates a quickly growing vocabulary. He has no significant medical illnesses or significant injuries. They tell you that Caleb seems happy outside of these episodes.

You ask to see Caleb alone, and he agrees to let his parents leave the room. On exam, Caleb seems shy, but then starts to push a toy truck around the room while he makes truck sounds. He colors on a sheet of paper and hands you a pen and asks you to draw a circle. He then draws several circles as well and smiles. He is able to build a nine-block tower, then knocks it over and laughs. He finds a Spider Man toy, and you respond "You found Spider Man." Caleb then starts to tell you how the superhero jumps and gets the bad guy. He jumps up and down himself. He tells you that he has a Spider Man at home that he sleeps with in his bed. He asks for his mother a few times during the exam, but is willing to keep playing. He makes good eye contact and shares smiles. He denies that anyone has ever hurt him or made him particularly scared (he does admit he's scared of the dark). When his parents return, he runs to his mother and hugs her.

Please proceed with the problem-based approach!

Case Vignette 2.1.3 Continuation

Caleb attends daycare 3 days a week for the past 6 months. The teacher told Caleb's mother that he did have difficulty sharing with the other kids initially. He would tantrum, sometimes to the point of hitting other children, if he had to share toys. He responded to counts to three and time-outs in the time-out chair at school. The teacher counts to three to give him time to calm down or facilitates a trading of toys when another child has what he wants. He can also choose to play with a different toy. If he does not make a trade, play with a different toy, or calm down by the count of three, then he gets a time-out. Initially he required several time-outs a day, but for the past 2 months has had only one time-out every few days. The teachers have not noted any other concerns.

Learning Issues

Caleb behaves like a normal boy of his age. His cognitive development is on track: he is using multiple word sentences and pronouns, he names objects, colors, and knows letters. His daily living skills are also well developed for his age. Nearly 3 years old, he is learning to use utensils, undress, and even dress himself and use the toilet. His motor skills are also on target, as he is able to effectively interact with and explore his environment. Socially, he demonstrates that he is able to communicate, appreciate personal boundaries, and share affect (Smidt, 2006). His play and conversations remain self-centered, but this is expected in toddlers and preschoolers. This self-centered perspective of the young child can be frustrating for many adults especially if they do not appreciate this developmental stage. Caleb is only focused on his interests and does not ask the examiner of her opinion or her interests. His attention span is limited to 5 or 10 minutes, and he changes activities frequently. It is clear, however, that the examiner's presence is important to Caleb. The adult provides a reference for the child and can serve to share experiences and encourage appropriate exploration, communication, and expansion on Caleb's own self-awareness during his play.

According to Erikson, a child of this age is in the midst of the developmental phase of autonomy versus shame and doubt (18 months–3.5 years), during which the child seeks to attain autonomy. As the young child becomes more aware of being a separate individual with differing wants/needs from the parents, he or she may start to strongly resist limits. "No!" is a common refrain heard by parents. There is a battle of the wills as the child attempts to exert initial control. Effective communication and established trust between the child and the caretaker are essential for how this stage is resolved. In fact, parents who learn to apply supportive interactions will have ongoing rewards, as the child's efforts toward greater separation may begin during this phase but will continue throughout childhood (Wiener and Dulcan, 2004).

It is also important to consider the neurodevelopment occurring in the preschooler's brain. At birth, the human brain already has a hundred billion neurons, but is still only a fraction of the size it will be in adulthood. As a child experiences life, these neurons branch dendrites and synapse to one another to form networks of great complexity that integrate their understanding of their environment and their control over their own abilities. The brain also develops by layering neurons with insulating myelin to increase the speed of conducted information. Finally, this process is completed by the neurons pruning themselves of less useful dendritic and synaptic connections (Higgins and George, 2007). Only one-fifth of neurons are programmed by the age of 2. Through exploration and testing of limits, the young child gathers data for programming the other 80 % of the brain. The child's desire for social and environmental interactions are paramount to learning (Lewis, 2002).

Most parents understand that they serve a critical role in providing a safe and interesting environment as well as rules and structure to help children learn without physical injury. Emotional development and learning affective (emotional) regulation also requires such interactive parenting. A child may push the limits of behavior in an attempt to further engage in exploration and continue his self-serving behaviors. A caregiver can acknowledge this desire and voice an understanding that the child desires to learn. ("I know that you want to go across the street and see how the garbage truck picks up garbage.") It is important to remain accessible to the child to help shape his or her expectations. The caregiver can clearly identify the child's desires versus the real and acceptable options for the child. ("We can't go near the truck, but we can watch it from over here or go home and read about trucks.") Offering the child options and time to make a decision helps the child develop self-awareness and problem solving.

When children resist and retaliate, it may be time for a brief and respectful consequence. If the child makes a good choice then it is helpful to immediately praise the child. Consistency in these ongoing interactions models appropriate emotional and behavioral regulation and also nurtures the child's security and attachment with the caregiver. Piaget noted that the 2- to 5year-old child is in a preoperational developmental phase, which is egocentric from a cognitive, affective, perceptual, and social standpoint. Sociocultural theorists describe, however, that children this age utilize significant social referencing. They offer the concept of scaffolding, in which problem solving for the young child occurs with helpful adults who are the child's primary tool for learning (Lewis, 2002).

Case Vignette 2.1.4 Conclusion

You reassure Caleb's parents that he is normal, bright and healthy. You offer your favorite resource for parenting: 1,2,3 Magic! (Phelan, 2003) and Your Child (Pruitt, 2000), as well as the American Academy of Child and Adolescent Psychiatry's website, with resources for parents. You strongly recommend that both parents observe the preschool teacher's techniques so that they can see what works at the school and be consistent at home. A local resource for parenting classes is reviewed. They are encouraged to return to the clinic if these initial recommendations are not effective for the family.

Case Vignette 2.2.1 Presenting Situation: Susana

Susana is a 10-year-old Hispanic girl brought to your Outpatient Clinic by her mother, who is worried that she has had difficulty concentrating and crying episodes in the past few weeks. The girl sits politely next to her mother with a sad expression and wide opened eyes. She is holding a rubber toy dinosaur close to her chest with her right hand and is touching her mother's arm with her left hand. Susana is an only child and has not had any major health problems in the past.

Please proceed with the problem-based approach!

Case Vignette 2.2.2 Continued

Susana's mother tearfully tells you that her husband, Susana's father, passed away from cancer last month. He had been sick for several months and in hospice care at their home. She says that even before he died, Susana had been having difficulty completing her work at school and her homework. Susana's teacher sent a note home that her worksheets are covered with drawings of clouds and the sky. Her mother tells you that Susana has been crying for about 20 minutes a few times a day for the past several weeks. One time she became frantic when she couldn't find the toy dinosaur that she has been carrying with her for the past 2 months—a gift from her father for her ninth birthday. She also has awakened her mother at night in a panic needing to find a particular T-shirt that her father used to wear. Once she finds the shirt, she goes back to sleep. Her mother notes that even though her sleep has been disturbed, her appetite has remained fine. You glance at the chart and see that Susana is slightly above the 50th percentile for weight.

Please proceed with the problem-based approach!

Case Vignette 2.2.3 Continued

When asked about their support system, Susana's mother tells you that they do not have much family, but they do attend a grief group at their church. They have been able to talk about the impact of the father's death.

You ask to speak to Susana alone. When asked about friends, Susana tells you about two close friends. She has been able to play with them and tells them her feelings about missing her father. Susana tells you that her grades continue to be good in school, and she enjoys riding bikes or playing computer games. She feels angry when she sees other kids with their fathers. She still feels that it is unfair that her father had to die.

Looking at the sky and the clouds are a comfort because she feels her father is "up there" and with her always.

 Please proceed with the problem-based approach!

Learning Issues

Grief is the emotional pain or anguish that one feels after the loss of a loved one. Anticipatory grief is a similar emotional pain that occurs before the impending death. Three categories, based on age and maturity, of a child's understanding of death have been described. Three to five-year-old children look at death as sleep or a long journey. Five to nine-year-olds accept that someone can die; however, they do not believe it happens to everyone and especially not to themselves. By 10 years of age, children know that death is inevitable and that it may happen to them. Normal bereavement is not considered a disorder, and loss of a close friend or relative occurs to up to half of all youths by the age of 21. Loss of a parent may occur to approximately 4 % of children by age 18 (Lewis, 2002).

Susana's developmental phase has been described by Erikson as industry versus inferiority (5–12 years old). This is a time during which a child develops a sense of competence and focuses on self-worth. The child learns how to become a friend and to identify with a peer group. He or she also gains satisfaction in experiencing hard work that leads to success and also learns to compensate for their weaknesses in some areas by noting accomplishments in other areas. The child not only learns to read but eventually "reads to learn." Motor development also progresses, and physical activity can be a positive way to engage with peers and master a talent (e.g., playground games such as tag; team sports such as soccer and softball). Piaget describes the cognitive stage of concrete operations. The child is able to conceptualize rather than simply perceive, but is not yet able to utilize abstract thinking. Thus, Susana may understand the irreversibility and inevitability of death, but may have difficulty in applying the concept generally. She may continue to have concerns about potential harm to her own body, not just her father's. Mastery of these thoughts may be seen in dreams or play. If the child becomes overwhelmed, however, he or she may feel vulnerable or even helpless.

Just as a child's body goes through a maturation process at puberty, her brain also undergoes regular maturation processes through the formative years. Susana is at an age where she is just between two peaks in brain development. Between the ages of 4 and 8, her brain continues the process of development. This occurs through gray-matter loss and by maturing the primary sensorimotor regions which consolidate basic sensory and motor function. Between the ages of 11 and 13 her brain will peak in development in the regions of spatial orientation and language (Toga et al., 2006). This process of gray-matter loss maturation will go on through adolescence. From the earliest studies on brain volumes, children between 8 and 10 have been shown to have significantly more cortical gray-matter relative to cerebral size than young adults do (Sowell et al., 2004). Thinning of specific regions in the brain represents focused maturation of the cognitive abilities associated with those regions. For example, thinning of the left dorsal frontal and parietal lobes in children aged 5–11 has been correlated with improved performance on a test of verbal functioning (Toga et al., 2006).

Further research is needed to clarify the psychiatric morbidity among adults who lost a parent in childhood. It helps to recognize complicated bereavement in children in order to minimize morbidity later in life for these individuals. Symptoms of complicated grief are: longing and searching for the loved one, preoccupation with thoughts of the loved one, purposelessness and futility about the future, numbness and detachment from others, difficulty accepting death, lost sense of control and security, and anger and bitterness over the death. The anger can lead to problems in interactions with family and friends, schoolwork, and other activities. Even 2 years after the parent's death, preadolescent girls were noted to have more anxiety, depression, and aggressive behaviors than controls, and adolescent boys were noted to be more withdrawn and have more social problems than their matched controls. Adolescent girls and preadolescent boys showed no differences from their matched controls. Overall, approximately 20 % of children who suffered the death of a parent had serious problems at 1 year that could require treatment such as counseling (Melham et al., 2007).

Case Vignette 2.2.4 Conclusion

You are able to reassure Susana's mother that she is experiencing normal grief. This can present in myriad ways—some children cry, some avoid, and others respond by denying that the death occurred. Susana and her mother were commended for their open communication and participation with community and peer groups that are supportive. It will be important to maintain open lines of communication to allow Susana to express sadness, anger, and memories of her father as she works to process grief. You advise Susana's mother to be aware of signs of pathological grief, as described above. Many cities have bereavement groups and resources for children who have lost a parent. This can be a wonderful source of support, because often a child can otherwise feel very alone in this experience.

Case Vignette 2.3.1 Brian

Brian is a 15-year-old male with a history of insulin-dependent diabetes who comes to your family medicine clinic with his mother. He is currently in the 10th grade at the local public high school and lives with his mother, 17-year-old-sister, and 11-year-old brother. Brian's parents divorced when he was 9. His father, who lives in town, sees Brian and his siblings every week. His mother brought him to see you for an evaluation due to concerns about some of his recent behavior. Over the past 6 months, he has changed from a "sweet, loving, and attentive son," to a "stranger." She tells you that he spends most of his time in his room, on the phone with friends, or on the computer. He used to be a conscientious student, but recently has been doing his homework at the last minute. The last semester he lost his 4.0-grade average and currently has three Bs on his report card. Brian has also been staying up late and sleeping in more on the weekends. His taste in music and dress has changed. She describes that he used to be very neat, but more recently has been wearing "skater" clothes, and he pierced his ear and eyebrow. He has been talking about getting tattoos. His eating habits have changed, and he has been more casual about managing his blood glucose levels.

 Please proceed with the problem-based approach!

Case Vignette 2.3.2 Continuation

You meet with Brian without his mother. He is soft-spoken and cooperative, with brown shaggy hair, a large hooded sweatshirt and baggy jeans. He tells you he doesn't know why his mother brought him in and that she "overreacts" to everything. Brian reports that he was diagnosed with diabetes when he was 10 years old, "so things were pretty stressful then." He says, "I know I should do better (managing his diabetes), but sometimes I just want to eat without thinking about it, and it's a pain carrying my insulin around all of the time." Brian used to spend more time at home in elementary and middle school because "I didn't have anyone my age to hang out with, so I hung out with my mom." He states that his mother is fairly strict. "It's unfair. My sister would never do anything my mom wouldn't like, so she now doesn't know what to do with me." He doesn't tell his mother too much about his girlfriend or his friends "because it usually turns into a lecture." Brian also has positive things to say about his family: "My mom is an awesome cook, and she would do anything for us. My sister is kind of a dork, but she always looks out for me."

Brian tells you that school has been going fairly well, though he could try harder. He skipped school a few times when the weather was warmer to go skateboarding with friends. He also has a girlfriend and says it's a serious relationship. He had few friends when he was younger and, until a couple of years ago, he was one of the shortest children in his class. Since starting high school, he has grown 11 inches and is now 5'9" tall. In high school he has established a large group of friends. When you ask him about substance use, he tells you that he has tried alcohol and marijuana at parties, but "they're not for me." He denies discipline problems in school, with the exception of getting detention in middle school for once having a water balloon fight during recess. He denies any history of stealing, fire setting, harm to animals, or running away. He has never been in trouble with the law.

He notes that his mood overall the past several months has been good. He has been sleeping well, but does stay up until 12 a.m. because he is either online or talking on the phone. When his parents divorced, he remembers that he was easily frustrated and somewhat angry at his father, but he continued to enjoy his usual activities and perform well in school. He has a good appetite and denies history of or current suicidal ideation or self-injury. In addition to skateboarding, he likes to write, listen to music, and play guitar. He works at an ice cream shop 10 hours per week, and reportedly his supervisor hopes he can work longer hours during his school breaks. Brian's ultimate goal is to become a professional skateboarder, but if that does not work out, he would like to eventually open his own skate shop or do "accounting, like my dad."

You invite Brian's mother to talk with you alone. Brian was diagnosed with diabetes after presenting to the emergency room in diabetic ketoacidosis. Brian's mother strictly managed his diet and blood glucose levels. Recently, Brian has wanted more responsibility, and his last hemoglobin A1C was 7 (previous levels had been in the normal range). She tells you that Brian is a "great kid," but points out that her own brother had some behavioral difficulties when younger, and started using substances during high school. Brian's mother was raised in a very religious household, and her brother was regularly in conflict with the family. Her brother continues to use substances, has irregular contact with the family, has spent time in jail related to his drug use, and has been unable to maintain steady employment. Brian's mother says, "I may be completely off base, but I just don't want to see what happened to my brother happen to Brian."

 Please proceed with the problem-based approach!

At this point the differential remains quite broad. Brian's change in behavior including being more isolative, change in school performance and sleep patterns could suggest possible substance use, depression, or even disruptive behavior disorder. It would be important to understand how Brian's change in behavior is affecting his function in other areas, such as with friends, school, or work.

Teenagers at risk for developing serious substance problems include those who: have a family history of substance use, are depressed, have low self-esteem, feel like they do not fit in or are out of the mainstream. Signs and symptoms of substance use may be physical fatigue, repeated health complaints, red or glazed eyes, and a lasting cough. Emotional complaints may be personality change, sudden mood changes, irritability, irresponsible behavior, low self-esteem, poor judgment, depression, and general lack of interest. The family may notice the teen argues more, breaks rules, and is more withdrawn. School concerns are decreased interest, negative attitude, drop in grades, many absences, truancy, and discipline problems. The teen may have new friends who are less interested in standard home and school activities, have problems with the law, and are interested in less conventional styles of dress and music.

It is important to discuss substance issues as well as screen for mental health disorders, as 10–15 % of the child and adolescent population have symptoms of depression at any one time (Smucker et al., 1986). The prevalence of major depression among children aged 9–17 has been estimated at 5 % (Shaffer et al., 1996) and substance use disorders are quite common.

Another consideration would be a normal variant of adolescent development. According to Erikson's stages of development, adolescence (12–17 years) is the period of identity versus identity diffusion. The adolescent's goal is the answer to the question "Who am I?" As the adolescent tries to figure this out, they may experiment with different identities and rebel against some adult expectations. This stage accompanies significant physical changes and further development of gender identity. The teen's social network increases in importance. The adolescent engages in various activities as he or she determines his or her own values and goals. The developmental goals during this time include not only solidifying one's own identity, but also separating and reconciling one's feelings for the family of origin, developing romantic relationships, and mastering one's bodily functions and impulses (Wiener and Dulcan, 2004). The normal process of separation and individuation can make this a challenging time for parents.

As adolescents approach adulthood their brains continue to develop in areas of greater and greater complexity. For example, the process of myelination to insulate neurons into greater conduction speed is already finished with ventral and deep brain structures that control primitive functions, but continues on in dorsal regions responsible for higher cognitive functions, like the prefrontal cortex, onward to adulthood. In the peak adolescence years after puberty the brain matures specific regions devoted to integrating senses and reasoning ("executive function") (Blakemore and Choudhury, 2006) (Toga et al., 2006). This picture of brain development matches with Erikson's stages of development, as it represents the brain developing in areas associated with response inhibition, emotional regulation, planning, and organization or, in other words, self-control and personal choices (Sowell et al., 2004).

Case Vignette 2.3.3 Conclusion

You discuss with Brian's mother that Brian (and she) are likely experiencing normal adolescent development. Though Brian may at times seemingly push his family away, he needs her to remain present and consistent while allowing him to explore as much as is safe (similar to in toddlerhood). It will be important to continue to express the family's values and expectations to him, though in a non-shaming way. Continuing to engage in activities as a family is also helpful to maintain open lines of communication. You refer Brian's mother to the AACAP website, particularly to the Normal Adolescent Development sections. You also meet a few months later with Brian and his mother together to discuss how each feels things are going in the family. You allow time for clarification of certain rules that are non-negotiable. It is helpful for Brian's mother to hear from him his perspective and overall positive feelings about the family.

Review Questions

1. What process of neurodevelopment is responsible for the great speed information travels in the brain?

   (a) Loss of unnecessary gray-matter.
   (b) Myelin insulation of neurons.
   (c) Pruning excess dendrite and synapse connections.
   (d) Forming new dendrite and synapse connections.

2. Which of these statements about a 3 year old would be developmentally unusual?

   (a) The child eats with a fork or spoon.
   (b) The child focuses conversations on an adult.
   (c) The child can ride a tricycle.
   (d) The child's attention span only lasts 5–10 minutes.

3. What would be a sign that a child's grief at the loss of a parent had become complicated bereavement?

   (a) Numbness and detachment from others.
   (b) Seeking out objects belonging to the deceased.
   (c) Bouts of crying between normal behavior.
   (d) Preoccupation with activities associated with the decreased.

4. What brain morphology change is correlated to improved verbal function test scores?

   (a) Thickening of the right dorsal frontal and parietal lobes.
   (b) Thinning of the right dorsal frontal and parietal lobes.
   (c) Thickening of the left dorsal frontal and parietal lobes.
   (d) Thinning of the left dorsal frontal and parietal lobes.

5. Which of these is associated with 15 year olds according to Erikson?

   (a) Satisfaction in hard work that leads to success.
   (b) Resisting limits to develop autonomy.
   (c) Learning to identify with a peer group.
   (d) Determining personal goals and values.

6. What percentage of the child and adolescent population has symptoms of depression at any one time?

   (a) 1–5%
   (b) 5–10%
   (c) 10–15%
   (d) 15–20%

Answers

1. b, 2. b, 3. a, 4. d, 5. d, 6. c

References

Blakemore, S. and Choudhury, S. (2006). Development of the adolescent brain: implications for executive function and social cognition. *J Child Psychol Psychiatry* 47(3/4), 296–212.

Higgins, E.S. and George, M.S. (2007). *The Neuroscience of Clinical Psychiatry*. Philadelphia: Lippincott Williams & Wilkins.

Lewis, M. (2002). *Child and Adolescent Psychiatry: A Comprehensive Textbook*. Philadelphia: Lippincott Williams & Wilkins.

Melham, N.M., Moritz, G., and Walker, M. (2007). Phenomenology and correlates of complicated grief in children and adolescents. *JAACP* 46(4), 493–499.

Phelan, T. (2003). *1-2-3 Magic: Effective Discipline for Children 2–12*. Glen Ellyn: Child Management, Inc.

Pruitt, D. (2000). Your Child: Emotional, Behavioral, and Cognitive Development from Birth through Preadolescence. New york: Harper Collins.

Shaffer, D. et al. (1996). The NIMH Diagnostic Interview Schedule for children, version 2.3 (DISC 2.3): Description, acceptability, prevalence rates, and performance in the MECA study methods for the Epidemiology of child and Adolescent Mental Disorders Study. J Am Acad Child Psychiatry 25, 865–877.

Smidt, W. (2006). *Nelson Essentials of Pediatrics*. Philadelphia: Elsevier Saunders.

Smucker, E.R., Craighead, W.E., and Green, B.J. (1986). Normative and reliability data for the Children's Depression Inventory. *J of Abnormal Child Psychology* 10, 277–284.

Sowell, E.R, Thompson, P.M., and Toga, A.W. (2004). Mapping changes in the human cortex throughout the span of life. *Neuroscientist* 10(4), 372–392. Review.

Toga, A.W., Thompson, P.M., and Sowell, E.R (2006). Mapping brain maturation. *Trends Neurosci* 29(3), 148–159. Review.

Wiener, J. and Dulcan, M. (2004). *The American Psychiatric Publishing Textbook of Child and Adolescent Psychiatry*. Arlington, VA: American Psychiatric Publishing.

Resources

www.aacap.org

Normal Adolescent Development Part I, No. 57; updated June 2001. www.aacap.org/cs/root/facts_for_families/normal_adolescent_development_part_i.

Normal Adolescent Development Part II, No. 58; updated June 2001. www. aacap.org/cs/root/facts_for _families/normal_adolescent_development_part_ii.

Normality, No. 22; updated July 2004. www.aacap.org/cs/root/facts_for_ families/normality.

When to Seek Help For Your Child, No. 24; updated July 2004. www.aacap.org/ page.ww?section=Facts+for+Families&name=When+To+Seek+Help+ For+Your+Child.

www.aap.org

Refer to *Caring for your Child* parenting books.

www.brightfutures.aap.org

Clark, L. (2005). SOS Help for Parents Bowling Green: SOS Programs and Parents Press.

Chapter 3
Effects of Experience on Brain Development

Jeffrey Raskin, Whitney Waldroup, Nikhil Majumdar, and Melissa Piasecki

The classic "nature–nurture" debate continues to stimulate research in human behavior. This chapter explores how experience (nurture) can modulate brain architecture and brain function. These cases illustrate how childhood experiences can have lifelong effects on behavior and well-being.

At the end of this chapter, the reader will be able to

1. Discuss the role of early experience on normal brain development
2. Identify early adverse effects of deprivation
3. Determine some common deficits which result from early deprivation
4. Describe resilience and differences in innate ability

Case Vignette 3.1.1 Peter Magellan

As the Chief Resident in a pediatrics outpatient office, you pause outside a patient's room to read the chart. You learn that inside the room there is a concerned couple and their adopted son. Having been unable to conceive naturally, the Magellans adopted a foreign-born child, Peter. They were assured at the time of adoption that Peter was 2 years old and had a normal gestation. He was born at term and is without congenital defect. Mr. and Mrs. Magellan have been waiting quietly in the exam room with their newly adopted son.

Good morning Mr. and Mrs. Magellan. My name is Dr. Sam and I will be working with you today. What brings you in? You notice Mr. Magellan remains quiet as his wife begins nervously.

Mrs. Magellan: Well, Doctor, we're very concerned because we adopted Peter four weeks ago and it seems that he just doesn't act like the other kids his age at the playground. We thought that maybe he was closed off just because of the change

J. Raskin
Medical Student, University of Nevada School of Medicine

A. Guerrero, M. Piasecki (eds.), *Problem-Based Behavioral Science and Psychiatry*,
© Springer Science+Business Media, LLC 2008

in location and language, and that it would probably pass, but . . . I don't know now. The social worker told us there may be some differences, but we just didn't anticipate this. He looks really small and he weighs less than the other kids too. Is this normal?

You notice that Peter has been quiet and still, sitting stiffly in a chair by himself, clutching a dirty looking teddy bear. He does not appear to have any interaction with his new parents. His eyes do not meet yours even when you approach him at his level. He appears frail and withdrawn. You see on the chart that Peter weighs 22 pounds and is 31 inches tall.

Mrs. Magellan: What's wrong with him?

You tell the parents that although Peter falls below the fifth percentile on the CDC growth chart for boys, this is not by itself a sign of a medical problem. You obtain more information on Peter's development. He uses one-syllable words and gestures to communicate. Although he uses the toilet, he cannot manage his clothing. He also is unable to climb down the stairs and must be carried. The Magellans bought a quantity of toys for 2-year-olds, but Peter does not show any interest in the puzzles or blocks.

Mrs. Magellan describes the adoption: Well, I read about how many orphans there were without proper care in Romania and we decided it would be best to try to save at least one of them. We looked at hundreds of babies and toddlers online and just fell in love with Peter's little cheeks. The orphanage in Romania seemed like a reputable place. There were so many babies to choose from . . . maybe we should have not gone to Romania or we should have used a different agency. She looks at Peter. Doctor, is there anything we can do that may make Peter more normal?

Please proceed with the problem-based approach!

Case Vignette 3.1.2 Continuation

The Denver Developmental Screening Test showed that, for a 2-year-old, Peter has significant areas of deficit including fine motor control, gross motor control, personal social skills, and language skills. Physical exam was negative for any abnor-

mal finding, including heart murmur, pallor, capillary refill delay, or respiratory problem.

You tell the parents: First we will run some simple tests on his blood and stool to make sure there isn't an organic cause for his size and behavior. You order the following: a Complete Blood Count (CBC), thyroid function tests (TFTs), a chemistry panel, a screen for lead poisoning, and a screen for tuberculosis. You recommend a multivitamin, offering a variety of foods and a follow-up visit in 2 months. You also recommend that the parents spend lots of time reading and playing with Peter. You encourage "sandbox time" at the playground with other 2-year-olds.

 Please proceed with the problem-based approach!

Case Vignette 3.1.3 Continuation

You search the Internet for Peter's adoption agency and learn about the protocol for adoptions. The website indicates that all prospective parents get counseling prior to the adoption and that there is a social worker who follows up as well. The website places emphasis on an orphan's special needs for "extra tender loving care."

You make a follow-up phone call to the Magellan's residence, 2 weeks later to let them know about the test results. All of the test results were normal. Mrs. Magellan picks up the phone and tells you, Hi Doctor! Peter smiled the other day and we found some foods he likes. It seems like he is already responding.

 Please proceed with the problem-based approach!

Case Vignette 3.1.4 Continuation

Three months later, when you pause outside the room to read over Peter's chart for his follow-up appointment, you hear the unmistakable sound of a child giggling. You enter to see Peter sitting on Mrs. Magellan's lap and Mr. Magellan tickling his feet.

You greet the parents. It looks like Peter is having some fun there. Sitting down on a low stool you look into Peter's eyes. How are you today Peter? Peter turns away, squirming back into his mother.

Mrs. Magellan: Oh, Hi Doctor. As you can see Peter is quite a bit more social with us. When we talked a couple of weeks ago it seemed that Peter was just coming out of his shell, but now he really does great. He'll point at things he wants and he seems to have a healthy appetite, though I don't know how much weight he has gained. He still doesn't use many words though, and sometimes he throws temper tantrums.

Dr. Sam: Well, the progress he has made already is phenomenal. You two really are great parents. According to his chart, he weighs 24 pounds and is 31 inches tall. He's gained two pounds and grown a half inch.

Mrs. Magellan: Did we do something wrong? I thought he was interacting so much better with us now—shouldn't he be up higher on the growth chart?

Dr. Sam: Well, typically a child will stay on one of the percentile lines once they begin being traced on it. It is possible that Peter will always be smaller than most boys his age. It is also possible that, given more time, Peter will start to grow more and move up the percentiles. Right now is it not possible to tell. A varied diet and home enrichment will be the best treatment. Later on, it may be helpful for Peter to be enrolled in a speech or language program to help his language acquisition. Let's see Peter again in a few months to make sure he continues on the right track. You are doing a fantastic job with Peter. Looking at Peter, you tickle his leg. Peter smiles shyly and turns toward his mother.

Please proceed with the problem-based approach!

Case Vignette 3.1.5 Conclusion

Two and a half years have passed since you last saw the Magellan's, and you have been very busy in your new practice. Somehow, you missed the Magellan's as you transitioned from Chief Resident to Attending. Today you look at the chart with amazement. Walking into the room, Mr. and Mrs. Magellan sit talking quietly while 5-year-old Peter creates a car out of connecting blocks.

Mr. Magellan tells you that Peter started a toddler program 2 years ago and then preschool last year. Peter's language and motor skills are up to speed with his preschool peers. You look twice at the growth chart: Peter is at the 25th percentile. Peter looks through his glasses at you, Hello Doctor. Grinning, he returns to his blocks.

Mrs. Magellan is beaming as she tells you "Peter knows his ABC's and can even count to twenty. He's ready for kindergarten next fall."

Learning Issues

Early Deprivation from Institutionalization

Although there is a degree of variability in standards of care within orphanages internationally, many are overburdened with children. With high staff to child ratios and inadequate resources, some children do not receive adequate nutrition, stimulation, personal contact, or education. These types of conditions lead more than half of orphans adopted from Eastern Europe to lie below the fifth percentile in length/height and weight scales (Judge, 2003). This statistic is exclusive of those children with yet undiagnosed medical conditions. After 6 months in enriched adoptive environments, the majority of adopted children significantly outgrow developmental and growth delays. The longer the stay in the orphanages, the more diverse and severe the deficits experienced by the child.

The Importance of Early Attachment

Infants of many species require a nurturing bond with an older member of the same species. Most often this bond is formed between infant and mother. The anecdotal baby duck hatchling forming an unchangeable nurturant bond with the local pig is well known and does occur due to imprinting. Attachment is another term for the bond between mother and child. Evidence of good attachment is attunement, where the mother and child respond to each other's cues. A well-attached child will be soothed by the mother after an upset and over time will learn to self-soothe. Healthy attachment allows for healthy development of the infant's motor and social skills as well as overall growth.

Perhaps the most famous research investigating the importance of bond formation was by Harry Harlow and his rhesus monkeys. Dr. Harlow was an American psychiatrist interested in defining the importance of early bond formation. Although his research is considered unethical and would never be performed in today's laboratories, he found that isolation of baby macaque monkeys from other monkeys for up to 24 months led to severe social disturbance. When a substitute mother monkey covered in either cloth-like material or wire was offered, the monkeys chose the cloth-like material surrogate over the wire surrogate. Baby monkeys only chose the wire surrogate if it offered food and the cloth-like mother did not. These early experiments provided a base for understanding the intricacies of early bond formation (Harlow et al., 1965).

Disrupted or unhealthy attachment can lead to problems in childhood and beyond. Such is the case in situations like orphanages, children in serial foster homes, or children in neglectful and abusive homes. Post-partum depression can also severely affect mother–child bond, consequently possibly leading to psychological disturbance in childhood and beyond (Miller et al., 2002). Anaclitic depression is a disorder in children separated from their caregiver and who then fail to thrive (grow and develop). Children with prolonged separation from a caregiver will experience deficits in one or more categories defined by the *Denver Developmental Screening Test*, such as fine motor control, gross motor control, personal social skills, and language skills. Children may also develop problems with trust that can affect social relationships later in life. Deprivation longer than 6 months worsens symptoms and can lead to long-term difficulties in social functioning.

Disruption of Early Attachment Affects Neural Circuitry

Successful formation of the caregiver (mother)–infant bond provides the basis for normal brain development. The potential difficulties that arise from abnormal brain development are problems such as depression, inability to self-soothe, and instability in relationships. Research has identified the right brain as the site of early emotional development. Research suggests that healthy attachment promotes development of emotional regulation centers in the right side of the brain during infancy and deficits in attachment (as well as abuse and neglect) disrupt the normal organization in the right brain during the first 3 years of life. Schore has documented EEG findings as evidence of changes in right brain development.

Maternal environmental conditions play a role in the brain development of the offspring. Animal studies reveal how stress during pregnancy or maternal separation can increase the seizure risk in the offspring or evoke psychological symptoms in the offspring consistent with anxiety and mood disorders. Compared to rats with non-stressed mothers, the offspring of the stressed mothers later had significantly increased the output of the hypothalamic–pituitary–adrenal axis (see Chap. 11) (Edwards, 2002).

People who suffer early trauma are at risk for other problems as well. Depression and anxiety occur at higher rates for people with early trauma histories (Heim and Nemeroff, 2001). Animal studies show that babies that are stressed by separation from their mothers later have problems with socialization and anxiety and are more likely to self-administer substances (Huot, 2001).

Resilience as a Basis for Different Child Response Rates

The formation of attachment between mother and child is subject to complicated interactions between nature and nurture. There is an innate temperament among babies that contributes to the formation of a successful bond. This innate difference between babies may underlie the property of *resilience*.

Resilience allows an individual to grow and develop, despite significant setbacks or disadvantages. The term resilience defines an ability to maintain, to prevail, and, in some cases, to thrive in the face of problems such as child neglect or mistreatment, exposure to violence, or mental illness in the home. Children who exhibit resilience

Table 3.1 Personality traits correlated with resilience

Intelligence	High intelligence is correlated with increasing abilities of children to succeed despite stress
Mutability	The extent to which personality can be molded in the long-term seems highly correlated with resilience
Charisma	An undefined trait in which some individual phenotypes are more socially acceptable
Easy going	Like the concept of mutability, but less rigidity in the everyday routine
Perseverance	As a more mature trait it really is a manifestation of resilience, but when present as a child it seems to be a harbinger of resilient ability

are more often described as charismatic, intelligent, easy going, or socially adept (Luthar, 2005). Resilience can be strengthened during child development by the presence of at least one strong relationship with a meaningful caregiver. Table 3.1 summarizes personality traits correlated with resilience.

Full Circle: Neuronal Circuitry Affects Global Development

As discussed, resilience is an adaptive behavior of an individual, and like all behaviors, it relates to a neural substrate. Many researchers are attempting to correlate biological functions with the development of resilience. Stress is correlated with biological responses, i.e., fear and increased heart rate, based on the physiological hypothalamic–pituitary–adrenal axis. Resilient children may have a lower biological response to the same stressors as cohorts. Extreme levels of stress may result in psychogenic dwarfism—a condition where psychological stress during childhood interferes with growth to the point of dwarfism despite adequate nutrition. Very high levels of cortisol are implicated as the neurohumoral mechanism underlying these severe growth deficits.

Covering Your Bases: Screening for Non-experiential Causes

As seen in this case, a variety of medical tests are used to differentiate medical, and possibly treatable, causes for delayed development. While a complete discussion of delayed development is likely beyond the scope of this textbook and more appropriately discussed in pediatric textbooks, it is important to note that knowledge of the etiology may give a better understanding of prognosis and help guide focused behavioral therapies to treat likely neurocognitive deficits (e.g., in the case of genetic or congenital conditions) or lead to specific preventive or curative treatments (e.g., in the case of malnutrition or heavy metal poisoning) (Table 3.2).

Table 3.2 Sources of delayed development

Classification	Condition	Effect on cognition
Perinatal	Anoxia, hypoxia	Lower cognitive performance
Infectious disease	*TORCH*	Hearing impairment, including deafness
	Toxoplasmosis	Mental retardation or other learning, behavioral, or emotional problems
	*O*ther: hepatitis B, syphilis, herpes zoster	Microcephaly, or small head and brain size
	*R*ubella	Low birthweight or poor growth inside the womb
	Cytomegalovirus	
	*H*erpes simplex, *H*IV	Blindness or other vision problems, such as cataracts
Environmental contaminants	Mental retardation	Mercury poisoning causes encephalopathy leading to permanent brain damage
		Lead poisoning is especially important to catch in young children because they absorb more lead than adults after ingestion. Lead poisoning is associated with a vast symptomology, but most seriously it causes permanent damage to the brain resulting in seizures, coma, and death
Nutritional deficiency	Iron deficiency anemia	Increased fatigue with anemia. Look for microcytic hypochromic anemia on peripheral smear, hx of heavy menses in teenage girl
	B12 deficiency	Neurological symptoms with B12 deficiency. Watch out for macrocytic anemia as a clue

Case Vignette 3.2.1 Presenting Situation: Jane and Sarah Jones

You are a second year resident in pediatrics and you notice the last exam room has two charts on the door. It is an intake evaluation for two new patients, twins Jane and Sarah Jones, aged 15. Looking over the history, you notice that Jane and Sarah were raised in separate households after their parents divorced. Jane grew up with her father in New York, and Sarah lived with her mother in Colorado. They are now both living with their mother in California.

The chart indicates that they are both in good health but Jane is having problems in school. You enter the room and see identical twin girls and their mother.

Hi, I'm Dr. Smith, it's great to meet you—all of you. Now, who is Sarah and who is Jane? You two look exactly alike! I bet you can play great tricks on your friends.

The girls giggle. Ms. Jones speaks up and points to the girls: This is Sarah and this is Jane.

So can you tell me what brings you in today?

Ms. Jones: We recently moved to the area and we need a doctor for the girls. Jane has been living with her father since she was born and I just recently got her back 2 months ago. I've noticed some differences between the girls which I thought was strange because they are identical. Sarah does extremely well in school, excels in band, and just scored in the 90th percentile on the PSAT. Jane is struggling in school and did not-so-well on the PSAT; I am worried that she is having a hard time in her new school.

You learn that the girls were born at 38 weeks by C-section and that the pregnancy was normal. Their mother did not smoke or drink. Sarah has always been a very healthy child outside of a broken leg from skiing. Jane and her mother don't know of any health problems.

You turn to Jane: Your mother says you are having a hard time in school. What can you tell me about this?

Jane looks down as she speaks: I don't know. It just seems like Sarah is better at school than me. She is probably smarter than me.

Jane's mother tells you Jane is behind her peers in basic skills such as math and reading and that she has a hard time answering questions in class. Otherwise, her teachers say that she tries hard, interacts well with her peers, and is very kind and polite.

What I would like to do today is examine both girls. I know that Jane and Sarah look identical but have they ever been checked to see if they are identical or fraternal? We can do a simple karyotype of their chromosomes as a first step. I would also like to check both the girls' hearing and vision.

 Please proceed with the problem-based approach!

Case Vignette 3.2.2 Continuation

At a follow-up visit 2 months later, you learn that Jane is still behind at school even though she works with a tutor four nights a week. The girls' chromosomes have the same banding pattern, which means that most likely they are identical genetically. Both Jane and Sarah have perfect hearing and vision. You ask about developmental experiences.

Ms. Jones: I have always tried to keep Sarah busy. As a single mom, I singed her up for lots of activities while I was working. She has always seemed to love music. I started her in piano lessons when she was 4 years old and she has had 11 years of lessons. She also plays the clarinet and is first chair in the school band.

Dr. Smith: Congratulations, Sarah. You must be very excited. Now what about Jane? Jane, what kind of things did you do outside of school when you were growing up?

Jane: My dad didn't have much money so I just went to after-school care at my school every day or watched TV at home. My dad didn't want to get me an instrument so I didn't get to play in the band when everyone else started in 4th grade. I like basketball—I am going out for the team next week.

Dr. Smith: That is excellent. Good luck. What I would like to do now, if you are agreeable, is refer the twins to a research center that specializes in twin studies. It might be that the environment that they grew up in is influencing the differences that you see between your daughters. There is a researcher who specializes in twins and I think he would be interested in adding your girls to a current study.

Please proceed with the problem-based approach!

Case Vignette 3.2.3 Conclusion

Dr. Davis is an expert on functional MRI and neuropsychological testing and specializes in twin studies. He is excited about the Jones twins as it is rare to have identical twins separated at birth, raised apart for 15 years, and then reunited. It was documented in the referral note that Sarah seems to have grown up in a more enriched environment and has had considerable musical training while Jane did not have the benefit of these early exposures.

Jane and Sarah (with their mother's permission) agree to undergo neuropsychologic evaluation including standardized intelligence testing. There is a follow-up visit 1 month later.

Dr. Davis: Welcome back Jones family! I have some thoughts on why Sarah may have an easier time in school. In the testing that we did, the girls' overall intelligence is very similar. It seems that Sarah, however, is better at remembering things that she learns verbally. One theory is that the differences between the girls are due to their different experiences as children. There have been some recent studies that show musical training at a young age may positively affect the brain and improve certain areas of functioning including those that relate to verbal learning. Sarah started playing instruments at a very young age and therefore the benefits of training on her brain may be more pronounced than if she had started later on in life. Jane had different experiences as a child and may benefit from learning differently. She and Sarah are both excellent visual learners and this should be emphasized in helping Jane catch up in school. I'll send a copy of the testing results to your pediatrician.

Learning Issues

1. Experience may modulate brain structure size and function

This case serves to illustrate how experience may change brain structure and function. Musical training is an example of a specific, measurable experience that has been well studied. Research suggests that training at an early age has a positive effect on verbal memory.

Magnetic resonance imaging has shown that specific regions of the brain, such as the left anterior corpus callosum, are larger in musicians than in non-musicians (Schlaug, 1995b). Because verbal memory is mainly a function of the left temporal lobe, and visual memory of the right, adults with music training should have better verbal, but not visual, memory than adults without such training. Adults who received music training before the age of 12 have a better memory for spoken words than those who did not. (Chan et al., 1998).

Motor-related regions in the cortex play critical roles in the planning, preparation, execution, and control of bimanual sequential finger movements. Researchers find significant positive correlation between musician status and gray matter volume in motor and somatosensory cortex as well as other brain areas. The gray matter volume is highest in professional musicians, intermediate in amateur musicians, and lowest in non-musicians (Gaser and Schlaug, 2003). From this research, we see the potential for experience to impact both brain structure and function.

Converse to the studies on the positive effects of music training, a great amount of research has been delving into the negative effects that early exposure to abuse or neglect has on brain function and structure. Studies have shown that childhood abuse is associated with a multitude of brain changes. These include a smaller hippocampus, corpus callosum, and prefrontal cortex, altered symmetry in some cortical lobes, and a reduction in neurons in the anterior cingulate cortex.

There is some controversy over whether differences in brain structure between abused and non-abused children are due to the abuse or a predisposing factor for the abuse. Because no ethical experimentation can be done to study the brain before and after abuse, this research must be compared to animal models of abuse to determine whether the structural and functional differences noted in abuse victims are caused by, or causes of, abuse.

Unfortunately, some research shows specific neurological changes dependent on the type of abuse, which may be difficult to develop an animal model for. Examples of this are recent findings that childhood sexual abuse is associated with a smaller primary and secondary visual cortex, while verbal abuse is associated with decreased size of small portions of the temporal gyrus that play a roll in processing language (Teicher et al., 2006). Still, all of these types of research offer insight into possible mechanisms for treatment of specific post-abuse psychiatric and behavioral symptoms.

2. Brain plasticity may have a critical period; ability to shape brain structure and function may be best at a young age

There are critical periods for types of learning, such as language learning. These critical periods reflect differences in brain plasticity during development. Our brains have the ability to learn and adapt more readily to some experiences at specific developmental periods—when the over-abundance of synapses are undergoing pruning in response to learning. In this example, early musical training may have impacted the patient's brain structure and function more than musical training in adolescence or adulthood.

Human brains are born with great potential to learn in response to the environment—plasticity. Impoverished or traumatic early environments can lead to abnormalities in development of brain structure and function. These abnormalities can have longstanding impact on relationships and risk of psychiatric disorders. Alternatively, enriched environments and exposure to experiences during key developmental periods may allow for optimal brain development. Plasticity of the child's brain represents the greatest vulnerability and the greatest opportunity of our species.

Review Questions

1. Evidence of good attachment between a mother and child includes

   (a) Each wishing the other well
   (b) Attunement to each other's cues
   (c) The child eating everything a mother offers
   (d) The mother crying when her child cries

2. Deficits in attachment are likely associated with early disruption in organization of what neurological function?

   (a) Left brain motor center development
   (b) Left brain emotional center development
   (c) Right brain motor center development
   (d) Right brain emotional center development

3. Which of these is a true statement about people trained in music from a young age?

   (a) They have better verbal memory than non-musicians.
   (b) They have better visual memory than non-musicians.
   (c) They have better verbal memory than they have visual memory.
   (d) They have better visual memory than they have verbal memory.

4. An English-speaking American child moving to China and learning to speak Mandarin as fluently as a native is indicative of

   (a) Resilience
   (b) Plasticity
   (c) Attunement
   (d) Training

Answers

1. b, 2. d., 3. a, 4. b

References

Chan AS, Ho YC, Cheung MC. Music training improves verbal memory. *Nature* 1998;396:128.

Edwards HE, Dortok D, Tam J, Won D, Burnham WM. Prenatal stress alters seizure thresholds and the development of kindled seizures in infant and adult rats. *Horm Behav* 2002 December;42(4):437–47.

Gaser C, Schlaug, G. Brain structures differ between musicians and non musicians. *J Neurosci* 2003 October 8;23(27):9240–5.

Harlow HF, Dodsworth RO, Harlow MK. Total social isolation in monkeys. *Proc Natl Acad Sci USA* 1965.

Heim C, Nemeroff CB. The role of childhood trauma in the neurobiology of mood and anxiety disorders: preclinical and clinical studies. *Biol Psychiatry* 2001;49(12);1023–39.

Huot RL, Thrivikraman K, Meaney MJ, Plotsky PM. Development of adult ethanol preference and anxiety as a consequence of neonatal maternal separation in Long Evans rats and reversal with antidepressant treatment. *Psychopharmacology* 2001;158(4):366–73.

Judge S. Developmental recovery and deficit in children adopted from Eastern European orphanages. *Child Psychiatry Hum Dev* 2003 Fall;34(1):49–62.

Luthar SS. Resilience at an early age and its impact on child psychosocial development. In: Tremblay RE, Barr RG, Peters RDeV, eds. *Encyclopedia on Early Childhood Development* [online]. Montreal, Quebec: Centre of Excellence for Early Childhood Development; 2005: 1–6.

Miller WB, Feldman SS, Pasta DJ. The effect of the nurturant bonding system on child security of attachment and dependency. *Soc Biol* 2002 Fall–Winter;49(3–4):125–59.

Schlaug G, Jancke L, Huang Y, Staiger JF, Steinmetz H. Increased corpus callosum size in musicians. *Neuropsychologia* 1995b;33:1047–55.

Sowell E, Thompson P, Leonard C, Welcome S, Kan E, Toga A. Longitudinal mapping of cortical thickness and brain growth in normal children. *J Neurosci* 2004;24:8223–31.

Teicher MH, Tomoda A, Andersen SL. Neurobiological consequences of early stress and childhood maltreatment: are results from human and animal studies comparable? *Ann N Y Acad Sci* 2006;1071(1):313–23.

Appendix

Table 3.1.1 Populated tables for Case Vignette 3.1.1 Peter Magellan

What are the facts?	What are your hypotheses?	What do you want to know next?	What specific information would you like to learn about?
Peter is in the fifth percentile in height and weight	Organic causes Anaclitic depression	*HPI:*	
		PMH:	
He is adopted from Romania		*FH:*	
There is no evidence that Peter is ill		*SH:*	

Table 3.1.1 (continued)

What are the facts?	What are your hypotheses?	What do you want to know next?	What specific information would you like to learn about?
The parents appear genuinely concerned		*Exam:*	
The doctor orders clinical tests to rule out organic causes			
Taking immediate action reassures the parents and suggestions for reversing any deficits are instituted		*Labs:*	
Contacting the social worker will give you more information and put the family at ease			

Table 3.1.2 Populated tables for Case Vignette 3.1.2 (continuation)

What are the facts?	What are your hypotheses?	What do you want to know next?	What specific information would you like to learn about?
Peter is in the fifth percentile in height and weight	Organic causes Anaclitic depression	*HPI:*	
		PMH:	
He is adopted from Romania		*FH:*	
The social worker agrees that there are commonly non-physical medical deficits		*SH:*	
Although orphanages are screened, the need for health care is overwhelming		*Exam:*	
Including the social worker will broaden the health care team and provide better care		*Labs:*	

Table 3.1.3 Populated tables for Case Vignette 3.1.3 (continuation)

What are the new facts?	What are your hypotheses?	What do you want to know next?	What specific information would you like to learn about?
Mr. and Mrs. Magellan sound like they are making extreme efforts to interact with Peter	Anaclitic depression An enriched environment is responsible for amelioration of developmental deficits	*HPI:* *PMH:* *FH:*	
Peter is starting to respond to the attention with smiles and wanting his favorite foods		*SH:* *Exam:*	
There is no evidence that Peter has an organic illness			
The parents appear relieved that Peter is responding positively			
Peter is scheduled to come into the office again in 5 months.		*Labs:*	

Table 3.1.4 Populated tables for Case Vignette 3.1.4 (continuation)

What are the new facts?	How do these facts help rule in or rule out previous hypotheses, and what are new hypotheses?	What do you want to know next?	What specific information would you like to learn about?
After 6 months of a balanced diet and an enriched home life, Peter seems to be reaching his developmental milestones in the areas of motor control and social skills	The enriched environment and balanced diet is abating several of the developmental milestone delays Peter may be delayed in communication because of the apparent neglect he suffered at the orphanage; alternatively, Peter may be suffering communicative delay because he was not exposed to English for 2 years	*HPI:* *PMH:* *FH:* *SH:*	

Table 3.1.4 (continued)

What are the new facts?	How do these facts help rule in or rule out previous hypotheses, and what are new hypotheses?	What do you want to know next?	What specific information would you like to learn about?
Peter is still unable to communicate with words, but is able to point		*Exam:*	
Peter remains very slight according to the American CDC growth curves		*Labs:*	

Table 3.1.5 Populated tables for Case Vignette 3.1.5 (continuation)

What are the new facts?	How do these facts help rule in or rule out previous hypotheses, and what are new hypotheses?	What do you want to know next?	What specific information would you like to learn about?
Three years have passed since implementing an enriched environment for Peter and he is thriving	Peter is currently of sufficient height and weight to not be too concerned	*HPI:*	
	Peter does not appear delayed in any of the areas in which he was initially	*PMH:*	
		FH:	
Peter is now able to communicate with his family and strangers		*SH:*	
Peter remains slight according to the American CDC growth curves, but has gained enough weight and height to reach the 25th percentile		*Exam:*	
		Labs:	

Table 3.2.1 Populated tables for Case Vignette 3.2.1 Jane and Sarah Jones

What are the facts?	What are your hypotheses?	What do you want to know next?	What specific information would you like to learn about?
Sarah and Jane are identical twins	Organic causes—lead exposure, iron deficiency anemia, B12 deficiency	*HPI:*	
The pregnancy and delivery were uncomplicated	TORCH infection Birth trauma, anoxic event	*PMH:* *FH:*	
The girls were raised in different environments	Vision or hearing deficit Depression Adjustment disorder	*SH:*	
There is no evidence that Jane is ill The mother appears genuinely concerned	Attention deficit disorder	*Exam:* *Labs:* Labs and vision and hearing screening to rule out organic causes	

Table 3.2.2 Populated tables for Case Vignette 3.2.2 (continuation)

What are the new facts?	How do these facts help rule in or rule out previous hypothesis, and what are new hypothesis?	What do you want to know next?	What specific information would you like to learn about?
Labs show genetically identical twins with no genetic reason for the difference in cognitive function	Less likely to be physiologic cause for apparent discrepancy in twin's cognitive environment	*HPI:* *PMH:* *FH:*	
The twins grew up with different environmental influences	Nature versus nurture—can environment influence academic abilties?	*SH:*	
Sarah grew up in a more enriched environment and was exposed to musical training at a young age	Are certain experiences related to improved cognitive function?	*Exam:* *Labs:*	

Chapter 4
Learning Principles of Human Behavior

David O. Antonuccio and Amber Hayes

Behavioral principles are powerful predictors of human behavior. When health care professionals understand these principles, they can be applied to changing health behaviors. In this chapter, we review the principles, which many of the readers will be familiar with from undergraduate and graduate classes. We apply the principles to PBL cases to illustrate behavioral principles in medical care.

At the end of this chapter, the reader will be able to

1. Define the important behavioral terms such as classical conditioning, operant conditioning, reinforcement, reward, punishment, reinforcement schedule, antecedents, consequences, stimulus control, modeling, and functional analysis
2. Apply behavioral principles to some common behavioral problems observed in medicine
3. Develop treatment plans for some common behavioral problems using behavioral principals

Case Vignette 4.1.1 Presenting Situation: Richard Smith

Richard Smith is a 58-year-old man who comes to see you, his primary care physician, for an annual exam. During the routine interview, you ask about tobacco use. He admits to being a smoker and smoking two packs of cigarettes per day for the last 40 years. Richard states that he wishes he could "quit this nasty habit," but has had difficulty in the past.

 Please proceed with the problem-based approach!

D.O. Antonuccio
Professor of Psychiatry, University of Nevada School of Medicine

A. Guerrero, M. Piasecki (eds.), *Problem-Based Behavioral Science and Psychiatry*,
© Springer Science+Business Media, LLC 2008

Case Vignette 4.1.2 Continuation

When you ask Richard why he wants to quit now, he says that he has been hearing about all of the bad health effects of smoking. His wife has been nagging him whenever he smokes because she is worried about his health so he has been sneaking cigarettes behind her back and now he feels guilty about this. Richard will soon be a grandfather and he is worried about the potential effects of second-hand smoke on babies. He also wants to make sure he is around to enjoy his grandchildren growing up. In the past, Richard says he has tried stopping "cold turkey," but the withdrawal symptoms and cravings drove him back to smoking after about 3 days.

 Please proceed with the problem-based approach!

Learning Issues

Functional Analysis

You request the patient perform a **functional analysis** of his smoking. A functional analysis is a systematic way to characterize a behavior by examining events that happen prior to (i.e., **antecedents**) the unwanted behavior (in this case, smoking) and the consequences of acting out that behavior. Richard will record each cigarette he smokes and the activities leading up to the cigarette to find out what types of triggers or **antecedents** cause him to want to smoke. Smoking a cigarette has been paired with some environmental stimuli many hundreds of times, causing them to become **classically conditioned**. For example, a patient who smokes after a meal to satisfy a craving may find that he has an urge to smoke after all meals. You also ask Richard to make a list of the **consequences** of smoking to help understand the role of **operant conditioning**. Not all consequences are bad, for example the feeling of relief after having smoked. Some consequences are powerful **reinforcers**, i.e., increase the probability of smoking.

Case Vignette 4.1.3 Continuation

Richard returns to your office 1 week later with a daily log of cigarettes and activities. Table 4.1 lists some antecedents and consequences for his smoking and identifies them as punishing (any consequence that makes smoking less likely) and reinforcing (any consequence that makes smoking more likely). You notice that Richard has a cigarette upon waking, with morning coffee, after every meal, while

Table 4.1 Functional analysis of Richard's smoking

Antecedent	Consequence	Punishing (P) versus reinforcing (R)
Waking	Feeling relieved	R
On phone	Wife nags him	P
Coffee	Costly	P
After meal	Smoker's cough	P
Driving	Satisfies boredom	R
Visiting with friends	Feeling socially accepted	R

driving, while on the phone, and while visiting with other smoking friends. Except for one cigarette, he smokes outside of the presence of his wife. Though her nagging serves as a punisher for his smoking, he feels resentful and tends to avoid talking to her about his smoking. You point out that by definition, punishment decreases the probability of a behavior but does not encourage appropriate alternatives. This may be why he feels angry and then avoids his wife. You invite Richard's wife to the session to educate her about the downside of nagging and other punishment and encourage her to be supportive or at least neutral when he is struggling with his smoking.

 Please proceed with the problem-based approach!

Learning Issues

Stages of Change

The stages of change can be seen in just about any behavior that one wants to modify including behaviors such as eating habits, compliance with treatment, and addiction (Zimmerman et al., 2000). The stages are divided into five phases: precontemplation, contemplation, preparation, action, and maintenance (DiClemente et al., 1991). It is important to note that a person may fluctuate back and forth between stages as they consider changing a particular behavior. Understanding a person's current stage will guide your treatment approach. Most smokers will exhibit the stages of change as they attempt to quit smoking.

Precontemplation stage. In this stage, one is not even considering changing the behavior. To assist people in this stage, it is appropriate to recognize and validate their unwillingness to change at this time, provide personalized reasons that the behavior puts them at risk, and provide an opportunity to revisit the idea of changing the behavior in the future.

Contemplation stage. In the contemplation stage, the idea of the behavior being a problem has crossed the person's mind more than once, but currently he or she lacks lack the commitment to take action. To assist people in this stage it is often helpful to make a list of "pros and cons" for continuing the behavior versus changing it. It is also important to highlight the benefits of changing.

Preparation stage. A person in the preparation stage has begun to "test the waters" and is much more serious about changing and developing a plan to change in the near future. A person in this stage will actually set some specific goals or target dates. To assist a person in this stage you can help him or her to identify possible roadblocks to changing the behavior, set up a support system, and identify "next steps" for changing the behavior.

Action stage. The action stage has begun when the person begins modification of the behavior. This may require assistance in changing the normal cues for the undesired behavior, continuing to build the support system and identifying obstacles to maintaining the change. It is important to note that persons in this stage may begin to feel a sense of loss for the old behavior.

Maintenance stage. In the maintenance stage, the behavior has been modified for some time but requires continued work to prevent a relapse. Your role is to help identify the situations in which a relapse could occur and as a team decide on how best to overcome them. It is important to stress that the occurrence of a relapse does not mean instant failure—more than likely it provides a learning opportunity for the future.

FYI: Smoking Cessation Tools (**Table 4.2**)

Table 4.2 The 5 A's approach to smoking cessation

The 5 A's approach
The U.S. Public Health Service recommends the "5 A's approach" to treatment of smoking (Fiore et al., 2000):
Ask about tobacco use. This also involves addressing myths about quitting. For example, it is a myth that past attempts decrease ability to quit or that older smokers do not benefit from quitting
Advise users to stop. Provide the patient with information on the medical benefits
Assess willingness to quit. An important factor is to match the intervention with the stage of quitting (see below)
Assist in quitting
Arrange for follow-up
(This five-step program could easily be adapted to any kind of habit change a physician is encouraging in a patient)

Case Vignette 4.1.4 Conclusion

Richard asks you what he should do next. You ask your patient if he is ready to pick a target quit date. He chooses his wife's birthday in 3 weeks. You suggest that he practice not smoking before his quit day by eliminating smoking during one of the easier situations he has identified. Richard decides to become a nonsmoker while driving his car. He plans to keep his cigarettes in the trunk of his car and to put sugarless candy in his ashtray as a substitute to help him achieve this goal. This is called a **stimulus control** *strategy, i.e., altering the environment to make it easier to disconnect the stimulus of driving from the behavior of smoking. By altering some of the environmental stimuli, hopefully, he can reduce his smoking (Antonuccio, 1992).*

Richard comes back to see his physician weekly to evaluate his progress and for support. On his wife's birthday, he begins using the nicotine patch you suggested. He chooses to reduce his patch each week so that 3 weeks after his quit date (e.g., Bolin et al., 1999) he is totally nicotine-free. He feels proud of himself and his wife tells him it is the best birthday present she has ever received.

Case Vignette 4.2.1 Presenting Situation: Samantha Brown

Samantha Brown is a 48-year-old woman who comes to the clinic today because of sleeping problems. She states that over the last 3 months she has not been sleeping well at all and wonders if there is anything that can be done.

Please proceed with the problem-based approach!

Case Vignette 4.2.2 Continuation

You take a sleep history using the BEARS (Bedtime, Excessive daytime sleepiness, Awakenings, Regularity and duration of sleep, Snoring) acronym. First you review bedtime rituals and what happens at sleep onset. You ask about the use of alcohol, nicotine, caffeine, and medications. You ask about how tired she gets during the day. Other questions you ask are, how well she sleeps through the night, how many hours of sleep she typically gets, and about snoring.

You ask Samantha to keep a log of her daily activities, emphasizing her nightly rituals before, during, and after sleep. Her log shows that she is having difficulty falling asleep and staying asleep. She details that it takes her over an hour to fall asleep and then she wakes up a short time later. Her average evening includes getting home from work at approximately 6 p.m. Then she usually goes to the gym and exercises on the elliptical machine for an hour. When she returns home, it's usually about 8:30 p.m., and she will have her dinner. At dinner, she usually tries to unwind by having a glass or two of wine. After dinner, she showers and goes to bed but notes that every night she feels as though she is not tired and often lies in bed thinking of tomorrow's duties and errands. To try to fall asleep, she will turn on the television and have another glass of wine. After approximately 1 hour she will fall asleep, but later at 3 or 4 a.m. she will be wide awake and have difficulty falling back asleep. Her alarm usually goes off about 6 a.m.

Please proceed with the problem-based approach!

Case Vignette 4.2.3 Conclusion

*You explain to Samantha that there are many causes of insomnia and that often they are the result of our own activities (antecedents) during the day. She is given a Sleep Hygiene handout that explains which activities, like exercising late and alcohol use, can lead to the adverse consequence of insomnia. You also discuss how her mood can influence her sleep. You ask her about her mood lately and if she has had any feelings that are consistent with depression. Samantha answers no, except to a question on worrying often. Instead of worrying about the next day while lying in bed, you suggest setting aside some "worry time" in which she can think over tomorrow's events and current stresses before she starts her bedtime rituals. You also ask her not to go to bed until she is actually sleepy in order to restrict her time in bed to actual sleep time. This is a **stimulus control** strategy to help make the bed a stimulus primarily for sleep. You suggest that she get out of bed if she is unable to fall asleep within 20 minutes. You also suggest that she get up at the same time each morning no matter what time she falls asleep the night before to help condition her body to waking up on a regular pattern. In fact, you would like her to look toward the horizon (not directly at the sun) each morning to get her biological clock started with broad spectrum light. In addition to limiting her alcohol intake, you ask Samantha to avoid caffeine after 6 p.m. You also suggest keeping her bedroom cool, dark, quiet, and conducive to sleep. You congratulate her on her exercise routine but advise never exercising less than 3 hours before she is planning to go to sleep. You reassure Samantha that most people don't actually need a full 8 hours of sleep per night to function adequately and even after a night of insomnia she is not likely to feel impaired all of the next day.*

Samantha decides to start her exercise routine in the morning. She also makes a commitment to limit her alcohol consumption to no more than one glass of wine before 7 p.m. on any given evening. She returns to your office after 1 month of adjusting her choices throughout the day, and the result is that she now is sleeping much better.

Case Vignette 4.3.1 Presenting Situation: Dennis

You are the pediatrician to Dennis, a 4-year-old boy with lots of energy. He is smart and is the only child in a loving family of older parents who are grateful to have him after years of infertility interventions. He is their "miracle baby." His parents have expressed the desire not to spoil him but they fear that they already have. He plays well with other children at preschool and his preschool teachers do not report any behavioral problems. Dennis's parents are happy he is adjusting well to preschool but they are concerned about some of his behavior when he is at home. They report that several times a week he will have a "melt down" during which he will throw a verbal and physical tantrum, often rolling on the floor screaming.

Please proceed with the problem-based approach!

Case Vignette 4.3.2 Continuation

*You request that Dennis's parents perform a **functional analysis** of their son's tantrums. After tracking the behavior for a week, the parents discover that he had three tantrums at the supermarket. A careful analysis of the tantrums revealed that it is common for Dennis to go shopping with his mother at the local supermarket and find a toy or candy that he wants. When his mother tries to say no, he will cry. If she continues to say no, he will escalate and start to throw a tantrum. If she continues to resist, he will often escalate to falling on the ground and screaming. At this point, his mother feels acute embarrassment and will do anything to make it stop, including giving him the toy or candy. He then quickly calms down and a smile returns to his face. Then his mother quickly leaves the store red-faced with the purchases. What are the antecedents and consequences of their son's behaviors? What consequences would be properly characterized as punishers or rewards? How would you characterize the **reinforcement schedule** for the tantrums?*

Please proceed with the problem-based approach!

Case Vignette 4.3.3 Continuation

Dennis's parents learn that they are continuously reinforcing their son's tantrums by giving him what he wants until he calms down. This is a pattern they would like to change. They also learn that Dennis is negatively reinforcing his mother's giving in to him by stopping the tantrum as soon as she gives in to his demand and agrees to buy the candy or toy. In other words, the child stops the aversive tantrum (negative) whenever the mother gives him what he wants, thereby increasing the *mother's behavior of giving in. By definition this is negative reinforcement of the mother's behavior. The parents learn that his preschool uses a system called 1-2-3 Magic (Phelan, 2004). This system involves giving the child a warning when his behavior is disruptive by telling him "You are on one." If he does not comply with the request, he is told, "You are on two." If he still does not comply with the request, he is told "You are on three" and there is a negative consequence of some kind. At school the negative consequence is sitting quietly by himself in a time-out room for 3 minutes. His parents unobtrusively observe the teachers **model** these techniques in the classroom. One of the teachers is an especially good **model** because she herself also struggled with her own child's tantrums issues and can relate to the parents' struggles. This teacher had to work at learning the system with her own child by practicing it repeatedly in the classroom. In that sense, she is a **coping model** (i.e., someone who had to learn to cope), an even more powerful **model** than a **mastery model** (i.e., someone for whom reward and time-out comes naturally). **Models** are also more effective if they are similar to the person observing, they are skillful in their implementation of the target behavior, they are attractive, and there is opportunity to practice the target behavior.*

Dennis's parents decide to use this system and make the consequence a 3-minute time-out in the corner of whatever room they are in. If he comes out of time-out, he will lose the privilege of dessert after dinner. His parents decide to build in some flexibility for him to earn back dessert with good behavior like helping his mother with a household chore. To reduce her embarrassment, Dennis's mother talks to the store manager and lets him know that she is trying to do a better job of setting limits with her son when he is in public. The store manager, who is also a parent, is completely sympathetic and understanding. He says it is fine with him if her son has a full-out tantrum on the next trip to the store and he supports her setting appropriate limits. He agrees to alert the cashiers of her plan the next time she comes in. She lets him know she will come in later that afternoon after preschool. What would you expect to happen the next time Dennis's mother goes shopping at the store with him?

*Dennis's mother explained to Dennis the new system of discipline she was planning to implement. She takes him shopping that afternoon as planned. The store manager gives her a wink when she arrives. Dennis finds some M&M candy-coated peanuts and within 5 minutes he is asking his mother for the candy. She says "No" because it will spoil his dinner. He begins to cry and it gets louder. She tells him he is "on one." He escalates to falling on the floor. She tells him he is "on two." He begins screaming, and she tells him he is "on three" and must sit on the floor in time-out until he calms down and that under no circumstances can he have M&Ms today. He screams louder and keeps it up for about 3 minutes, much longer than he usually does when she gives in to his demands. This is called an **extinction burst**, i.e., a burst of behavior following the withdrawal of an expected reinforcer. She tells him that when he is calm for 30 seconds, he can come out of time-out. Another mother whispers to her that she is totally supportive and admires her limit setting. Eventually Dennis calms down and they leave the store together holding hands. The mother, though still somewhat embarrassed, is proud of herself for sticking to her boundary.*

Please proceed with the problem-based approach!

Case Vignette 4.3.4 Conclusion

*Dennis's mother implements the same strategy the next time she goes to the store and notices that Dennis's tantrum only lasts about 30 seconds. The third time in the store together he doesn't tantrum at all. His tantrum behavior is **extinguishing**.*

Case Vignette 4.4.1 Presenting Situation: Nana

Phyllis White ("Nana") is a 75-year-old grandmother who loves to come to Reno to gamble and visit her adult grandson, in that order. Her grandson is concerned because she goes from casino to casino in a bus with her fellow senior citizens but doesn't even take time out to eat sometimes. Her favorite game is the pull slot machine. She feels she is getting good exercise but her grandson is concerned that she can't afford to spend long hours gambling in smoky rooms, both physically and financially (Unwin et al., 2000).

Please proceed with the problem-based approach!

Case Vignette 4.4.2 Continuation

You are a family medicine doctor who has been working with Phyllis on general health maintenance and treatment of arthritis and acid reflux. You meet with her and her grandson at his request and learn of the concerns about the trips to Reno. You ask Phyllis to track her gambling behavior and to write down exactly what games she plays and exactly how much time she is gambling. You also ask her to write down other activities she enjoys on her trip to Reno. You find that she gambles as much as 20 hours on a 2-day trip to Reno. Although she does not skip any meals, she does delay them sometimes. She also enjoys seeing her grandson and his young children play baseball when they have a little league game scheduled.

Please proceed with the problem-based approach!

Case Vignette 4.4.3 Conclusion

*In an application of the **Premack Principle**, you encourage her to socialize with her grandson and his children before she goes gambling at the casino with her friends. In order to accomplish this, she stays at her grandson's house instead of the casino. After a morning brunch and afternoon baseball session, her grandson drops her off at a casino with her friends from about 7 p.m to 9 p.m. After that she is ready for bed. Her tracking shows that she has reduced her gambling from 20 hours per weekend visit to only 5 hours. She has more quality time with her grandson and great grandchildren in the process.*

Learning Issues

1. Premack Principle

The Premack Priniciple (named for the theorist David Premack) is that animals have baseline levels of engaging in different behaviors (e.g., eating, drinking, running, playing). The Premack Principle postulates that humans and other animals will work at a less probable behavior for the opportunity to engage in a more probable behavior. In this case, Phyllis collaborated with you to plan to do other things that were important to her, like spend time with her grandson and great grandchildren and get proper nutrition, before she allowed herself her guilty pleasure of gambling. This is an important and simple principle of self-reinforcement, i.e., work before play or eating vegetables before dessert.

2. Reinforcement schedules

The pattern of reinforcement is called a reinforcement schedule (Beaton, 2001). Reinforcement schedules can vary according to the number of responses before a reward is delivered (ratio schedule) or in the time elapsed between rewards (interval schedule). A ratio schedule or an interval schedule can be fixed or variable. In a fixed ratio schedule, a reward is delivered after a certain number of responses. For example, a factory worker might receive a bonus for every 10 cars manufactured by his or her team. In a variable ration schedule, a reward is delivered after an average number of responses. For example, the slot machines that Phyllis enjoys are usually set to deliver a payoff after an average number of pulls. Ratio schedules tend to result in a high response rate and a variable ratio schedule results in a pattern of responding that is the most resistant to extinction (i.e., a dropping off of the response when the reinforcer is removed).

Receiving a paycheck every 2 weeks is an example of a fixed interval schedule. A variable interval schedule might involve a fisherman who catches his limit of 10 fish over the course of 5 hours of fishing. Some of the fish are caught within 5 minutes of each other while others might be caught several hours apart.

3. The neurobiology of reinforcement

The neurobiology of anticipation, reward, and reinforcement has been studied at molecular, cellular, genetic, systems, behavioral, and computational levels. Though there are still many things we do not understand about the neurobiology of human learning, research in this field is richly productive and rapidly expanding. The neurobiology of addiction (see Chap. 20) appears to be pathologic use of the same brain structures as normal behavioral adaptation (seeking food, water, and opportunity to mate). These structures are collectively referred to as the "mesolimbic reward circuit" and utilize dopamine primarily as the neurotransmitter or chemical messenger (Haynes, 2004). This circuit is composed of dopamine-producing neurons of deep brain structures (the ventral tegmentum that forms projections to the nucleus accumbens and amygdala) and the prefrontal cortex (Vetulani, 2001).

We can better understand normal behavior by dividing the behavior systems of the brain into three major categories: arousal, reward, and cognitive systems. The arousal system is further subdivided into general arousal (regulating overall central nervous system excitability) located in the ascending reticular system, directed or goal-oriented arousal (providing motivation and emotion) located in the hypothalamus and parts of the limbic system, and peripheral arousal (linking up the brain to other organ systems) made up of the autonomic nervous system and hormonal systems. All of these systems interact to allow the organism to adapt to the environment although the directed arousal system is involved most substantially in voluntary behavior. The directed arousal system provides a ranking of goals and initiates the behavior needed to attain the goal and then processes whether or not the goal was met. If these goals aid in the organism's survival or survival of the species, it is properly rewarded and we say that the goal is reinforced. In the case of the brain, this reward is dopamine (Vetulani, 2001). Research has also shown that dopamine is released at a basal tonic rate in anticipation of a previously received pleasurable, reinforcing event, such as sugar water presented to monkeys after a paired stimulus. If the reward is given sooner than expected, it is perceived as "better than expected" and there is a burst of dopamine release. If there is no reward when one is expected there is a pause in the dopamine release indicating "worse than expected." It is believed that these bursts and pauses of dopamine release encode a "prediction-error signal" that will help the animal to *learn* the new relationship and reinforce behavior that results in the reward. This is termed the "Reward Prediction-Error Hypothesis." With addictive drug intake, the signal may be always "better than expected," resulting in an overriding of all other goal-directed behavior (Hyman, 2005).

Better understanding of these brain mechanisms may open doors in the future for treatment of drug addiction as well as other behavioral problems.

Review Questions

1. Two new parents wake up quickly to the sound of their 1-year-old baby crying in the middle of the night. Every night when this occurs, they immediately bring the baby to bed with them to comfort her. The baby immediately settles down to sleep. This is an example of

   (a) Intermittent reinforcement
   (b) Extinction
   (c) Continuous reinforcement
   (d) Shaping
   (e) Successive approximations

2. A resident observes a skilled surgeon conducting a heart bypass. Based on what you learned about MODELING in the text, the likelihood of learning and retention is UNRELATED to

   (a) The attractiveness of the surgeon
   (b) The practice opportunities for the resident
   (c) The manual dexterity of the resident
   (d) The acclaimed skill of the surgeon
   (e) The age of the surgeon

3. Pick the FALSE statement about punishment:

   (a) Punishment does not teach appropriate behavior.
   (b) The punisher (i.e., the person doing the punishing) may model verbal or physical aggression.
   (c) The punisher may increase the target behavior (i.e., the behavior that is being punished).
   (d) People learn to avoid the punishment.
   (e) Punishment tends to generate more emotional behavior.

4. In behavioral approaches to treatment, behavior is thought to be UNRELATED to

   (a) Reinforcement history
   (b) Current contingencies
   (c) Genetic endowment
   (d) Ego functioning
   (e) Reinforcement schedule

5. A patient notices some anxiety while driving following a serious car accident. She notices some relief of her anxiety if she avoids driving on the freeway, causing her to avoid freeway driving entirely. The relief of anxiety she experiences from avoiding freeways is an example of

   (a) Negative reinforcement
   (b) Positive reinforcement

(c) Punishment

(d) Conditioned stimulus

(e) Generalized reinforcer

6. An adult patient comes to you with stomach pain that does not appear to have an underlying biological basis. You decide to use your skills in functional analysis to help correct the problem. You ask the patient to

(a) Keep track of their dreams.

(b) Focus on available punishers in their environment.

(c) Keep track of the antecedents of the pain, the pain itself, and what happens after the pain occurs.

(d) Take an in-depth history of childhood, focusing on toilet training.

(e) Focus on cognitions, and reward systems in the environment.

7. Behavior analysis is characterized by all EXCEPT one of the following:

(a) Identifying antecedent events

(b) Evaluating consequences

(c) Measuring duration of behavior

(d) Determining a DSM-IV diagnosis

(e) Measuring the frequency of behavior

Answers

1. c, 2. e, 3. c, 4. d, 5. a, 6. c, 7. d

Possible Answers to Behavioral Principles Tables

Case table 1.1 Richard Smith 1

Facts	Hypotheses	Information needed	Learning issues
58-year-old-male 80 pack-year smoker wants to quit	Given the patients extensive heavy smoking history, he will need lots of assistance to quit	Why does he want to quit now? What has RS tried in the past? When does he usually smoke? What is his longest period of prior abstinence? How does he deal with stress?	Principles of functional analysis

Case table 1.1 (continued)

Facts	Hypotheses	Information needed	Learning issues
		What is the functional relationship between the patient's environment and his smoking?	
		What are typical antecedents to smoking for this patient?	
		What are the typical consequences of smoking for this patient?	

Case table 1.2 Richard Smith 2

Facts	Hypothesis	Information needed	Learning issues
R.S. identifies the **antecedents** and the **consequences**	Changing the antecedent behavior may change the likelihood of smoking	What type of follow-up plan will he need?	Stages of change Smoking cessation tools

Case table 2.1 Samantha Brown 1

Facts	Hypotheses	Information needed	Learning issues
48-year-old female complains of insomnia for 3 months	Possible medical reason? Possible stress? Mood disturbance? Substance use?	What part of sleeping does she have trouble with? What is her bed-time routine like?	How to take a sleep history Typical antecedents for a good or poor night of sleep What are the consequences of a good or poor night of sleep

Case table 2.2 Samantha Brown 2

Facts	Hypotheses	Information needed	Learning issues
Difficulty falling asleep Difficulty staying asleep	Changing her routine may have an impact	How does the patient's sleep change after the intervention?	Sleep hygiene causes for insomnia

Case table 2.2 (continued)

Facts	Hypotheses	Information needed	Learning issues
Antecedent behaviors include exercising late, eating late, alcohol intake, staying in bed and worrying, and watching television in bed			
Consequences include feeling fatigued the next morning and inability to concentrate at work			

Case table 3.1 Dennis 1

Facts	Hypotheses	Information needed	Learning issues
4-year-old boy	Parents actions are reinforcing tantrums	What type of activities lead to tantrums (antecedents)?	Reinforcement schedules
Parents complain of tantrums			
No problems in school		How do the parents react to the tantrums (Consequences and reinforcers)?	
Plays well with peers			

Case table 3.2 Dennis 2

Facts	Hypotheses	Information needed	Learning issues
Antecedents to their son's tantrums: Dennis sees a small toy or piece of candy he wants	Changing the consequences may alter the behavior	What happens to the behavior after implementing the intervention?	Reinforcement schedules
Dennis realizes he is in a public place that will be embarrassing for mom if he throws a fit			What are some tools to modify behavior in children?

Case table 3.2 (continued)

Facts	Hypotheses	Information needed	Learning issues
Consequences of his tantrums: Mom gets embarrassed by Dennis's tantrum Mom gives him the toy or candy he wants and Dennis calms down immediately			

Case table 4.1 Nana 1

Facts	Hypotheses	Information needed	Learning issues
75-year-old female grandson concerned about gambling to point of exhaustion	Gambling may be out of control	How much does Nana actually gamble?	Gambling addiction
	Reinforcement schedule of slot machines makes it difficult to extinguish the gambling behavior	How much time does she devote to gambling? Does she skip meals?	Reinforcement schedules of slot machines
		What else does she like to do besides gambling?	

Case table 4.2 Nana 2

Facts	Hypotheses	Information needed	Learning issues
20 hours in 2 days	Using gambling as a consequence for other activities like adequate socialization and nutrition will help her have better balance	What happens to Nana's gambling after the intervention?	Premack principle
Delays meals			Reinforcement schedules
Enjoys seeing her grandson and watching his young children play baseball			

References

Antonuccio, David O. (1992). Butt out, A Compassionate Guide to Helping Yourself Quit Smoking, with or Without a Partner. R&E Publishers, Saratoga, CA.

Beaton, J.M. (2001). Learning Theory and Human Behavior in Behavior & Medicine, edited by D. Wedding. Hogrefe & Huber Publishers, Toronto.

Bolin, L., Antonuccio, D.O., Follette, W., and Krumpe, P. (1999). Transdermal nicotine: the long and the short of it. Psychol. Addict. Behav., 13, 152–156.

DiClemente, C.C., Prochaska, J.O., Fairhurst, S.K., Velicer, W.F., Velasquez, W.F., and Rossi, J.S. (1991). The process of smoking cessation: an analysis of precontemplation, contemplation, and preparation stages of change. J. Consult. Clin. Psychol., 59, 295–304.

Haynes, Thomas L. (2004). The Neurobiology of Addiction and Its Implications for Treatment—Drug-Seeking Behavior and the Transition to Dependence. http://www.medscape.com/viewarticle/472498.

Hyman, Steven E. (2005). Addiction: "A Disease of Learning and Memory." Am. J. Psychiatry, 162, 1414–1422.

Phelan, T.W. (2004). 1-2-3 Magic: Effective Discipline for Children. Parent Magic Inc.

Unwin, B., Davis, M., and DeLeeuw, J. (February 1, 2000). Pathologic Gambling. AFP, 61(3).

Vetulani, Jerzy (2001). Drug addiction. Part II. Neurobiology of addiction. Pol. J. Pharmacol., 53, 303–317.

Zimmerman, G., Olsen, C., Bosworth, M. (March 1, 2000). A stages of change approach to helping patients change behavior. AFP, 61(5).

Chapter 5
Sexuality Throughout the Life Cycle

Kevin Allen Mack and Anthony P.S. Guerrero

There are few topics in medicine that blur the boundaries of science and morality more than *sexuality*. The "culture war" keeps our courts busywith cases involving hate crimes, marriage equality, and gay-lesbian-bisexual-transgender (GLBT) rights, while churches, synagogues, and mosques look for ways to interpret the ancient writings and instruct their faithful. Public health departments and state governments construct databases to capture information about persons and practices that may inadvertently transmit HIV.

This chapter aims to provide a basic discussion on sexuality throughout the life cycle. At the end of this chapter, the reader will be able to

1. Distinguish between the terms: sex, gender, gender identity, and sexual orientation
2. Identify normal sexual development in children, adolescents, and adults
3. Describe the human sexual response cycle
4. Discuss issues in sexuality for elderly and medically ill patients

Case Vignette 5.1.1 Baby Pat

As a busy family physician in a diverse community, you are called by the certifiednurse-midwife to see Baby Pat, a newly born infant who was noted, at birth, to have ambiguous genitalia. No additional pre- or perinatal risk factors were identified. The family histories of both parents were negative for any prior genetic abnormalities.

The patient's vital signs and physical exam were entirely within normal limits with the exception of the genitourinary exam, which showed a 1 × 1 cm phallus. Labioscrotal folds were present bilaterally, with some hyperpigmentation and rugae. A perineal opening was present. No gonads were palpable in the labioscrotal folds.

K.A. Mack
Assistant Professor, University of California, Berkeley/San Francisco

A. Guerrero, M. Piasecki (eds.), *Problem-Based Behavioral Science and Psychiatry*,
© Springer Science+Business Media, LLC 2008

With the assistance of a pediatric endocrinologist, you obtain laboratory studies, which yield the following results (with normal range in parentheses):

Electrolytes:
Sodium = 127 mmol/l (132–142)*
Potassium = 6.4 mmol/l (4.0–6.2)*
Chloride = 94 mmol/l (95–110)*
CO_2 = 21 mmol/l (18–27)
Glucose = 66 mg/dl (60–115)
Calcium = 9.0 mg/dl (8.0–10.5)
Capillary blood gas (CBG): normal
Urinalysis:
Clear, straw colored
Specific gravity = 1.003 (1.007–1.030), pH 8.0 (4.5–8.0), otherwise normal

Urine chemistries:
Sodium = 24 mmol/l (0–40)
Potassium = 13.1 mmol/l (7.0–18.1)
Chloride = 21 mmol/l (2–9)*
17a-OH progesterone: 11,767 ng/dl (0–200)*
Other steroid studies:
Cortisol—decreased
24-hour urine for pregnanetriol—increased
24-hour urine for 17-ketosteroids—increased
Plasma testosterone—increased
Plasma dehydroepiandrosterone—increased
Plasma renin—increased
Plasma and urine aldosterone—decreased
Ultrasound of pelvis: Confirms presence of uterus and ovaries
Karyotype: XX female

State-required PKU and hearing tests for newborns were entirely normal.

You review the laboratory studies with the family and begin answering their questions about whether they have a "girl" or a "boy," and whether their "son" or "daughter" will be "normal" and what impact this condition will have on the child's future sexual orientation.

 Please proceed with the problem-based approach!

The industrious PBL student will have little problem identifying the likely diagnosis for this clinical presentation. More challenging, however, will be identifying the clinical and social science issues that will need to be addressed from the very onset of the child's presentation to caregivers. What is at issue here? The child's sex? The gender? The sexual orientation? How much family education needs to occur to facilitate an informed medical decision regarding the child's treatment? What is the role of the family's values in directing the medical intervention? Is there sufficient consensus about the relationship between sex determination, gender identity, and sexual orientation to constitute a "standard of care" for this child?

At this point, while a complete discussion of the biology of sex determination is beyond the scope of this chapter, it is worth reviewing a few basic definitions, which are summarized in Table 5.1.

While these terms may seem relatively straightforward, sexual development is complex enough to be associated with various concerns and questions that may be presented to the physician throughout the life cycle of a patient.

Case Vignette 5.2.1 Mike

In your outpatient practice, you see children of all ages. One of your patients is Mike, a 6-year-old boy, who is brought in by his mother because of "behavior problems in school that might cause him to get kicked out." According to the principal, he once exposed his penis to a group of his male and female classmates in the playground. While the other children found what he did to be outrageously funny, several parents lodged complaints that they would pull their children out of this school if the teachers couldn't contain the "immorality" of "other troubled children." He also tends to make "lewd comments" about people depicted in bathing suits in various magazines.

 Please proceed with the problem-based approach!

Following awareness of gender identity, and with the further strides in cognitive development that occur at around the preschool age, children become naturally curious about matters pertaining to sex and sexual organs. Common behaviors include sexually themed play, exploration of one's own body and the bodies of others, and enactment of adult sexual roles (e.g., being mommy or daddy), often within the safety of the family. While many of these behaviors are "normal" (as is often the best choice in multiple-choice exams on sexual development), the clinician should certainly consider other conditions and situations that may predispose to behaviors that are either quantitatively or qualitatively inappropriate for the given age of development. Consider Table 5.2.

Table 5.1 Basic definitions

Term	Definition	When determined or manifested	Mechanism of determination	Examples of clinical concerns relevant to this concept
Chromosomal sex	Whether the human is male (XY) or female (XX)	At conception	Fertilization: fusion of mother and father's genetic material	Phenotypic males with multiple copies of either the X or the Y chromosome
				Phenotypic females with either three or more copies of the X chromosome or only one X chromosome
Assigned gender	Whether a baby is identified as a girl or boy, usually based on the appearance of genitalia	Traditionally at birth, though determinable in utero with ultrasound technology	Expression of genes and action of hormones that influence the development of sexual organs	Androgen insensitivity syndrome (genetic male with tissues unresponsive to male hormones; hence with female-appearing genitalia)
				Congenital adrenal hyperplasia (genetic female with overproduction of androgens; hence with male-appearing or ambiguous genitalia), illustrated in the case above
				Numerous other intersex conditions: while it had been traditionally taught that sexual reassignment surgery should occur before gender identity (defined below) is established, the implications of this condition are much more complex because of the reality that sexual behavior is determined by more than just the outward appearance of one's genitalia

Table 5.1 (Continued)

Term	Definition	When determined or manifested	Mechanism of determination	Examples of clinical concerns relevant to this concept
Gender identity	A child's awareness of being male or female	Usually at around age 2 years	Likely complex interplay between awareness of assigned gender, what is taught and reinforced by caregivers, and biological influences on sexual brain development	In gender identity disorder (described further in Chap. 29), there is discomfort with one's own gender; may be seen as early as preschool years, and more commonly in boys than in girls
Gender role	Culturally proscribed roles associated with each gender	Usually by preschool age	What is taught and reinforced by caregivers and the community	In gender identity disorder, there may be a preference for the roles associated with the opposite gender
Sexual orientation	Preference for males, females, or both as sexual partners	Usually by adolescence	Genetic and other biologically mediated influences on development; likely an interplay between bio-psychosocial factors	Psychological distress around either being in roles that are contrary to one's basic sexual orientation or experiencing the social stigma attached to a non-majority sexual orientation

Case Vignette 5.2.2 Conclusion

You talk to Mike and his mother. Mike conveys regret over what he had done and says that he'll try to be "good" in school. You learn that, while he may have seen some kissing and adult sitcom shows while being babysat by a teenage cousin and her boyfriend a few months ago, he has not had any other exposure to inappropriate sexual material. While your general behavioral screening questionnaire, the 17-item Pediatric Symptom Checklist, suggests that he may have a possible attentional problem, specific questions do not suggest that he has a bipolar, obsessive-compulsive, or pervasivedevelopmental disorder. You provide counseling about

Table 5.2 Examples of normal and potentially concerning sexual behavior in a preschool or school-age child

Examples of probably normal sexual behavior in a preschool or school-age child	Examples of behavior that suggest either inappropriate exposure to sexual activity or other psychopathology
Fascination and glee with pictures of half-clothed bodies or of people kissing	Detailed knowledge about specific sexual acts
Manually exploring one's own body or attempting to manually explore the bodies of family members and close friends	Attempted or actual sexual behaviors that involve penetration, propositioning strangers, and other inappropriate sex talk
Masturbation (possibly aided by toys or other objects) that does not appear to be associated with psychological distress or physical injury and that does not interfere with other developmentally appropriate tasks	Compulsive masturbation associated with psychological distress and/or physical injury and that is so time-consuming as to interfere with other developmentally appropriate tasks

developmentally appropriate supervision and refocusing on developmentally appropriate tasks.

Obviously, what is "normal" sexual behavior is different for different ages and different stages of development. In general, sexual development closely follows development in other areas, including cognitive development, social development, and physical development. Consider the following cases.

Case Vignette 5.3.1 Mary Jane

Your next patient is Mary Jane, a 14-year-old high school freshman, who is brought in by her mother, who requests that Mary Jane be tested for HIV and "anything else that can be sexually transmitted," placed on the "birth control shot," and given "that new cervical cancer vaccine and anything else that can prevent sexually transmitted diseases." The mother learned that Mary Jane slept with a boy classmate at band camp and is now worried that she will catch something from "being promiscuous." Mary Jane explains that she previously had never had sexual intercourse, other than having "experimented" with fondling a close female friend who is lesbian (even though she herself is "straight.") She denies ever having had any other sexual experiences. Mary Jane comes from a "traditional family" that, she believes, would not otherwise condone any premarital sexual activity or any homosexual behaviors.

 Please proceed with the problem-based approach!

Adolescence is a time when hormonal influences lead to the development of secondary sexual characteristics and heightened interest in sexual activity. Key

Table 5.3 Highlights of adolescent development

	Male physical development	Female physical development	Cognitive and social developments
Early adolescence	Testicular enlargement	Breast bud formation	May still have concrete thinking Same-sex peer groups are common
Middle adolescence	Peak in height growth, spermarche	Peak in height growth, generally followed by onset of menses	Emergence of abstract thought, questioning, and risk-taking
Late adolescence	Mature biological sex characteristics	Mature biological sex characteristics	Independence, potential commitment to career, stable partner, etc.

milestones in adolescent development (that often are asked about in standardized tests) are summarized in Table 5.3.

The influence of hormones, primarily testosterone (in both males and females), leads to heightened sexual interest in adolescence. Statistics suggest that sexual activity, including intercourse, is common in adolescence and should prompt the clinician to assist youth in preventing sexually transmitted disease and unwanted pregnancy. According to the Centers for Disease Control and Prevention (2005) youth risk behavior surveillance, 46.8 % of high school students have had sexual intercourse. Among the 33.9 % of high school students who are currently sexually active, 62.8 % reported that they or their partner had used a condom during their last sexual intercourse.

Case Vignette 5.3.2 Conclusion

You examine Mary Jane and find that she is at sexual maturity rating (SMR) stage 4. You perform a pelvic exam with Papanicolau smear and cultures for gonococcus and chlamydia. You also offer blood testing for HIV and syphilis. You insure that her hepatitis B immunizations are up to date and administer the first of the human papillomavirus vaccine series. You counsel her on effective methods of preventing sexually transmitted diseases (including abstinence). Even though the mother states she is "still grieving" over the loss of her daughter's "sexual innocence," she is nevertheless very grateful for your care.

Sexual development continues to be influenced by developmental issues at other phases of the life cycle, as illustrated by the following case.

Case Vignette 5.4.1 Presenting Situation: Phil Robinson

Mr. Phil Robinson is a 58-year-old male with a history of panic disorder and hypertension. He reports that for the past 6 months he and his 49-year-old wife have had sex less and less frequently. While they continued to have a satisfying sex life even

after the birth of their three children, they have recently had more difficulties getting
"in sync" with each other: either she has little sexual interest (which she relates to
"pre-menopause") or she is sexually interested but he has difficulty maintaining an
erection.

 Please proceed with the problem-based approach!

While a decline in libido-promoting hormones may occur in later adulthood for
both women and men, healthy sexuality remains an important priority for most older
adults. Familiarity with Table 5.4 is often helpful when approaching clinical situations involving the human sexual response cycle.

While "normal sexual development" (once again) may be consideredin the differential, the above case may suggest the diagnosis of male erectile disorder in
Mr. Robinson and the possibility of a hypoactive sexual desire disorder in his wife.
Given Mr. Robinson's medical history, it would be important to further inquire about
the specifics of his health condition and any medications he may be on. Any health
condition or medication that can affect any aspect of sexual physiology (including
blood supply and innervation to the sexual organs or anything at all related to brain
functioning) could be a culprit in any disorder of the sexual response cycle.

Case Vignette 5.4.2 Conclusion

In reviewing Mr. Robinson's chart, you discover that he is currently on a beta-
blocker for hypertension and a serotonin-selective reuptake inhibitor along with
a benzodiazepine for panic disorder. He denies any past history of sexual difficulties

Table 5.4 Characteristics of the human sexual response cycle

Stage of cycle	Characteristics	Examples of conditions involving this stage of the sexual response cycle
Desire	Fantasies	Hypoactive sexual desire disorder, sexual aversion disorder
Arousal	Lubrication in female, erection in male	Female sexual arousal disorder, male erectile disorder
Plateau		
Orgasm	Intensified pleasure, rhythmic contractions, ejaculation in males	Orgasmic disorder (male and female), premature ejaculation
Resolution		

other than what he reports as "premature ejaculation" earlier in his adult life. He thinks it is possible that he had more erectile difficulties ever since his serotonin-selective reuptake inhibitor dose had been increased. He also believes that the increased anxiety symptoms he had been having around that time (hence the dose increase) may have played a more important role and may have contributed to what he feels may be a "vicious cycle" of performance anxiety around sexual intercourse. You work to optimize his medication regimen and insure that he has no new medical problems. At a future visit, you provide education to him and his wife about the various factors that can affect the sexual response cycle. You encourage Mrs. Robinson to follow up with her physician. In the meantime, you encourage them to focus on enjoying emotional and physical closeness with each other, with a de-emphasis on sexual intercourse. A few months later, he is happy to report that they have enjoyed their sex life once again.

Sexual issues are encountered in all specialties of medicine and in patients of all age groups. In this chapter, we have reviewed sexual development throughout the life cycle. A further discussion of clinical disorders that involve sexual behavior is found in Chap. 29.

Review Questions

1. An adolescent girl who presents with primary amenorrhea and otherwise normal-appearing pubertal development is found to have an XY karyotype. The most likely diagnosis is

   (a) Normal development
   (b) Polycystic ovary syndrome
   (c) Congenital adrenal hyperplasia
   (d) Androgen insensitivity syndrome
   (e) Turner's syndrome

2. All of the following patients likely are exhibiting normal sexual development EXCEPT for

   (a) A married couple in the mid-50s who engage in sexual intercourse several times per week
   (b) A 5-year-old male who makes two attempts in the office to peek under his mother's dress
   (c) A 16-year-old female who presents with flight of ideas, seductiveness toward the physician, and her fifth episode of pelvic inflammatory disease, which she said she caught from "sleeping with the whole football team"
   (d) A 12-year-old female who is accidentally caught stroking her genital area while in her bedroom
   (e) An 18-year-old male who presents with a urinary tract infection, which he believes he might have caught from his male partner, whom he has been with for the past year

3. Which of the following represent the earliest signs of puberty in males and females?

   (a) For males: testicular enlargement; for females: breast bud development
   (b) For males: spermarche; for females: height spurt
   (c) For males: testicular enlargement; for females: menarche
   (d) For males: spermarche; for females: breast bud formation
   (e) For males: testicular enlargement; for females: height spurt

4. Which of the following represents the correct temporal sequence of the sexual response cycle?

   (a) Plateau, desire, arousal, orgasm
   (b) Desire, arousal, plateau, orgasm
   (c) Arousal, desire, plateau, orgasm
   (d) Plateau, arousal, orgasm, plateau
   (e) Orgasm, plateau, arousal, desire

Answers

1. d, 2. c, 3. a, 4. b

Bibliography

Bright Futures, Tool for Professionals. Pediatric Symptom Checklist. http://www.brightfutures.org/mentalhealth/pdf/professionals/ped_sympton_chklst.pdf.

Centers for Disease Control and Prevention. Morbidity and Mortality Weekly Report Youth Risk Behavior Surveillance—United States, 2005. Surveillance Summaries June 9, 2006/Vol. 55/No. SS-5, http://www.cdc.gov/mmwr/PDF/SS/SS5505.pdf.

Sadock B.J. and Sadock V.A.. (2003). Kaplan and Sadock's Synopsis of Psychiatry: Behavioral Sciences/Clinical Psychiatry. 9th Edition. New York: Lippincott Williams & Wilkins.

Chapter 6
Adaptation and Coping in a Medical Setting

Maria-Christina Stewart

Coping adaptively in the face of medical adversity is a critical advantage. This chapter illustrates the importance of adaptive coping and how physicians can help patients develop skills. This chapter, like the sample vignette in Chap. 1, uses graphics in the vignette text to help identify key facts for the PBL process. While this chapter does not cover all of the psychiatric illnesses that may occur following the diagnosis of a medical illness (as these are covered in the specific chapters), it highlights both healthy and potentially unhealthy behaviors.

At the end of this chapter, the reader will be able to:

1. Define and identify methods of coping and adaptation
2. Determine neurobiological, psychological, social, and spiritual variables affecting coping and adaptation
3. Classify and distinguish among functional and dysfunctional methods of adapting to and coping with stressful situations such as medical adversity
4. Identify methods of intervention to facilitate adaptive coping

Case Vignette 6.1.1 Presenting Situation: Paul Davis

Paul Davis is a 75-year-old African-American male who recently presented with "cognitive difficulties." *Accompanying him at every medical appointment and assisting in decision-making processes is his wife: his number "one supporter" and partner in life. Paul is scheduled today for cognitive testing. He arrives with his wife and shares with you his comfort with end-of-life issues, claiming to be "keeping a stiff upper lip" and endorsing a stoic disposition in the face of stress. During the testing process, his wife leaves to run errands and then returns to bring*

M. Stewart
Department of Psychology, University of Hawai'i, Currently a Research Fellow at the Center for Anxiety and Related Disorders, Boston University

A. Guerrero, M. Piasecki (eds.), *Problem-Based Behavioral Science and Psychiatry*,
© Springer Science+Business Media, LLC 2008

him home. Paul is $\boxed{silent}$ *during the majority of cognitive testing, including after his wife returns to bring him home.*

 Please proceed with the problem-based approach!

Adaptation and Coping Defined

Adaptation

Adaptation refers to efforts and processes aimed at managing demands of stressors. It involves the use of resources, coping, and problem-solving strategies, with the ultimate goal of altering an individual's state of functioning. As we will see, this new state may be positive or negative (e.g., a positive adaptation of using external resources to aid in coping with cancer may become negative if it is the only process of adaptation employed and the individual does not learn to use inner resources). The process of adapting involves making changes to (Friedman, Bowden, & Jones, 2003):

- Established patterns of functioning
- Internal resources
- Resources within the family and community
- Appraisal of how demands are being and should be met
- World views
- Problem-solving skills
- Coping methods

Coping

Coping refers to problem-specific efforts aimed at preventing, avoiding, or controlling specific external and/or internal stressors that are impairing an individual's well-being (e.g., emotional distress and/or solving problems). More specifically, coping refers to behaviors that can or are being employed, rather than resources that could be of use (Friedman et al., 2003). As patients adapt to and cope with medical visits, diagnoses, and procedures, it is normal for them to experience transient emotions. When such emotions become persistent or uncontrollable, however, they may hinder adaptive coping and adaptation behaviors and result in a psychiatric disorder.

Table 6.1 Considering the facts, examining hypotheses, and identifying specific information

What are the facts?	What are your hypotheses?	What do you want to know next?	What specific information would you like to learn about?
Age 75 Male Married Cognitive difficulties Receiving cognitive testing Claims to be comfortable with end-of-life issues Stoic disposition Considers wife to be a source of support Silent	1. He relies on his wife for significant support 2. He is facing and considering end-of-life questions and issues 3. His silence and stoic disposition may be a sign of underlying difficulties in adapting to and coping with his cognitive deficits 4. His silence and stoic disposition may be related to an underlying medical/neurological or psychiatric condition (e.g., major depression, dementia, etc.) 5. Cognitive deficits, in particular, may be difficult for him to accept because of stigma	*HPI* Medication? Sleep? Appetite? Hopelessness? Fear? *PMH* Has he had any previous medical or psychiatric diagnoses, including substance abuse? *FH* Any history of psychiatric illness? *SH* Social support besides wife? *Exam* Physical exam? Vital signs?	1. How are adaptation and coping defined? 2. What are the major neurobiological and psychosocial correlates of adaptation and coping? 3. How does social support affect adaptation and coping? 4. What are the interventions for coping deficits?

Neurobiological Correlates of Adaptation and Coping

As we start to formulate our case conceptualization of Paul and consider which methods of adaptation and coping, if any, he may be employing or may be beneficial (see Table 6.1 to review our problem based approach), let's keep in mind the physiology behind two primary emotions often associated with medical adversity: fear and sadness (summarized in Table 6.2, for a detailed review, see Carlson, 2006). While a detailed discussion of the physiology of stress is beyond the scope of this chapter and is more comprehensively covered in Chap. 11 (Stress and Health), it is important to consider the ways in which the primary medical illness being adapted to can, in itself, pose a biological risk to maladaptive coping.

Table 6.2 Examples of neurobiological correlates of persistent fear and sadness

Oversensitive norepinephrine system in the locus coeruleus
Abnormal function of serotonin system
Over-secretion of corticotropin-releasing factor and subsequent long-term reduction in cortisol
Reduction in hippocampal volume

Effect of Social Support on Adaptation and Coping

Support from external sources such as extended social support networks and the community can significantly aid in both adapting to and coping with major stressors through alleviating much of the associated burden and preventing additional stress and negative consequences. Individuals and families with support from social networks tend to cope with medical crises and illness better than individuals or families employing only internal strategies, and absence of social support can engender feelings of vulnerability—especially among individuals whose cultural norms include relying on extended kin for assistance (Friedman & Ferguson-Marshalleck, 1996). As a result, active participation in and promotion and maintenance of relationships in the individual's immediate and larger social network (e.g., neighborhood, town, society) are vital.

Types of Social Support

Individuals in crisis may benefit from short-term crisis management or longer-term support for general life issues (e.g., adjusting to loss of a child or parent). Families often play key roles in providing all types of support, and extended resources aid in meeting those needs that the family cannot address. Types of social support include (House & Kahn, 1985):

- Instrumental support (e.g., offering direct assistance)
- Informational support (e.g., sharing information about the illness)
- Appraisal support (e.g., aiding in assessing the illness and/or decision-making)
- Emotional support (e.g., providing counseling)

Barriers to Seeking Social Support

Though empirical literature repeatedly demonstrates the value of employing external sources of support, individuals and/or families especially from Anglo-Saxon communities may interpret such use as a marker of weakness and/or failure to independently cope with the stressor. Additionally, individuals may wish to utilize professional services but be unable to afford them (Walsh, 1998).

Case Conceptualization of Paul

Now that we've examined the meanings behind *adaptation* and *coping*, the neurobiological correlates of fear and sadness, and the role of social support in handling medical adversity, let's take another look at what we know thus far about Paul. His cognitive difficulties may have neurobiological underpinnings that may, in turn, relate to his silence. At this point, however, it is unclear to what extent his quiet presentation is reflective of his personality. He described his wife as a significant source of support, and it is possible that her absence during most of the visit related to Paul's silent disposition. He also claimed to be comfortable with end-of-life issues but did not define "issues" or rate his comfort level on a meaningful scale.

Case Vignette 6.1.2 Continuation

Paul returns to the hospital the following day to continue testing. He arrives again with his wife, who stays during today's visit and anxiously asks several questions about the meaning behind these "cognitive difficulties."

Paul has been healthy for most of his life, with the exception of essential hypertension currently well controlled with diet and medication and osteoarthritis. He denies any personal history of a psychiatric illness and assures you with a chuckle that he's not crazy and can hold it together just fine. He denies any definite problems with his sleep or appetite.

Paul is again quiet *and looks at the ground as his wife chastises him about being a difficult patient, says he is to blame for being sick, and lectures him about the necessity of taking better care of himself. You are in the room as they talk to their daughter and overhear Paul* suddenly start screaming *that she can be as cool and comfortable as she wants to be about his cognitive difficulties and can leave the entire family and never talk to him again if she chooses.*

Adaptive and Maladaptive Methods of Adapting to and Coping with Medical Adversity

Emotional, cognitive, and behavioral strategies of adaptively or maladaptively coping with medical adversity are person-, problem-, and situation-specific and can either develop within an individual or group or be drawn externally from social networks and the larger community. Having a pool of adaptive strategies from which to select is best in effectively coping with stressors. Several such strategies are summarized in Tables 6.3 and 6.4. (For a detailed review, see Friedman et al., 2003; McCubbin & McCubbin, 1993.)

Adapting to and Coping with Illness in the Context of the Family

Families can also play a significant role as agents of social change during medical adversity (Burr et al., 1994; McCubbin & McCubbin, 1993; Walsh, 1998). The success of adaptation is determined by the family's ability to function and adapt to change; the situational pile-up of demands, transitions, strains, and stressors; and family communication. Those families with affirming and/or stress-reducing communication (e.g., calm, soothing support) are more likely to adapt to stress compared

Table 6.3 Adaptive methods of adapting to and coping with medical adversity

Cognitive coping strategies

Normalizing involves focusing thoughts, attention, and behaviors on the normal aspects of life and may be achieved through maintaining rituals and routines that preexisted the stressor, defining life as normal, participating in activities that reflect the normalcy of the individual and/or family, and minimizing attention to any negative social effects of the stressor (e.g., stigma)

Cognitive reframing and passive appraisal describes adjusting the meaning of a situation and viewing stressors as something that will care for themselves

Joint problem solving involves identifying and communicating in an effort to isolate, select, carry out, and monitor solutions based on shared input from everyone involved in the problem-solving process

Becoming educated about medical adversity is an easy method for individuals to both increase the feeling of control in uncertain situations and better evaluate situations when making decisions. It offers medical teams a means of communication with patients and families and is associated with effective coping and decreased stress

Effective communication

Sharing ideas and feelings, being honest and clear, and using humor significantly effect coping during medical adversity

Table 6.4 Maladaptive methods of adapting to and coping with medical adversity

Individual methods

Denial is a defense mechanism that allows individuals to disbelieve that a situation or some aspect thereof exists

Emotional distancing describes an inability to cultivate close, emotional relationships and may occur during periods of extreme stress

Creation of myths involves suspension of reality by altering belief systems. Myths are produced when wishes and expectations have not been fulfilled and may serve as reflections of both inner and outer states of an individual

Group methods

Scapegoating involves a group negatively labeling, blaming, and displacing tensions, hostilities, guilt, and stress on one member while appearing to have achieved group harmony and cohesiveness

Triangling gives the illusion of limiting and diminishing group tensions by welcoming additional members on whom the stress is displaced

Threats involving permanent ostracism, self-destructive acts of other members of the group (e.g., suicide), and emotional withdrawal may be posited when one group member appears to display autonomy and independence from the group and the group fears losing cohesiveness

Dissolution and Addiction: During periods of extreme stress, attempts to reduce tension may result in separation from loved ones (e.g., divorce), addiction (e.g., gambling, substance use), or violence

to families with conflict-escalating communication (e.g., yelling, blaming), which elevates tension (Friedman et al., 2003). Adaptive relational methods of coping with medical adversity are summarized in Table 6.5. (For a detailed review, see Walsh, 1998).

Table 6.5 Adaptive relational methods of adapting to and coping with medical adversity

Family group reliance involves increased structure and organization in the family and home (e.g., chores, visits, mealtimes) and more rigid time schedules and routines. It can lead to increased integration, cohesion, strength, and predictability, thereby leading to increased coping with the stressor

Increased family cohesion may be achieved through involvement in shared leisure-time activities and rituals, especially when these rituals maintain and foster shared identity and world views among group members and increase integration, cohesion, morale, satisfaction, and resilience. Among families, cohesion is characterized by emotional bonding among family members and is considered to be a central attribute to the family unit

Role flexibility describes the ability for family members to share and change roles during times of stress. It is essential for maintaining the equilibrium between stability and change and thereby increases adaptive coping with developmental, environmental, and life stressors

Case Conceptualization of Paul

Now that we have discussed how the family can influence a patient's ability to adaptively or maladaptively cope with and adapt to medical adversity, let's take another look at Paul. We cannot yet be sure about the nature of his quiet disposition; however, but we know that he has been quiet both on his own and while being chastised by his wife, who appears anxious. We have also caught a glimpse of him screaming threats at his daughter, suggesting that his and his family's methods of coping and adaptation are dysfunctional. He appears to have some stigma toward mental illness, suggesting that he may not be very receptive to acknowledging having difficulty coping with his current medical situation.

Case casevignette 6.1.3 Continuation

Paul was cooperative and forthcoming during a semi-structured interview and mental status exam, which was remarkable for blunted affect and tearfulness *. He denied any substance use, including coffee and cigarettes. Paul revealed having* **served in the Korean War** *and having* **grown up Black in the United States before the Civil Rights Movement.** *He indicated having a* **troubling relationship with each of his six children** *and admitted to being "too hard" on them and unnecessarily screaming at them too often. He* **denied having much of a support network outside of his family.** *Paul denied feeling suicidal and expressed his hopes to live as long as possible, reiterating feeling comfortable with the concept of death and attributing these feelings to his Christian faith and daily prayer.*

Please proceed with the problem-based approach!

Factors Influencing Coping and Adaptation

Sociocultural Values

Important variables in understanding and considering adaptation and coping strategies are culture and society. A significant amount of research has demonstrated wide variation in the use of the strategies discussed in this chapter, and it is imperative that medical staff sensitively respond to the patient's and family's values and norms. For example, the extent to which individuals rely on internal and external coping and adaptation strategies varies across cultures, and medical staff are advised to take cultural values and background into account when assisting patients and their families in adjusting to illness (Friedman et al., 2003; Friedman & Ferguson-Marshalleck, 1996).

Similarly, many individuals and families may find that spirituality and/or religious beliefs lie at the core of coping with and adapting to medical adversity. However, reliance on these beliefs varies across developmental, cultural, and socioeconomic groups (Clark & Heidenreich, 1995).

Gender Differences

Methods of coping tend to vary across genders. Women use more strategies that involve closeness and intimacy, such as reaching out, sharing concerns with family members and friends, openly expressing emotions, cognitive reframing, delegating, and taking time for self-care; men, on the other hand, tend to withdraw more, keep emotions hidden, and use alcohol (Burr et al., 1994).

Development

Special consideration and attention should be given to the effect of developmental stage on coping and adapting to medical illness and trauma. This is particularly true for children, whose experiences are especially influential in shaping future reactions to hospitals and medical procedures. Further discussion on the role of development in adjusting to various transitions is provided in Chap. 4, Learning Principles of Human Behavior.

Bio-psycho-social-cultural-spiritual Conceptualization

Now that we have garnered information pertinent to most of our learning issues, let's review the neurobiological, social, psychological, and spiritual information relating to Paul's case conceptualization so that we can identify its impact on his psychiatric presentation:

Biological

Past: Genetics (no known history of psychiatric illness in patient or family), history of hypertension
Presenting problem: Cognitive difficulties

Psychological

Past

Trauma (United States War Veteran; history as a racial minority in the United States before the Civil Rights Movement)
Personality (stoic disposition)

Present

Affect (blunted; tearful; quiet/silent)
End-of-life issues (eager to live as long as possible; comfortable with death; no suicidality)
Possible stigma about mental health problems, including cognitive difficulties

Social/Cultural/Spiritual

- Married to wife whom he describes as supportive and who appears anxious
- Six children; troubled relationships; none live in same city; use of threats toward them
- No support network outside of family
- Scapegoating and blame from wife
- Christian/prays daily

As we conceptualize Paul's case and consider effective interventions, it may be helpful to continue the inquiry process outlined in Table 6.1 and summarize the current hypotheses in a diagram (Fig. 6.1).

Psychosocial Interventions to Facilitate Adapting to and Coping with Medical Adversity

Developing and practicing adaptive coping when facing medical crises can be challenging for many patients, especially when they are used to employing maladaptive coping strategies in their daily lives. As a result, psychotherapy for individuals and families is often recommended and has been empirically demonstrated to benefit patients struggling to cope with medical adversity.

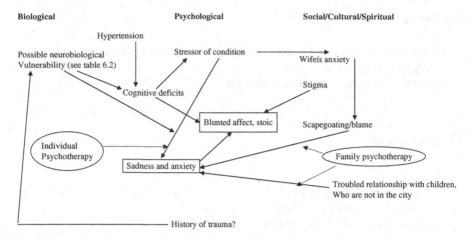

Fig. 6.1 Bio-psycho-social-spiritual case conceptualization model of our sample client Paul. This model demonstrates the interrelated nature of biological, psychological, social, and spiritual variables relevant to case conceptualizations, as demonstrated through the case sample of Paul. *Solid arrows* represent mechanisms underlying clinical hypotheses; presenting symptoms are in *boxes*; potential therapeutic interventions are in *ovals* and linked with *dotted arrows*; and proximal etiological variables are *underlined and asterisked*

Additionally, several psychosocial models have been developed to guide medical staff in both addressing maladaptive coping and facilitating in the development of adaptive coping methods. Specific psychosocial strategies include: reviewing the event that led to the injury; processing the sensory experience of the event; assessing beliefs related to the event; and using desensitization, relaxation techniques, and pain management for medical interventions. Specific strategies for pediatric patients include using drawings and play to symbolize and elaborate the event further, explaining medical interventions carefully to the child, increasing the child's sense of control over their own bodies, and assisting the parents to manage their own affect relating to the event and subsequent injury.

Case Conceptualization of Paul

When we examine Paul's story, though still incomplete, we can see the great extent to which biological, psychological, social, and spiritual factors interact and influence his presenting symptoms of cognitive deficits and quiet, blunted, and tearful affect. It remains unclear whether these symptoms reflect underlying depression and/or anxiety. However, because Paul's personal history and family presentation reflect the use of some maladaptive methods of coping with his cognitive deficits (e.g., silence, screaming), it is possible that his daily life and family relations would improve from psychosocial interventions. Let's take a look at a psychosocial assessment conducted 6 months following the end of a psychosocial intervention.

Case Vignette 6.1.4 Conclusion

Following a 3-month intervention of weekly family therapy and individual therapy focused on processing Paul's experience with his cognitive deficits, reviewing previous and current family relations, and increasing family cohesion, reliance on one another, and role flexibility, Paul arrives for a 6-month follow-up assessment. His wife is accompanying him and stays during the entire appointment. Together, they indicate that the amount of screaming in their family has significantly decreased, while the amount of support and communication has increased. They both become tearful and link arms as they admit that they continue to struggle with Paul's cognitive difficulties and unknown diagnosis and sometimes lash out at each other. Overall, though, they express gratitude for their therapy.

Conclusions

As Paul's case illustrates, adaptive coping with medical illness is influenced by many different factors, especially those related to biology, psychology, social support, and spiritual beliefs (e.g., the type and onset of the illness, individual and family coping styles). It is imperative to assess patients and, when possible, their family members not only on their medical illness but also on their adjustment to the illness.

Review Questions

1. Maladaptive methods of coping with and adapting to medical adversity include

   (a) Addiction
   (b) Triangulating
   (c) Threat
   (d) All of the above

2. Adaptation involves

   (a) Specific behaviors aimed at preventing, avoiding, or controlling specific stressors
   (b) Changing external situations to improve internal responses
   (c) Use of internal and external resources, coping, and problem-solving strategies aimed at managing demands of stressors
   (d) Selection of only one effective strategy to adjust to stressors

3. Which of the following is recognized as a specific type of support?

   (a) Instrumental
   (b) Informational
   (c) Appraisal
   (d) Emotional
   (e) All of the above

4. Assessing beliefs related to medical trauma has been discussed as one method of

   (a) Maladaptive coping
   (b) Facilitating adaptive coping
   (c) Both of the above
   (d) Neither of the above

Answers

1. d, 2. c, 3. e, 4. b

References

Burr, W., Klein, S., Burr, R., Doxey, C., Harker, B., Holman, T., et al. (1994). *Reexamining family stress: New theory and research*. Thousand Oaks, CA: Sage.

Carlson, N. (2006). *Physiology of behavior* (9th ed.). New York: Allyn & Bacon.

Clark, C., & Heidenreich, T. (1995). Spiritual care for the critically ill. *American Journal of Critical Care, 4*(1), 77–81.

Friedman, M. M., Bowden, V. R., & Jones, E. G. (2003). Family stress, coping, and adaptation. In M. M. Friedman, V. R. Bowden, & E. G. Jones (Eds.), *Family nursing: Research, theory, and practice* (5th ed.). Upper Saddle Ridge, NJ: Prentice Hall Health.

Friedman, M. M., & Ferguson-Marshalleck, E. (1996). Sociocultural influences on family health. In S. Hanson & S. Boyd (Eds.), *Family health care nursing: Theory, practice & research* (pp. 81–98). Philadelphia: Davis.

House, J. S., & Kahn, R. L. (1985). Measures and concepts of social support. In S. Cohen & S. L. Syme (Eds.), *Social support and health* (pp. 83–108). Orlando, FL: Academic Press.

McCubbin, M. A., & McCubbin, H. I. (1993). Families coping with illness: The resiliency model of family stress, adjustment and adaptation. In C. Danielson, B. Hamel-Bissell, & P. Winstead-Fry (Eds.), *Families, health, and illness: Perspectives on coping and intervention* (pp. 21–63). St. Louis: Harcourt Health Services.

Walsh, F. (1998). *Strengthening family resilience*. New York: The Guilford Press.

Chapter 7
Violence and Abuse

Jeanelle J. Sugimoto and Anthony P.S. Guerrero

This chapter reviews conditions that are among the leading causes of morbidity and mortality throughout the life cycle, yet remain under-recognized and under-addressed in clinical practice.

At the end of this chapter, the reader will be able to

1. Discuss typical presenting signs and symptoms of patients who are victims of various types of violence or abuse
2. Define the different types of violence and abuse
3. Discuss resources and treatments for victims of violence and abuse

Case 7.1.1 Presenting Situation: Mary Infante

Mary Infante is a 32-year-old married woman who is 20 weeks pregnant and having severe cramps. She has had two miscarriages in the past and is worried that she may be having another one. Previous laboratory tests were remarkable. Upon physical examination, she has bruising on the upper arms and abdomen. The bruising is not noticeable on any areas of the body that are not covered by her clothing.

Ms. Infante is a secretary at a local law firm. Her husband was recently laid off from his position with a construction company and is seeking another company to work with. He has apparently been let go from a number of positions since they have been together. They have been married for approximately 3 years, but have not yet been able to have children. A psychiatric consultation was requested by her physician to evaluate the situation.

 Please proceed with the problem-based approach!

J.J. Sugimoto
Program Manager, Asian/Pacific Islander Youth Violence Prevention Center, Department of Psychiatry, University of Hawai'i John A. Burns School of Medicine

A. Guerrero, M. Piasecki (eds.), *Problem-Based Behavioral Science and Psychiatry*,

Abuse and Neglect of Adults

Although further information must still be gathered from the patient and her husband, spousal abuse should be a strong consideration in this case. All physicians in all specialties must be aware of the physical and emotional signs of violence and abuse. As can be seen in this case study, the obstetrician discovered the symptoms in the context of a recent miscarriage. Injuries and bruising can be discovered during any physical examination, and key statements that may reveal underlying problems can be elicited during any patient interview. It is up to the physician to make the initial identification and refer the patient to an appropriate specialist.

Family violence is a general term that includes acts of violence between family members or other individuals with close relations (Director & Linden, 2004). Domestic violence is a specific type of family violence, and includes acts between intimate partners (therefore the term is also interchangeable with "intimate partner violence") (Director & Linden, 2004). It includes acts that may coerce, control, or demean the victim (Director & Linden, 2004). The American College of Emergency Physicians outlines domestic violence as "... part of a pattern of coercive behavior which an individual uses to establish and maintain power and control over another with whom he or she has or had an intimate, romantic, or spousal relationship. Behaviors include actual or threatened physical or sexual abuse, psychological abuse, social isolation, deprivation, or intimidation" (American College of Emergency Physicians, 1995). The DSM-IV-TR notates abuse and neglect under "Other Conditions that May be a Focus of Clinical Attention" and categorizes these diagnoses as follows: (1) physical abuse of child, (2) sexual abuse of child, (3) neglect of child, (4) physical abuse of adult, and (5) sexual abuse of adult.

According to the July 2000 National Violence Against Women Survey, 7.7 % of women surveyed reported having experienced rape from an intimate partner at some point in their life. Twenty-two percent reported having been physically assaulted, 4.8 % reported having been stalked, and 25.5 % reported having been victimized in some other way, all by an intimate partner (Tjaden & Thoennes, 2000). The effects of domestic violence are varied and widespread. Not only do the victims suffer physically and emotionally, but family and friends become involved. The situation is especially taxing on children who may witness the abuse. These secondary victims may in turn show their own signs and symptoms, including behavior changes, sleep disturbances, and increased aggression (Director & Linden, 2004). They may also be at risk for posttraumatic stress disorder, acute stress disorder, adjustment disorder, and other conditions (please refer to Chaps. 23 and 30).

Case 7.1.2 Continuation

You interview Ms. Infante individually. You talk to her about her career. She received a merit-based raise, and her co-workers even put together a small dinner to thank her for such good work. When asked about her husband's career, she comments that he was recently laid off from his job. Apparently, the construction company he worked for was restructured. She thinks he feels cheated out of a position, and even wrote an angry letter to the president of the company.

After further inquiry, she reveals that the miscarriages might have been caused by spousal abuse while she was pregnant. You suspect that her husband also abuses her when she is not pregnant. She says that he is a very caring husband when in the presence of others, but his temper "gets the best of him" when they are alone. He relates his temper to the severe physical and emotional abuse he had experienced while growing up.

You then call the husband into the room to discuss your concerns with the current pregnancy. Overall, he is cordial and polite and seems attentive to his wife. You note that he often interrupts his wife while she is attempting to answer a question. You politely ask him to refrain from answering questions directed at his wife, but he continues to answer questions for her.

 Please proceed with the problem-based approach!

While there are no definitive tests that can determine with 100 % accuracy that an individual is a victim of domestic violence, there are certain risk factors and signs/symptoms the physician can consider (Director & Linden, 2004).

- Risk factors

  - Being female
  - Being younger
  - Being single, separated, or divorced

- Physical signs and symptoms

  - Initial signs may be vague and nonspecific
  - Injuries

    - Injuries that are not consistent with the patient history or complaints that are not consistent with the problem
    - Recurrent injuries with increasing severity over time
    - Multiple injuries in different stages of healing
    - Injuries to central body areas (breasts, abdomen, chest) in addition to the face and extremities
    - Injuries to normally protected areas (inner thigh, inner arm)
    - Injuries suggesting defensive posture

  - General health concerns

    - Higher rates of general health problems (headache, back pain, vaginal infections, gastrointestinal complaints)

- Frequent exacerbations of chronic illnesses (asthma, diabetes, hypertension)
- Increased use of the health care system, but delay in seeking treatment for the actual problem
- Lack of prenatal care
- Injury during pregnancy

- Emotional signs and symptoms

  - Frequent reporting of emotional symptoms (depression, low self-esteem, increased daily stressors, anxiety)
  - Feelings of guilt and isolation
  - Possible substance abuse, eating disorders, posttraumatic stress disorder
  - Possible suicidality

- Characteristics of the abuser

  - Substance abuse
  - Lower educational achievement
  - Intermittent employment
  - Victimization as a child
  - Feelings of inadequacy
  - Personality disorders (antisocial, borderline)
  - Younger
  - Hovering, domineering presence in spite of cordial/attentive appearance to outside parties
  - Verbal abusiveness

The physician's first step toward treatment is screening. The screening process not only pushes all parties toward the end goal but also lets the patient know that the physician is concerned for his/her welfare and safety. The patient should be interviewed alone and in a supportive, nonjudgmental, confidential setting (Director & Linden, 2004). There are a number of protocols available to physicians. Overall, most of the literature suggests using simple, open-ended questions. Below are some suggested questions, ranging from less to more invasive.

- Simple and open-ended (Director & Linden, 2004)

  - How does your partner treat you?
  - Are you or have you been in a relationship in which you felt you were treated badly?
  - We all fight at home; what happens when you and your partner fight or disagree?
  - Do you ever feel afraid of your partner?
  - Has your partner ever prevented you from leaving the house, seeing friends, getting a job, or continuing your education?
  - Has your partner ever destroyed things you care about?

- More direct questions

    - The Partner Violence Screen—65–71 % sensitivity (Feldhaus et al., 1997)

        - Have you been hit, kicked, punched, or otherwise hurt by someone within the past year? If so, by whom?
        - Do you feel safe in your current relationship?
        - Is there a partner from a previous relationship who is making you feel unsafe now?

    - The "StaT" Screening Tool—97 % sensitivity (Liebschutz & Paranjape, 2003)

        - Have you ever been in a relationship in which your partner has pushed or slapped you?
        - Have you ever been in a relationship in which your partner threatened you with violence?
        - Have you ever been in a relationship in which your partner has thrown, broken, or punched things?

Case Vignette 7.1.3 Conclusion

You decide to admit Ms. Infante for threatened miscarriage and for further assessment and intervention for domestic violence. You consult a social worker, who meets with her individually and provides her with information on spousal abuse and women's shelters. A safety plan is formulated that includes cash, a cell phone, and keeping the car tank full of gas. You involve Ms. Infante's sister, as well as two of her closest friends. She will stay in the hospital for a few days, and then with her sister. The social worker also assists Ms. Infante with a referral to legal counsel, in case she wishes to file a formal restraining order against the husband.

You and the social worker meet with her and her sister about a month later. She states that she and her husband will attempt marriage counseling with a psychologist the social worker recommended. During this period however, she will still stay with her sister to maintain her personal safety.

After the initial screening, there are some general steps that should be taken to help abuse victims (McLeer & Anwar, 1987):

- Obtain history
- Diagnose and treat injuries
- Evaluate the emotional safety of the patient
- Determine the risk to the victim
- Determine the need for legal intervention
- Develop a follow-up plan
- Document findings

Brown (1997) applied the Trans-theoretic Model of Change to the process of a victim's emergence from the cycle of violence. This model is discussed in Chaps. 4 and 10.

There are many reasons why victims are unable to break out of the cycle of violence. If the physician has a good understanding of the victim's reasoning, he or she is more likely to make an appropriate referral.

Below are some common scenarios.

- Common reasons for the victim staying in an abusive relationship:

  - Nonrecognition that he or she is being abused
  - Fear of the abuser, or fear of retaliation
  - Desire to fulfill predetermined cultural or gender roles
  - Fear of losing financial or childcare support

- Common physician-related reasons why the victim may not disclose information to the physician

  - Failure of the physician to inquire
  - Discomfort with talking to patients about this topic
  - Lack of confidence in ability to diagnose abuse
  - Perceived inability to offer appropriate referrals if diagnosed
  - Fear of offending the victim or crossing a cultural barrier
  - Lack of time or privacy with the individual
  - Personal experiences with abuse

- Common patient-related reasons why the victim may not disclose information to the physician

  - Low self-esteem
  - Lack of trust toward the physician
  - Fear that disclosure will involve the police or child protective services
  - Fear of being judged
  - Language or cultural barriers

The Community Coalition on Family Violence (CCFV) notes that five statements can provide important encouragement to an abuse victim (Williams, 2005):

- You're not alone.
- No one has the right to hit you.
- Domestic violence is not your fault.
- It's against the law.
- Help is available and I'll be here when you need me.

Physicians should also be aware of other specific types of abuse among adults, including rape or sexual assault, and elder abuse.

There are several misconceptions about rape, including that it involves a sex-deprived young male attacking an attractive female, that it is not a violent crime, and that it is a street crime (rather than one that may even occur between partners and spouses). According to Englander (2007), there are various types of perpetrators, including violent rapists (who may engage in brutal beatings, who view sex as secondary, and who are chronically angry) and power rapists (who typically use only enough force to complete the act and who have underlying feelings of inadequacy). In general, perpetrators of rape often demonstrate a lack of empathy and an acceptance of cognitive misperceptions (e.g., that the victim deserved it or is making too big a fuss about it). Alcohol or substance abuse (on either the part of the perpetrator or victim) can be a risk factor (though by no means an excuse) for rape to occur.

Elder abuse can include physical abuse (including over-medicating, under-medicating, force-feeding, inappropriately using physical restraints, and exposing to the elements) and emotional abuse (including treatment like a child and isolation from family and friends, neglect, sexual abuse, and financial abuse) (Muehlbauer & Crane, 2006).

Given the unfortunately high prevalence of victimization and the potential serious sequelae, it is critical for physicians of all specialties to screen all patients of all ages for abuse. The next section is focused on abuse and neglect of children.

Case Vignette 7.2.1 Nicholas Head

An emergency room physician refers Nicholas Head, a 5-year-old boy, to your care. Nick's mother reported that he was running in the house and tripped and hit his head on the corner of their dining room table. Upon examination it was clear that Nick's left eye and the left side of his face are badly bruised. During the complete full-body examination, the ER doctor saw bruising on his upper arm and tenderness when palpating his abdomen. He orders several X-rays, one of which indicates that the boy has a healing fractured humerus. His mother reports that he was roughhousing on the playground with some other children at school and fell off the jungle gym. You are called to join the case to perform a psychiatric consultation on the child.

 Please proceed with the problem-based approach!

Abuse and Neglect of Children

At this point, child neglect and/or abuse is a valid suspicion. Child abuse is one of the leading causes of injury-related mortality in infants and children (McDonald, 2007). According to the Centers for Disease Control and Prevention, among all children confirmed by child protective service agencies in 2002 as being maltreated, 61 % experienced neglect, 19 % were physically abused, 10 % were sexually abused and 5 % were emotionally or psychologically abused (www.cdc.gov). In 2002, an estimated 1,500 children died from maltreatment, 36 % from neglect, 28 % from physical abuse, and 29 % from multiple maltreatment types (www.cdc.gov).

The Child Abuse Prevention and Treatment Act (CAPTA) defines abuse as "... a recent act or failure to act that results in death, serious physical or emotional harm, sexual abuse or exploitation, or imminent risk of serious harm; involves a child; and is carried out by a parent or caregiver who is responsible for the child's welfare (McDonald, 2007)." Child abuse can be categorized as neglect, emotional abuse, physical abuse, and sexual abuse, and each of these can be further categorized according to the definitions below (McDonald, 2007).

Child neglect

- Physical neglect—basic needs for food, clothing, shelter, hygiene, protection, supervision not met
- Emotional neglect—lack of love and affection
- Educational neglect—failure to enroll child in school
- Medical neglect—failure to seek medical assistance to upkeep child's well-being

Emotional abuse

- Several subtypes, including rejection, isolation, terrorism, ignorance, psychological unavailability, corruption, and inappropriate expectations of or demands on the child.

Physical abuse, of which typical findings may include

- Bruises, including

  - Handprints (typically adult-sized)
  - Unusually distributed lesions
  - Lesions at various stages of healing

- Bites (also, typically adult-sized)
- Burns

  - Cigarette burns
  - Burns with clear demarcation and uniform depth (e.g., submersion burns)

- Fractures

  - Posterior rib fractures
  - Long bone fractures in children under 2 years of age
  - Scapular, spinous process, sternal fractures

- Abdominal trauma
- Head trauma

  - Retinal hemorrhages

- Trauma that is inconsistent with the reported mechanism of injury

Sexual abuse

- The Child Abuse Prevention and Treatment Act (CAPTA) defines sexual abuse as "The employment, use, persuasion, inducement, enticement, or coercion of any child to engage in, or assist any other person to engage in, any sexually explicit conduct or simulation of such conduct for the purpose of producing a visual depiction of such conduct; or the rape, molestation, prostitution, or other form of sexual exploitation of children, or incest with children (McDonald, 2007)."

Children who experience any of these types of abuse may demonstrate emotional symptoms, which include social withdrawal, anger or aggression, feeding disorders, developmental delay, or emotional disturbances.

A number of risk factors for child abuse and neglect have been identified. They can be categorized by caregiver, child, and family/environmental factors (McDonald, 2007).

- Caregiver factors

  - Criminal history
  - Inappropriate expectations of the child
  - Mental health history
  - Misconceptions about child care
  - Misperceptions about child development
  - Substance abuse

- Child factors

  - Behavior problems
  - Medical fragility
  - Nonbiologic relationship to the caretaker
  - Prematurity
  - Special needs

- Family and environmental factors

  - High local unemployment rates
  - Intimate partner violence in the home
  - Poverty
  - Social isolation
  - Lack of social support

Abusive parents or caregivers may demonstrate the following characteristics (Lau, Valeri, McCarty and Weisz, 2006; McDonald, 2007):

- They may exaggerate the child's behavior, or even put blame on the child for the family's problems.
- They have low tolerance of behaviors that would otherwise not be seen as serious.
- They will make few statements or gestures that positively support the child.
- They are more likely to be critical in interactions with the child.
- They possess overall negative impressions of their child and the child's behavior.
- They may describe their child as bad, burdensome, or even "evil."

- They do not explain the child's injuries.
- The history changes over time or history of self-inflicted trauma does not correlate with development.

Case Vignette 7.2.2 Continuation

*You and a hospital social worker interview Nick and his mother. Currently they live
in a low-income housing complex. Nick's father is not around, and likely left the
city before the boy was born. Therefore, the mother is forced to work two jobs to
make ends meet. While she is at her second job in the evenings, the mother's live-in
boyfriend watches over her son.*

*You question the mother about Nick's living conditions at home. She states that
Nick receives the three meals a day that he deserves and has a roof over his head.
When asked how many hours of the day she spends with her son, she becomes defensive and goes on about her two jobs and how little sleep she gets each night. When
questioned about the incident that produced Nick's black eye, she alleges that she
was not home at the time of the accident.*

*You manage to question Nick independently of his mother. When asked about his
home he says that he usually goes to school without eating breakfast and is lucky to
have dinner at night. On certain nights, his mother's boyfriend will order pizza or
purchase fast food from the convenience store around the corner from their house
and give him a portion. On other nights, however, the boyfriend is not around, and
so Nick is forced to fend for himself. On certain mornings, he will see his mother
getting ready for work and inquire if any breakfast is available. When probed on
what her response is, he looks down at the floor and states that occasionally his
mother will become angry at his question so recently he has stopped asking. Nick
won't answer any more questions about the boyfriend.*

 Please proceed with the problem-based approach!

Because of the apparent neglect and abuse, the assessment of this child requires
both medical and legal investigation. Assessment must include history of the alleged
abuse, assault, or neglect; a medical history; a psychosocial history (including family composition, substance use in the home, and previous involvement with Child
Protective Services); a review of systems; a comprehensive physical exam (including an anogenital exam if sexual abuse is possible); and a collection of forensic
evidence and forensic interviews (Laraque, DeMattia, & Low, 2006). Especially
in sexual abuse cases, examinations should be done by a health care professional
trained in forensic examination techniques. Documentation is crucial during all
assessments (interviews and physical assessments). Comprehensive evaluation is

time-consuming, but statistics show that 50 % of abused children will likely be abused again (McDonald, 2007).

The following are general guidelines for interviewing and examining youth who are possible victims of abuse or neglect (Laraque, DeMattia, & Low, 2006; McDonald, 2007).

- Setting the tone

    - Initiate general rapport-building
    - Explain who you are and why you are there
    - Ask if the child knows why he/she is there
    - Clearly state that confidentiality will be upheld
    - Explain any physical exams you will conduct
    - Allow child to handle any equipment you will be using
    - Obtain consent for each part of the exam, and for the presence of anyone else who will be allowed in the room during the exam (it must be explained to parents/caregivers if the child requests that they not be in the room)
    - Establish ground rules prior to commencing the exam (stop at anytime, etc.)

- Type of environment

    - The examination should be in a safe, neutral place if possible
    - Only one interviewer should be present; multiple adults and multiple interviews are discouraged
    - If possible, interview the child separately from the parents/caregivers
    - Offer the option of writing answers down or making a sketch

- When speaking

    - Use short and simple sentences, concrete terms, proper names, direct questions
    - Do not be biased, leading, presumptive
    - Determine the child's language and development
    - Verify the child's statements; rephrase questions if needed; ask if the child understands the question

The evaluation process should not further traumatize the child. In certain instances, it may be helpful for a nonoffending parent (usually the mother if she is not suspected in the abuse) to be present for the exam (Laraque, DeMattia, & Low, 2006). Below are the recommended exams and assessments that should be done even in the middle of a hectic emergency room. While each case will be different and have several contributing factors, failure to conduct an exam properly can in the end devastate a criminal case and cause lifelong trauma for the child.

- Photography of all injuries (preferably taken by a forensic investigator or medical photographer)

    - Obtain informed consent if possible, although it is not required in child maltreatment cases

- Use a color or digital camera, with the highest resolution possible
- Photograph injuries before treatment
- Photograph from different angles and take at least two photos of each injury
- Use a ruler or coin to give perspective of the injury's size
- Include the patient's face in at least one photograph
- Document the patient's name, location of injury, date, photographer, names of those present on the back of the photo
- Place photos in a sealed envelope, mark as confidential, and attach to the medical record. Maintain chain of custody

Guidelines for further assessment in cases of suspected sexual abuse:

- General principles

  - Should be done by a medical professional trained in forensic examinations.
  - Should be done promptly if child complains of dysuria, anal or vaginal bleeding, vaginal discharge, or pain with defecation; or if alleged incident occurred less than 72 hours prior to presentation.
  - If alleged incident occurred more than 72 hours prior to presentation, child can be scheduled for an examination at a center specializing in sexual assault examinations.
  - Most sexual abuse cases do not show findings upon physical examination unless the child is examined within 24 hours of the incident; therefore, obtaining a history is especially critical.

- Examination should include collection of

  - Victim clothing, debris, stains on skin (dried secretions), oral swabs and smears, vaginal/penile swabs and smears, rectal swabs and smears, pubic hair brushings/combings, head hair combings, genital swab, saliva and blood specimen, reference head and pubic hair, fingernail scrapings or clippings, and nasal mucous
  - Condoms, tampons
  - Tests for sexually transmitted diseases
  - Linens and other clothing

Guidelines for further diagnostic studies:

- Recommended in most cases

  - Ophthalmologic studies—dilated, indirect ophthalmoscopy performed by an ophthalmologist to detect retinal hemorrhages in children younger than 2 years
  - Radiological studies—head CT to detect subarachnoid, subdural, or intraparenchymal injury; skeletal survey radiography (e.g., of the spine, extremities, skull)—suspected old or new fracture
  - Laboratory studies—evaluation of amylase, complete blood count, hepatic transaminases, lipase, partial thromboplastin time, prothrombin time, fecal occult blood test, urinalysis, urine toxicology—to detect genitourinary or abdominal trauma and to ensure no underlying blood disorder

- Optional

  - Abdominal CT—if history, examination, or laboratory results suggest abdominal trauma
  - Bone scan—to find occult fractures up to 2 weeks after injury
  - Dental consultation—if there is a bite present, dentists can determine the source
  - Magnetic resonance imaging of the head—if CT of the head is inconclusive

Case Vignette 7.2.3 Conclusion

The social worker calls CPS and expects a return call. You admit Nick to the hospital pediatrics unit for his safety and to ensure that his immediate medical needs are addressed first, such as possible malnutrition.

You learn later from an "auntie" that Nick has been more disruptive and aggressive in school. You hope that the boy, a victim of violence, does not go on to become a perpetrator of violence as an older child or adolescent. You wonder what interventions could prevent such an outcome.

Of course the next step is arranging for involvement of a social worker who makes plans with CPS for a safe discharge. The following are some online resources about child abuse that may be helpful to the physician.

- Recognition and management

  - Visual Diagnosis of Child Abuse (available through http://www.aap.org)
  - Tennyson Center for Children (http://www.childabuse.org)
  - Child Abuse Evaluation and Treatment for Medical Providers (http://www.ChildAbuseMD.com)
  - MedlinePlus: Child Sexual Abuse (http://www.nlm.nih.gov/medlineplus/childsexualabuse.html)
  - Child Welfare Information Gateway (http://www.childwelfare.gov)

- Crisis counseling

  - Childhelp USA (http://childhelpusa.org)

- State statutes

  - Child Welfare Information Gateway (http://www.childwelfare.gov/systemwide/laws_policies/search/index.cfm)

- Protocols and forms

  - California Governor's Office of Emergency Services, OES 900 Forms (http://www.oes.ca.gov/Operational/OeSHome.nsf/CJPD_Documents? OpenForm)

In this age of seemingly increased interpersonal youth violence being reported in the media, some consideration must be given to this topic. The literature shows an increased number of youth perpetrators. Therefore, assessment techniques must also adapt to this type of evaluation. The following are statistics from the 2006 Juvenile Offenders and Victims National Report:

- More than one-third of juvenile victims of violent crime known to law enforcement are under age 12.
- In 2002, 1 in 12 murders in the USA involved a juvenile offender. One-third of murders committed by a juvenile offender also involved an adult offender.
- On a typical day in 2004, about 7,000 persons younger than 18 were inmates in adult jails. Nearly 9 of 10 were being held as adults.
- Law enforcement agencies made 2.2 million arrests of persons under 18 years in 2003. The most serious charge in almost half of all juvenile arrests in 2003 was larceny-theft, simple assault, a drug abuse violation, disorderly conduct, or a liquor law violation.

The following are recommended priorities from the Commission for the Prevention of Youth Violence [2000]:

1. Support the development of healthy families.
2. Promote healthy communities.
3. Enhance services for early identification and intervention for children, youth, and families at risk for or involved in violence.
4. Increase access to health and mental health care services.
5. Reduce access to and risk from firearms for children and youth.
6. Reduce exposure to media violence.
7. Ensure national support and advocacy for solutions to violence through research, public policy, legislation, and funding.

Hopefully, with care for this patient's physical and emotional well-being and careful implementation of the above guidelines, this patient will not become one of the above statistics and will not suffer the same fate of the perpetrator in the first case vignette.

Review Questions

1. In the first case vignette, what signs were identifiable in both the wife and husband that would cause suspicion of spousal abuse?
2. Which of the following physical findings would raise the highest degree of suspicion for child abuse or neglect?

   (a) Retinal hemorrhages in a 2-year-old with head trauma, reportedly from falling out of bed
   (b) Second-degree burns in the shape of a splash mark on the leg of a 9-year-old, who reportedly spilled hot soup on himself
   (c) A fractured forearm in a 10-year-old girl who fell on outstretched hands while playing on the jungle gym

(d) "Picky eating" and being below the fifth percentile for height and weight in a 3-year-old child

(e) A child-sized bite mark on the shoulder of a 5-year-old who claims that the wound was inflicted by the 4-year-old sister during an episode of roughhousing

3. Which of the following are recommended strategies to prevent violent behavior in youth:

(a) Increase access to health and mental health care services
(b) Reduce access to and risk from firearms for children and youth
(c) Reduce exposure to media violence
(d) All of the above
(e) a and c only

Answers

2. a, 3. d

Bibliography

American College of Emergency Physicians (1995). Emergency medicine and domestic violence. *Annals of Emergency Medicine, 25*, 442–443.

Brown, J. (1997). Working toward freedom from violence: The process of change in battered women. *Violence Against Women, 3*, 5–26.

Commission for the Prevention of Youth Violence. (December 2000). *Youth and violence: medicine, nursing, and public health: Connecting the dots to prevent violence.* http://www.ama-assn.org/ama/upload/mm/386/fullreport.pdf. Accessed September 19, 2007.

Director, T. D., & Linden, J. A. (2004). Domestic violence: An approach to identification and intervention.*Emergency Medical Clinical of North America, 22*, 1117–1132.

Englander, E. (2007). *Understanding Violence.* Mahwah: Lawrence Erlbaum Associates.

Feldhaus, K., Kozoi-McLain, J., Amsbury, H., Norton, I., Lowenstein, S., & Abbott, J. (1997). Accuracy of 3 brief screening questions for detecting partner violence in the emergency department. *Journal of the American Medical Association, 277*, 1357–1361.

Laraque, D., DeMattia, A. & Low, C. (2006). Forensic child abuse evaluation: A review. *The Mount Sinai Journal of Medicine, 72*(8), 1138–1147.

Lau, A. S., Valeri, S. M., McCarty, C. A., & Weisz, J. R. (2006). Abuse parents' reports of child behavior problems: Relationship to observed parent–child interactions. *Child Abuse & Neglect, 30*, 639–655.

Liebschutz, J., & Paranjape, A. (2003). How can a clinician identify violence in a woman's life? In J. Liebschutz, S. Frayne, & G. Saxe (Eds.), *Violence against women: A physician's guide to identification and management* (pp. 39–69). Philadelphia: American College of Physicians— American Society of Internal Medicine..

McDonald, K. C. (2007). Child abuse: Approach and management. *American Family Physician, 75*(2), 221–228.

McLeer, S., & Anwar, R. (1987). The role of the emergency physician in the prevention of domestic violence. *Annals of Emergency Medicine, 16*, 1155–1161.

Muehlbauer, M., & Crane, P. (2006). Elder abuse and neglect. *Journal of Psychosocial Nursing,* *44*(11), 43–48.

Snyder, H., & Sickmund, M. (2006). *Juvenile Offenders and Victims: 2006 National Report.* Retrieved April 19, 2007, from http://ojjdp.ncjrs.org/ojstatbb/nr2006/index.html

Tjaden, P., & Thoennes, N. (2000). Extent, nature, and consequences of intimate partner violence: Findings from the National Violence Against Women Survey, July 2000.

Williams, B. (2005). Domestic violence: Medicine's response. *Tennessee Medicine, 98*(10), 477–480.

Part III
Healthcare Principles

Chapter 8
The Physician–Patient Relationship

My Kha and Melissa Piasecki

Among the many skills every student must learn in medical school, communication skills are far and away the most important. Effective communication helps with diagnosis and allows for solid physician–patient relationships. When patients feel their doctors understand and are honest with them, they are more likely to adhere to treatment. There is also some evidence that malpractice risk can be lessened with good communication skills. In this chapter, the problem-solving table columns have questions that specifically address the physician–patient relationship.

At the end of this chapter, the reader will be able to

1. Discuss some of the factors that influence patient behavior
2. Describe the impact of physician–patient relationship on malpractice risk and its outcome
3. Determine specific factors affecting alliance
4. Identify the role of apology in medicine
5. Describe a model for the communication of bad news

Case Vignette 8.1.1 Miriam Phillips

Mrs. Phillips is a widowed, overweight woman in her late 70s. She has been suffering from abdominal pain for several days prior to her same-day appointment. You are a few months out of residency working for an HMO. Your administrator recently acknowledged your excellent work but asked that you speed up the rate of patients seen and order less unnecessary tests as you are generating more costs than expected.

First outpatient clinic visit:

Mrs. Phillips had a 10:30-AM appointment. It has been a busy morning and as usual you are running behind.

M. Kha
Resident in Psychiatry, University of Nevada School of Medicine

A. Guerrero, M. Piasecki (eds.), *Problem-Based Behavioral Science and Psychiatry*,
© Springer Science+Business Media, LLC 2008

You call out to the waiting room: Mrs. Phillips?! You're already turning away as you see an elderly, slightly overweight and smartly dressed lady slowly get out of her seat. You glance quickly at her chart and note that she has a history of NIDDM, her temperature is 38.5°C and her pulse is 98. With brief eye contact, you introduce yourself, "I'm Dr. Smith and I'll be taking care of you today." You lead the way to the examination room. She settles in her seat, anxiously looking around the room. You stand, leaning against the sink and continue to read her chart as you introduce yourself. "What can I do for you today?"

Mrs. Phillips: *Well doctor, I know you're very busy and I don't want to take up too much of your time. I don't know where to start, doctor. I guess I have been feeling this pain in my belly (pointing to her RUQ) and my son finally made me come in.*

Have you had this pain before?

Mrs. Phillips: *Well, no, but . . .*

(Interrupting.) What is the quality of the pain?

Mrs. Phillips: *Quality? Why I don't know, it sort of comes and goes. I've been so sick to my stomach . . ..*

Is it associated with meals? Does it occur more after eating fatty foods? How long does it last?

Mrs. Phillips: *I'm sorry doctor, you're going too fast (she is visibly flustered). I've never been too good at this medical talk. Sometimes the pain is worse after breakfast . . ..*

You continue writing in the chart as Mrs. Phillips talks. When did the pain start?

As the interview progresses, you learn that Mrs. Phillips has abdominal pain in her RUQ, an associated abdominal tenderness, nausea and vomiting, and a positive Murphy's sign on physical exam.

You appear to have signs consistent with acute cholecystitis. You'll need to get some labs and an ultrasound done for the diagnosis. You circle orders for a WBC, HbA1C, serum bilirubin, serum amylase, LFTs, and an abdominal ultrasound on a lab sheet, and hand this to Mrs. Phillips while saying, I think this will take care of things today. We'll call you if the tests return abnormal. You can check out with the assistant at the front.

Mrs. Phillips *appears even more anxious. What is cholecystitis?*

It's an inflammation of your gallbladder. Many people get it. Why don't we get the results of the tests and then discuss it further.

Mrs. Phillips: *Well, okay doctor, you know best. Thank you for your time.*

 Please proceed with the problem-based approach!

Case Vignette 8.1.2 Continuation

*Mrs. Phillips gets the labs drawn but could not get the abdominal ultrasound sched-
uled until the following week. During the week, she developed worsening fever and
chills. However, she did not know to call your office with these symptoms. You call
her to come in when you receive her lab results showing a WBC of >15,000/μl.*

> *Telephone call: Mrs. Phillips, we just received your lab results and they are con-
> cerning. You need to come to the hospital right away as a direct admit.*
> *Mrs. Phillips: What's wrong? Am I going to die?*
> *I've seen hundreds of patients with your condition. You will be fine. I will see you
> in the hospital.*
> *Mrs. Phillips goes to the hospital and finds that she has a temperature of 40°C.
> She appears toxic with shaking chills. An abdominal plain film was ordered
> and results were consistent with suppurative cholecystitis. She starts intravenous
> antibiotics and is scheduled for surgery.*
> *You enter the hospital room, flipping through the medical chart. Mrs. Phillips, you
> have a condition called suppurative cholecystitis. I have ordered some antibiotics
> and we scheduled you for emergency surgery. Your surgeon will be by to discuss
> the procedure further with you.*
> *Mrs. Phillips: How did this happen? I thought you said that my condition is not
> serious. She starts to cry. I know you're busy, doctor, and you know what's best
> but my son had some questions for you. He's in the cafeteria right now. Will you
> come by later? He can wait until you're free.*
> *Unfortunately, sometimes people with an inflammation of the gallbladder develop
> an associated infection. Once you get the antibiotics and surgery, you should be
> as good as normal. Your surgeon can give you and your son more specifics. I will
> be back to check on you after your surgery.*

*During Mrs. Phillips surgery, she developed a cardiac arrhythmia that did not
respond to emergency treatment and she did not survive. The surgeon communicates
this news to her son.*

 Please proceed with the problem-based approach!

Case Vignette 8.1.3 Conclusion

*You get a call from the Risk Management office of the hospital advising you that this
case is under review and though you may express your condolences to the family, you
may not discuss any of the details of the case or admit wrongdoing by apologizing*

for her death. Her son attempts to contact you in the following weeks asking you to return his calls. Though you fully intend to call him, your long days and uncertainty about how to proceed keep you from making the call.

A month after Mrs. Phillip's death, you receive a notification of a malpractice lawsuit from her son. It alleges malpractice resulting in wrongful death.

Case Vignette 8.2.1 Jared

You have recently completed a residency in pediatrics and a fellowship in pediatric hematology–oncology.

You are consulted at Children's Hospital on an 8-month-old infant (Jared) with a rapidly enlarging abdominal mass. He initially presented to his pediatrician with irritability, vomiting, and failure to thrive. You review the chart, imaging studies, and laboratory results and speak with the referring physician about the infant prior to meeting with the infant's parents for the first time in the hospital. You enter Jared's room to see a young mother comforting the infant while the father sits anxiously on a chair by the mother's side. They both look up as you enter the room; a mix of fear and hope fill their eyes.

Mr. and Mrs. Nguyen?
Mr. Nguyen: Yes. Are you the cancer doctor?
Yes. You approach the Nguyens as you pull up a chair and reach out to shake both their hands in turn. My name is Dr. Smith. Jared's doctor asked me to help in his care. I understand that this is a very difficult time for your family and I want you to know that I will try to answer your questions and be as honest with you as I can. You then settle back in the chair and continue. Why don't we start with what your current understanding of Jared's illness is?
Mrs. Nguyen: There is something in his liver. They think it might be cancer. Can you take the cancer out?

You sit with the Nguyens, educating them on the differential diagnosis and the steps that will be taken in the evaluation of this hepatic mass. You reassure them that the medical problem is completely unrelated to their parenting. The parents listen intently. You examine Jared carefully and point out and educate his parent's on the physical exam findings as well as the imaging results. You answer the Nguyens' questions and leave them with the direct office number where you could be reached.

Case Vignette 8.2.2 Continued

After a full workup, Jared was diagnosed with hepatoblastoma. You discuss the options, including the risks and benefits of surgery, chemotherapy, and other alternative treatments. The parents consent to surgical treatment, but the initial attempt at a complete resection was unsuccessful because the tumor was too large. You meet with the parents after the surgery and explain that it is now necessary to start Jared on a chemotherapy regimen designed to shrink the tumor and make it resectable.

*You warn the parents of the risks of these agents. Though concerned and fatigued,
they express confidence in your recommendations and decide to proceed.*

*The appropriate chemotherapy protocol was ordered. Your pager goes off on the
morning of Jared's first round of chemotherapy and Jared's nurse notifies you that
Jared has a fever and just had a seizure. You ask the nurse to stop the chemotherapy,
and you rush to the infusion room. There, an irritable and uncomfortable looking
infant awaits you. However, it appears that Jared has stabilized. Looking through
the notes, labs, and orders, nothing appears amiss. However, on closer examination,
you note that the chemotherapy agent's dose was calculated based on a weight of
9.3 kg. Someone had misread your 6.3 kg for 9.3 kg!*

*After rechecking the calculations and confirming that the incorrect dose was
infused, you ask the Nguyens to step into a private room. The Nguyens appear
frightened. You ask them to sit and pull up a chair up to them.*

*Jared appears to be doing okay right now. He just had a seizure and developed a
fever after the chemotherapy was started.*

Mrs. Nguyen: What happened? Why did he have the seizure? Will he be okay?

It appears that Jared was given the wrong dose of medicine . . ..

Mr. Nguyen: What?! How could he be given the wrong dose? Who made the mistake?

*I know you are both upset and you have a right to be. I am so sorry that this
happened. I don't know where the mistake was made. However, I assure you I
will personally investigate this and keep you informed on what the results are.*

Mrs. Nguyen: Will Jared be okay?

*The infusion has been stopped and the dose has been corrected. I will personally
ensure that everything possible be done to prevent something like this happening
again with your son. We will bring our findings up with the quality management
team of our hospital to make sure it does not happen again with any other
patients. Again I am very sorry and I take full responsibility for the mistake.*

Mr. Nguyen: We appreciate your honesty. We are just so concerned about our son.

*I understand, and if I was in your position, I would also be upset. We will check his
labs and monitor him closely.*

Mr. Nguyen: When will you restart his chemotherapy?

*If he is still doing well tomorrow, we will restart his chemotherapy regimen then.
You are welcome to call me at my direct office number when you have questions
or concerns. I will come by and see you all tomorrow morning. Do you have any
more questions at this time?*

Mrs. Nguyen: No. Thank you for your time.

Case Vignette 8.2.3 Conclusion

*Jared's chemotherapy infusion was restarted the next day at the correct dose.
Though he did suffer from expected side effects, his regimen was successful. He
went on to have a complete resection of his tumor and was discharged home to his
grateful parents. At a 12-month follow-up appointment, the Nguyens confide to you*

that their friends had urged them to consider a malpractice suit after the incorrect chemotherapy dose was given. They did not pursue any legal action.

Learning Issues

1. Psychological and social factors influencing doctor–patient communication
   A patient's style of interaction with his or her physician can be a reflection of his or her culture. The effect of a patient's culture and family values on the patient–physician relationship has been well studied. While most Latin Americans may welcome a warm handshake and direct eye contact from their physician, many Asian Americans may feel uncomfortable with this display of familiarity. Thus it is important for all healthcare professionals to become familiar with the cultural norms of the populations they most commonly encounter. Please refer to Chap. 14 for a further discussion of culture in medicine.
   There are three general models of physician–patient interactions.

	Active–passive	Guidance–cooperation	Mutual participation
Physician	Makes and implements all decisions	Makes many of the decisions	Works with patient to make decisions and achieve goals
Patient	Unwilling or unable to participate in decisions	Patient's actions guided by physician	Works with physician to make decisions and achieve goals

The active–passive model was more common in the past. There is a movement toward the mutual participation model.

2. The impact of relationship on malpractice risk
   Research has shown that practicing patient-centered medicine can reduce the risk of litigation against physicians. Physicians who are able to communicate effectively, display appropriate empathy, and collaborate with their patients have higher patient satisfaction. Higher patient satisfaction correlates with decreased malpractice-lawsuit intentions.

Improves patient–physician relationship	Hurts patient–physician relationship
Timeliness	Perceived unavailability, perceived "hurry"
Empathy	Perceived lack of caring
Personal responses	Dismissing patient's concerns
Positive collaboration	Lack of collaboration

3. Physician–patient alliance and its effect on outcome
   Many studies have shown a correlation between a positive physician–patient alliance and a good outcome. The quality of the relationship and the existence of a personal connection between the doctor and the patient affect the patient's

compliance with care. Strong alliance is associated with increased compliance and thus reduced symptom severity and improved health (Brock & Salinsky, 1993; Neale & Rosenheck, 1995; Tongue, Epps & Forese, 2005). Conceptually, the physician–patient alliance involves mutual respect, attentiveness, and effective communication. There is a multitude of data that support that good communication leads to better alliance, and better alliance is linked to improved adherence to the physician's recommendations, including medications, treatment regimen, and follow-up.

4. Specific factors affecting alliance
   A number of researchers have studied physician–patient alliance. Some studies ask patients to rate their satisfaction with their doctor. Other studies record the physician–patient encounter and study the recorded dialog. Bernstein and Bernstein (1980) found that the expression of concern by the physician is important to patients in forming rapport. Explanations of the purpose behind tests and the rationale of treatment are also important (Cormier, Cormier and Weisser, 1984). Improving communication skills of physicians can lead to increased time efficiency with visits. Patients respond more positively to physicians trained in communication skills and express higher levels of satisfaction.

   The amount of time that physicians allow patients to describe their medical concerns also affects alliance. Numerous studies have found that physicians' verbalizations take up the majority of the sessions. Patients sometimes speak less than one tenth of the time spent with the physician. One study revealed that when physicians asked an average of 27 questions, patients were allowed to ask only 1.5 questions per visit (Waitzkin, Cabrera, Arroyo de Cabrera, Radlow & Rodriquez, 1996). Many physicians also believe that they spent 50 % of their time explaining, informing, and educating. Studies consistently have shown that physicians spend less than 10 % of their interaction time performing those activities (Bain, 1976; Davis, 1971; Fremon, Negrete, Davis & Korsch, 1971; Stiles, Putnam, Wolf & James, 1979; Waitzkin, 1984, 1985). Physicians also self-disclose information about their personal or professional experiences. Patients view these self-disclosures as generally unhelpful and at times disruptive (McDaniel et al., 2007). As many as 45 % of the patients are highly dissatisfied with the level of information their physician gave them regarding their diagnosis (Phillips, 1996).

   The literature suggests that physicians need to improve their communication patterns by offering patients more opportunities to clarify their concerns and ask questions. Physicians also need to avoid interruptions, give patients more information on their diagnoses, and have increased awareness regarding the impact of their interpersonal style and self-disclosures on patient satisfaction.

5. Apology
   Medical errors occur fairly often. After a medical professional detects an error or makes a mistake, should he or she apologize to the patient? Apologies in medicine are sometimes controversial because some physicians (or their lawyers)

believe that an apology is the same as an admission of malpractice and may be used against them in a lawsuit.

Although research has not yet answered the question about increased risk of malpractice in individual cases, there are several compelling reasons for a physician to consider apologizing to patients and families when he or she makes a mistake that harms a patient. Because an apology communicates an acknowledgement that the doctor made a mistake and intends to do better in the future, it maintains the trust between the doctor and the patient. If the patient becomes aware of a mistake and the doctor avoided talking about it, the patient may wonder if this doctor can be trusted to be open and honest in the future. Open and honest communication is the hallmark of a healthy and effective doctor–patient relationship.

Another reason for a doctor to consider an apology for an error is for his own well-being. Doctors are caring people and can be deeply affected when a patient is harmed by a mistake. An apology allows the doctor to express his regret and know that, despite the error, he did the honorable thing by offering a sincere apology. Sometimes a heartfelt apology will allow the doctor and the patient to talk about the problem in ways that deepen their relationship and allow the doctor to become more effective in the future.

Recent government rules require hospitals to inform patients of errors in their care. Some doctors and hospitals have started physician-support programs to assist doctors with the skills required for disclosing a medical mistake and making an effective apology (see references).

6. Communication of bad news

Because of the legal and ethical ramifications, bad news (such as testing and diagnostic information) should be delivered with sensitivity and skill. An article published by Medical Economics (Grandinetti, 1997) describes a six-step process with the mnemonic FRAMES used in difficult patient encounters. The following is an illustration of the FRAMES model.

As a family doctor, you examine a 4-year-old child brought in by her mother for required preschool immunizations. You notice the mother appears anxious asking you to just give the child the shots because they have to catch the bus. She promises to bring the baby back next month for an exam. You tell her that you understand her concerns but in order to document that the child is healthy enough for school, you need to do a quick examination. As you remove the child's clothes, you notice two large bruises encircling both upper arms and a few marks on her back resembling cigarette burns.

F (Feedback): "These bruises and scars on your child are very concerning to me. Last time you came in for your exam, you had a black eye and some bruises on your leg. You've denied any abuse or physical aggression before. But I cannot ignore what is happening to your child. Has someone been hurting Amanda?"

R (Responsibility): Allow the patient to take responsibility by responding to your feedback.

A (Advice): Offer patient advice. "I am very concerned for you and your child's safety. I encourage you to speak with a social worker today who can offer you some assistance and safe resources."

M (Menu): Offer patient a menu of options. "I will have to call child protective services regarding Amanda's injuries. They may be able to offer you additional resources and advice as well. Would you like a representative to meet with you in the office? Or would you prefer to see a social worker from our clinic first?"

E (Empathy): Provide patient with empathy as they will need to feel supported during this stressful time. "This must be an extremely difficult and scary time for you and Amanda. I admire your resilience."

S (Self-Advocacy): "You have made it through some very difficult times in your life and have had to make some tough decisions. I know you'll be able to do what's best for you and Amanda."

Review Questions

1. Which of the factors listed is the most likely barrier to effective communication in the following vignette?

   Physician: How are you Maurice?

   Patient: Fine doctor. I'm a little nervous about the test results though.

   Physician: That is understandable. You have been in a lot of pain. What do you think the problem is?

   Patient: I really don't know doc. What did the tests show?

   Physician: The results indicate that you have peripheral artery disease. The pain you experienced is due to intermittent claudication. We'll start you on Adalat and that should help.

   Patient: What is intermittent claudication?

   Physician: Peripheral arterial disease is a common manifestation of atherosclerosis. Intermittent claudication is a symptom of peripheral arterial disease . . ..

   (a) The physician did not demonstrate sensitivity to gender, racial, and cultural diversity
   (b) The physician attempted to elicit the patient's view of the health problem
   (c) The physician utilized medical terminology to explain a patient's health problem
   (d) The physician used silence and nonverbal facilitation to encourage the patient's expression of thought and feelings
   (e) None of the above

2. In case vignette 8.1.1, which of the following could the doctor have done to reduce his legal risk? He should have

   (a) documented more thoroughly
   (b) rectified medical errors to the patient in a timely manner

(c) provided false reassurance to prevent her from worrying unnecessarily
(d) provided inadequate information
(e) dismissed patient's concerns

Answers

1. c, 2. b

Case table 8.1.1 Miriam Phillips 1

What are the facts?	What are your hypotheses about this relationship? How does the patient feel?	What do you want to know next?	What specific information would you like to learn about?
Running an hour late with no explanation	Poor rapport		
Limited eye contact	Patient feels anxious		
No greeting			
No instruction			
Doctor stands instead of sitting at eye level of patient			
Doctor interrupts frequently			
Doctor uses doctor speak			
Does not explain diagnosis or procedures (pt may not know what an ultrasound is or why the labs are needed). Hands pt the lab sheet without explaining what she needs to do next			
Asks several questions before allowing patient to answer			
Poor follow-up instructions (did not explain what to expect or look out for)			
Not accounting for age and culture (do not respond well to rapid fire questions)			
Hurries patient out of office			
Dismisses patient's anxiety			

Case table 8.1.2 Miriam Phillips 2

What are the facts?	What are your hypotheses about this relationship? How does Mrs. Phillips feel?	What do you want to know next?	What specific information would you like to learn about?
Dismisses patient's anxiety			
False reassurance (reactive)			
Poor follow-up directions (should patient go to ER? Admission?)			
No greeting			
No eye contact			
No expression of medical concern			
Does not explain why the surgeon is needed			
Previous reassurance backfires on Dr. Smith (you said my condition was not serious)			
False reassurance again			

Case table 8.1.3 Miriam Phillips 3

What are the facts?	What are your hypotheses about this relationship? How does the son feel?	What do you want to know next?	What specific information would you like to learn about?
Poor follow-up with son			
Lost opportunity to establish rapport with family			

Case table 8.2.1 Jared Nguyen 1

What are the facts?	What are your hypotheses about this relationship? How do the parents feel?	What do you want to know next?	What specific information would you like to learn about?
Gathers information prior to seeing patient			
Introduces self and greets parents			
Demonstrates compassion			
Invites questions			

Case table 8.2.1 (continued)

What are the facts?	What are your hypotheses about this relationship? How do the parents feel?	What do you want to know next?	What specific information would you like to learn about?
Finds out current level of understanding of illness			
Examines level of prior knowledge			
Conserves time by not re-explaining parents already know			
Does not make assumptions about what patient knows			
Performs education			
Explains things during the examination Answers questions			
Provides parents with number and contact info			

Case table 8.2.2 Jared Nguyen 2

What are the facts?	What are your hypotheses about this relationship? How do the parents feel?	What do you want to know next?	What specific information would you like to learn about?
Explain options, risks, and benefits			
Parents kept informed			
Doctor responds to patient's emergency in a timely manner			
Doctor admits and explains mistake immediately and tells them how it was corrected			
Initiates investigation and keeps communication open			
Assures the family that a lesson has been learned from this mistake and the quality management team will be consulted to prevent future incidents			
Takes full responsibility for the mistake			

Case table 8.2.3. Jared Nguyen 3

What are the facts?	What are your hypotheses about this relationship? How does the patient feel?	What do you want to know next?	What specific information would you like to learn about?
Friends urged Nguyens to file a malpractice lawsuit Parents did not sue			

Bibliography

Bain, D. J. G. (1976). Doctor–patient communication in general practice consultations. *Medical Education, 10*, 125–131.

Bernstein, L., & Bernstein, R. S. (1980). *Interviewing: A guide for health professionals* (3rd ed.). New York: Appleton-Century-Crofts.

Brock, C. D., & Salinsky, J. V. (1993). Empathy: An essential skill for understanding the physician–patient relationship in clinical practice. *Family Medicine, 25*, 245–248.

Cormier, L. S., Cormier, W. H., & Weisser, R. J. (1984). *Interviewing and helping skills for health professionals.* Belmont, CA: Wadsworth.

Davis, M. S. (1971). Variation in patients' compliance with doctors' orders: Medical practice and doctor–patient interaction. *Psychiatry in Medicine, 2*, 31–54.

Engel, G. L. (1997). From biomedical to biopsychosocial: Being scientific in the human domain. *Psychosomatics, 38*, 521–528.

Fremon, B., Negrete, V. F., Davis, M., & Korsch, B. M. (1971). Gaps in doctor–patient communication: Doctor–patient interaction analysis. *Pediatric Research, 5*, 298–311.

Grandinetti, D. (Ed.) (1997). Handling patients you wish you didn't have. *Medical Economics, June 9*, 142–164.

Lazare, A. (2004). On apology. Oxford: Oxford University Press.

McDaniel, S. H., Beckman, H. B., Morse, D. S., Silberman, J., Seaburn, D. B., & Epstein, R. M. (2007). Physician self-disclosure in primary care visits: Enough about you, what about me? *Archives of Internal Medicine, 167*, 1321–1326.

Neale, M. S., & Rosenheck, R. A. (1995). Therapeutic alliance and outcome in a VA intensive case management program. Psychiatric Services, 46, 719—721.

Phillips, D. (1996). Medical professional dominance and client dissatisfactions. A study of doctor–patient interaction and reported dissatisfaction with medical care among female patients in 4 hospitals in Trinidad and Tobago. *Social Science and Medicine, 42*, 1419–1425.

Sorry works coalition: sorryworks.net.

Stiles, W. B., Putnam, S. M., Wolf, M. H., & James, S. A. (1979). Interaction exchange structure and patient satisfaction with medical interviews. *Medical Care, 17*, 667–681.

Tongue, J. R., Epps, H. R., & Forese, L. L. (2005). Communication skills for patient-centered care. *The Journal of Bone and Joint Surgery, 87A*, 652–658.

Waitzkin, H. (1984). Doctor–patient communication: Clinical implications of social scientific research. *Journal of the American Medical Association, 252*, 2441–2446.

Waitzkin, H. (1985). Information giving in medical care. *Journal of Health and Social Behavior, 26*, 81–101.

Waitzkin, H., Cabrera, A., Arroyo de Cabrera, E., Radlow, M., & Rodriguez, F. (1996). Patient–doctor communication in cross-national perspective. *Medical Care, 34*, 641–671.

Chapter 9
Ethics and Professionalism

Jacob Doris and Marin Gillis

Ethics and morality are features of human life, thinking, and concern. Questioning how one should rightly act and how one can be a good person and live a good life are compelling because as human beings we do not act simply on impulse or instinct and we do not live alone: how we act and what we believe about right and wrong cannot help but affect others. The study of ethics helps us in two ways: to understand the reasons that medical practice has developed as it has and to be able to defend our actions if called upon to justify them.

It is important to note the distinction between law and morality or ethics. Consider that the Supreme Court's Roe v. Wade decision did not settle the question of whether abortion is morally permissible. Whatever the law may be, we can always ask what the law should be. Law codifies society's majority practices, and practices as well as majorities change. Furthermore, not every act that is illegal is also immoral, for example, civil disobedience; and conversely, not every act that is immoral is also illegal, for example, lying to your spouse. Codes of professional ethics, for example, the AMA Code of Medical Ethics, are basically sets of rules and tend to be much the same as standards of good practice, such as, physicians maintaining a commitment to medical education. Sometimes codes do include moral imperatives, for example, "a physician shall support access to medical care for all people" (Council on Ethical and Judicial Affairs, 2007).

At the end of this chapter, students will be able to

1. Identify two reasons why the study of ethics is important
2. Conceptually distinguish ethics and the law
3. Describe four domains of ethical assessment
4. Identify four conceptual tools to construct ethical assessment
5. Distinguish the four principle of bioethics
6. Understand the ethical guidelines when principles of bioethics conflict
7. Apply the four principles of bioethics to clinical cases
8. Apply the ethical guidelines in a clinical case of conflicting bioethical principles

J. Doris
Resident in Psychiatry, University of Nevada School of Medicine

A. Guerrero, M. Piasecki (eds.), *Problem-Based Behavioral Science and Psychiatry*,
© Springer Science+Business Media, LLC 2008

The following cases illustrate how actions in medical practice may be ethically assessed according to the four principles of bioethics.

Case Vignette 9.1.1 Robert Sanchez

You are a neurologist seeing Mr. Roberto Sanchez, a financially stable, frail 48-year-old veteran whom was referred to you by his primary care physician after complaining of weakness over the past few months. He has been experiencing a gradually progressive weakness that has gradually involved both his arms and legs. On his first office visit, Mr. Sanchez notes complaints of twitching, muscle cramps and that his muscles appear to be "going away." On neurological exam, you note hyperreflexia, upgoing babinski reflex, and a completely intact sensory exam. You order a battery of tests, including heck and head MRIs, CSF analysis, and electromyelography (EMG).

Mr. Sanchez returns to your clinic, where you inform him that the tests support your suspicion that his diagnosis is amyotrophic lateral sclerosis, or ALS, commonly called Lou Gherig's disease. This is a progressive degeneration of motor neurons with no cure and a 3- to 5-year prognosis. Mr. Sanchez learns during the next few visits that eventually he will not have the strength to breathe adequately on his own, and that he will require long-term mechanical ventilation to sustain life. Over the proceeding months he undergoes treatment with the drug riluzone and remains in a positive attitude. He also continues to display intact mentation and makes clear on numerous occasions that when the time comes, he does not wish to be placed on long-term mechanical ventilation.

Please proceed with the problem-based approach!

Case Vignette 9.1.2 Continuation

Eventually, Mr. Sanchez's condition deteriorates, and his weakness progresses to include the muscles of respiration. He initially elects to continue with his decision about life-sustaining measures and receives only nasal positive-pressure ventilation. In his most recent office visit, Mr. Sanchez looks to be in rapid decline. At the previous visit, you helped make arrangements for hospice care, but at this visit, he asks what his options are to extend his life. You gently explain that no intervention will extend his life beyond a few days to weeks, and that once this decision is carried through, he will no longer be able to survive off the ventilator. He tells you that he is "not ready to say goodbye." His life expectancy is days to weeks, and the quality of his life is very poor.

Please proceed with the problem-based approach!

Case Vignette 9.1.3 Conclusion

You make arrangements for an immediate tracheostomy for mechanical ventilation. He is admitted to the VA hospital ICU and placed on mechanical ventilation and parenteral nutrition. His family visits him daily. Although he is unable to speak, he is able to make eye contact with the family. He dies 13 days later.

Learning Issues

There are four domains of ethics assessment: (1) action; (2) consequences of action; (3) the character of the person (moral agent) who is acting or contemplating action; and (4) the agent's motives for acting or contemplating action. In order for an agent or an action to be the object of ethical assessment, that is, in order to be able to evaluate whether the agent acts from beneficial, malicious, or neutral will, or whether the agent's actions are determinable as morally permissible, obligatory, or prohibited, the agent has to be responsible for his or her actions. To be responsible for one's actions, motives, or character, to be considerable as a moral agent, one has to be autonomous. To be autonomous is to be free from coercion and compulsion, to be able to act and think voluntarily, and to act rationally, in other words, to have logical reasons for what one does.

When we ethically assess action, decision, and motivations in medicine, we rely on the following tools: (1) logic, to assess the reasoning behind the determination of the morality of an action, motive, or character; (2) conceptual analysis, which involves defining, elucidating, comparing, and contrasting the ethical concepts of the cases; (3) consistency and case comparison, where we treat like cases alike unless a morally relevant difference is found; and (4) reasoning from principles (Hope, 2004).

In medical ethics, reasoning from four principles, dubbed the Four Principles of Bioethics by Thomas Beauchamp and James Childress, is a common way to start ethical assessment in medical practice. The four principles are (1) respect for patient autonomy; (2) beneficence, acting to promote what is best for patient (the standard of due care is grounded by this principle); (3) nonmaleficence, acting not to harm the patient; and (4) justice, including distributive justice, for example, the equal distribution of benefits and burdens, respect for the law, rights, and retributive justice, that is, punishment (Beauchamp & Childress, 2001).

Principles often conflict, such as when a patient autonomously refuses a treatment that the physician believes would have the best health outcomes. This conflict is between the imperative to respect a patient's autonomy (right to refuse treatment) and the principle of beneficence (acting to promote what is best for the patient). The following guidelines are broadly recognized as central in navigating conflicts.

1. The interests of the patient count most (interests = autonomy, beneficence, and nonmaleficence)
2. Respect for patient autonomy outweighs beneficence and nonmaleficence toward a patient (autonomy > beneficence, nonmaleficence)
3. The interests of others may outweigh respect for patient's autonomy
4. If harms and benefits are proportionate, duties of nonmaleficence outweigh those of beneficence (Mahowald, 2006).

In this case, as a physician you have acted to respect the autonomy of the patient. First, Mr. Sanchez appears to have made a decision about his treatment with informed voluntary consent. You explained the treatment alternatives to the patient, including the risks and benefits of each option, Mr. Sanchez indicated that he understands what he was told, Mr. Sanchez has no symptoms of depression, and he does not appear to be coerced into making this decision because neither family nor finances appear as relevant to his considerations. Second, you acted on the patient's decision.

This case can also be related to the question of health care rationing: a distributive justice issue. Health care resources are scarce, and health care costs are rising due to new medical technologies and population growth. Because much of the expensive health care technologies are used to prolong the lives of the critically ill, usually elderly people in the last years of their lives, the question of rationing health care resources, to allocate a certain amount of resources that can be accessed by any particular person, arises. Those in favor of distributive justice advocate a policy that balances an equal share for all people against a fair distribution of health care resources among those in need. This raises issues such as the merit of allocating health care resources only to health care or also to other areas that promote healthy lifestyle decision-making. It also implies the existence of a minimal acceptable amount of health care for all members of society.

Case Vignette 9.2.1 Presenting Situation: Mark Handon

You are a family physician who has been seeing Mr. Mark Handon, 48, whose medical problems include hypertension and stable angina, for which he takes, among other things, a nitrate drug medication. He is in your office for a routine follow-up visit. Accompanying him on this and prior visits is his wife, Nora Handon. On this office visit, she tells you that her husband has a "problem" for which he would like help. Mr. Handon appears sheepish while speaking, and his wife interjects a description of symptoms consistent with erectile dysfunction. Mr. Handon's wife

*states that their relationship has suffered due to this problem and that she would
like him to have a medication to help. His wife asks that you prescribe him that
medication "in the commercial with the football and tire" for his problem. Having
seen the commercial yourself, you know she is referring to a medication prescribed
for erectile dysfunction. While looking at Mr. Handon's chart, you notice that this
medication in combination with his nitrate medication could drop his blood pressure
and cause a heart attack.*

 Please proceed with the problem-based approach!

Case Vignette 9.2.2 Conclusion

*You indicate to Mr. Handon at this time that you will not prescribe him this drug due
to the risks of drug interactions that could endanger his health. You offer to refer
him to a urologist who can better assess his erectile dysfunction and make clear that
you can offer additional resources (reading, a psychology referral) if he would be
interested in other approaches.*

Learning Issues

The physician has acted according to the principle of nonmaleficence. The physician acted intentionally to not create a needless harm or injury to the patient, either through acts of commission or omission. In common language, an action is regarded as negligent if one imposes a careless or unreasonable risk of harm upon another. The physician may have felt conflicted, since most people in service-oriented professions want to please the people they serve, and withholding a desired treatment may disappoint or anger the patient. Clarity about the physician's duty to nonmaleficence can guide clinicians through those types of conflicts. At first glance, a case such as this may seem to act against patient autonomy in favor of nonmaleficence, but in actuality, autonomy has not been an issue for it.

Patients' autonomy is based in their right to control over their own body by leaving it unchanged except at their discretion. This case does not conflict with a patient's right to autonomy because it does not have the physician forcing an action on the patient, but rather withholding an action that could cause him great harm. A patient with decision-making capacity has a right to refuse having a beneficial treatment affect their body, but does not have the right to demand a detrimental treatment be used on them. In the first situation, they are *maintaining* their body unchanged as they see fit. In the second, they are requesting an *alteration* in their bodily process. With many treatment options, there is a balance between possible benefits and harms and, as noted above, when benefit and harm are equal, physicians should act to maintain nonmaleficence.

Case Vignette 9.3.1 Willa McTavish

You are an ER physician presented with a 46-year-old adult woman, Ms. Willa McTavish, brought into the ED by EMS after a motor vehicle collision. Your physical exam reveals that in addition to severe hypotension and tachycardia, she is pale with signs of an acute abdomen, most notably, extreme tenderness to palpation and distension. You suspect internal bleeding. A stat CBC shows a critically low hematocrit. The best chance of saving her life is a blood transfusion treatment. You explain the situation to Ms. McTavish, and she tells you that her religious principles require that she not accept the transfusion and that she is willing to die to follow her religion.

 Please proceed with the problem-based approach!

You speak with Ms. McTavish's family. They report that she has no psychiatric history suggestive of problems with depression or psychosis. They confirm that Ms. McTavish was baptized into the Jehovah Witnesses a few years ago and practices that religion actively. You use the Internet to confirm the church standards on refusing blood transfusions.

 Please proceed with the problem-based approach!

Case Vignette 9.3.2 Conclusion

You initiate infusion of blood alternatives and do not give her a blood transfusion. Ms. McTavish undergoes emergency surgery for internal injuries and survives the surgery. After a lengthy hospitalization, she is discharged to a rehabilitation center and eventually, home.

Learning Issues

The physician has been confronted with a conflict in this case. The principle of respect for patient autonomy would direct the physician to respect the patient's right to refuse treatment and therefore not give her the transfusion. But since this treatment appears critical to saving her life, and the physician is committed to the principle of beneficence, which is to act to benefit the patient and avoid harm, the physician would give her the transfusion. Further, the physician is also committed to the principle of nonmaleficence and not administering the transfusion would cause the patient grave harm. When such a conflict arises, the patient' right to autonomous control over her own body outweighs the principles of beneficence and nonmaleficence, even when the consequences of this respect are likely to cause the patient grave harm.

In the second installment of this case, the physician clarified that the patient was not making a decision to refuse potentially life-saving treatment as a result of psychotic thinking or depression. He took further steps to ensure that the patient's wishes were consistent with her behavior and beliefs. The physician in this case acted according to the principle of respect for patient autonomy.

Case Vignette 9.4.1 Presenting Situation: George Greely

Mr. Greely is a 58-year-old homeless man well known to the emergency room due to his frequent admissions related to alcohol intoxication. Tonight he comes in by ambulance because he was found face down in the street. He smells heavily of alcohol and poor hygiene. The intern on call for the ER, Norm, is watching the World Series in the on-call room when gets a page. When the nurse tells him it is Mr. Greely, he groans and decides he doesn't even need to put on a scrub shirt over his heavy metal band t-shirt since it's Mr. Greely.

Mr. Greely is not very responsive to questions and uncooperative with Norm's brief screening physical exam (listening to heart and breath sounds). Mr. Greely has an abrasion on his forehead and some blood in his hair. Norm decides to order some labs and to have the nurse page him in the call room when the labs come back. He also orders "Shower patient when awake."

Please proceed with the problem-based approach!

Case Vignette 9.3.2 Continuation

A few hours later, Norm is asleep and the nurse pages him again. He calls her phone number and crossly asks, "What is it that is so important?" She tells him that the labs show an alcohol level of 0.22, hypokalemia, elevated liver function tests, and an elevated white blood cell count. She reports Mr. Greely is sleeping peacefully in a quiet corner of the ER. Norm asks her to call the internal medicine resident and tell him that "Our friend Mr. Greely is coming in for a tune up and he doesn't smell good."

Please proceed with the problem-based approach!

The next morning, Norm receives a stat page to the morning report conference room. Mr. Greely has a subdural hematoma with midline shift and is currently in surgery for evacuation of the hematoma. The internal medicine chief resident is furious that Norm did not detect the brain injury last night and says so in front of all of the internal medicine residents present. In addition, she tells the entire room "Norm really blew it in the ER. I'm sure Greely's family will want to know who to sue."

Learning Issues

Professionalism is a term that describes a collection of physician duties. Some of these duties are put into the form of "rules" but many are considered to be so basic to the function of the physician that they are felt to be implicitly understood. In this case, we note several deviations from professional standards.

An obvious problem in the care of Mr. Greely is that the patient was not put first. The intern cut corners with the exam and assessment in order to watch the World Series and to sleep. Other lapses on the part of the intern include lack of professional appearance in the clinical setting, the disrespectful tone used to describe the patient and his disrespectful phone manners with the nurse. Another significant lapse in professionalism is that the intern delegated a communication responsibility to a nurse instead of making the call to the admitting resident himself. Professionalism standards are particularly important when transferring care of a patient. The physician who initiates the transfer has an obligation to let the receiving party know about the patient's problems and to continue to take responsibility for the patient if the transfer is unsuccessful. The Federal Government passed the Emergency Medical Treatment and Labor Act to ensure that transfers between hospitals follow these principles.

The next morning, the chief resident violated principles of professionalism, by impugning Norm's reputation and failing to maintain a professionally composed demeanor when addressing an important patient care problem. She appeared to intend to publicly shame him instead of providing respectful feedback. There are many additional aspects of professionalism that are important in every day interactions with patients, colleagues, and outside entities. The table below offers some examples of these considerations. Thoughtful publications on professionalism have been developed by the American Board of Internal Medicine (see references).

Elements of professionalism: Duties to patients, colleagues, self and everyone in work environment

Respect	Examples
Appearance	Neat, professional
Demeanor	Composed, friendly
Language	Not overly familiar, no swearing
Consideration	Attention to the needs and feeling of others; discretion in discussing differences with colleagues
Responsibility	
Put patient first	Defer own needs when in conflict with patients needs
Follow-through	Following up on labs, reports, patient follow-through on treatment plans
Conscientious	Comprehensive patient exams, getting records/ communicating with other providers
Follow rules	Institutional bylaws, professional standards, state laws
Honesty	Clear communication of the facts and what is unknown; disclosing error
Up to date	Maintaining current knowledge and skills; self-study
Accountability	Accepting responsibility for performance and outcomes
Responsiveness	
Timely	Responding to requests in a timely manner, avoid delays
Alacrity	Express willingness if available
Service	Working to meet the needs of the community, institutions, and profession
Support	Supportive of colleagues and institution

Review Questions

1. Which of the following statements most closely correlates to respecting patient autonomy?

   (a) Withholding information temporarily from a patient because the said information may worsen his or her clinical condition
   (b) Doing what is right for the patient
   (c) Allowing a patient to choose to withhold life-sustaining treatment for their condition
   (d) Informing patient of relative risks versus benefits of an indicated treatment

2. Which of the following is not one of the four main principles of biomedical ethics components as originally described by Beauchamp and Childress?

   (a) Beneficence
   (b) Respect for autonomy
   (c) Justice
   (d) Duty to warn

3. You decide not to prescribe a potentially beneficial medication because of the large potential for an injurious negative outcome. What principle of medical ethics would most closely correlate with this decision?

   (a) Duty to patient
   (b) Nonmalificence
   (c) Autonomy
   (d) Beneficence

4. Which of these is not a tool physicians use to assess ethical choices?

   (a) Case comparisons
   (b) Reasoning from principles
   (c) Anecdotal evidence
   (d) Conceptual analysis

5. A new law is passed stating that a certain commonly prescribed pain medication can only be prescribed by a board-certified pain specialist. You have a patient who has previously been found to gain pain relief from this drug and failed to gain relief from any other. If this patient is waitlisted to see a pain specialist for 2 months past his last refill, what is the ethical choice regarding his prescription?

   (a) Do not prescribe the drug because it is illegal and the law is never unethical
   (b) Do not prescribe the drug because it is not in the patient's best interest for you to go to jail
   (c) Prescribe the drug to prove a point about an unjust law as a method of civil disobedience
   (d) Prescribe the drug because it is in the patient's best interest and they will suffer harm without it

6. Which of these is most important to a health care decision for a psychologically fit patient?

   (a) The likelihood of an action hurting a patient
   (b) The likelihood of an action benefiting the patient
   (c) The patient's desire for a certain course of action
   (d) The patient's family's desires for a certain course of action

7. Which of these is not an ABoIM Element of Professionalism?

   (a) Responsiveness
   (b) Respect
   (c) Responsibility
   (d) Relationships

Answers

1. c, 2. d, 3. b, 4. c, 5. d, 6. c, 7. d

Suggested Readings

American Board of Internal Medicine Professionalism Project. (2001). http://www.abim.org/pdf/profess.pdf.
Beauchamp, T. L., & Childress, J. F. (2001). *Principles of biomedical ethics* (5th ed.) New York: Oxford University Press.

Council on Ethical and Judicial Affairs (CEJA). (2007). *AMA code of medical ethics.* http://www.ama-assn.org/ama/pub/category/2498.html. Retrieved August 20, 2007.

Hope, T. (2004). *Medical ethics: A very short introduction.* New York: Oxford University Press.

Jonsen, A. R., Siegler, M., and Winslade, W.J. (2002). *Clinical ethics: A practical approach to ethical decisions in clinical medicine* (5th ed.) New York: McGraw-Hill.

Mahowald, M. (2006). *Bioethics and women.* New York: Oxford University Press.

Kayhan, P. (2006). *Healing as vocation: A medical professionalism primer (practicing bioethics).* Lanham, MD: Rowman & Littlefield.

Tong, R. (2007). *New perspectives in healthcare ethics: An interdisciplinary and crosscultural approach.* Upper Saddle River, NY: Prentice Hall.

Chapter 10
Adherence in Medicine

Maxwell Takai Frank and Eriko Takai Frank

Most health care providers become frustrated with non-adherent patients early in their training. This chapter examines the problems associated with adherence and offers insights into possible interventions to improve adherence.

At the end of this chapter, the reader will be able to

1. Discuss the epidemiology of non-adherence within different patient populations and with respect to specific health domains
2. Understand the importance of maintaining healthy habits with respect to the prevention and treatment of chronic medical conditions (e.g., diabetes, obesity)
3. Recognize clinical situations where non-adherence with treatment recommendations (e.g., lifestyle changes, medication regimens, follow-up appointments) is an important reason for poor clinical outcome
4. Develop clinical evaluation strategies in order to discriminate between different causes of non-adherence
5. Discuss ways of preventing treatment non-adherence and how to successfully intervene when the diagnosis of non-adherence is made

Case Vignette 10.1.1 (Presenting Situation) Kelii

Kelii is a 17-year-old male high school senior from Hawaii who has come to your family medicine clinic for a physical exam, which is a requirement for a private college program that he wants to attend this summer. You have not seen Kelii in nearly 3 years. He is a tall but overweight young man, and while asking about HEADSS (i.e., Home, Education/Employment, Activities, Diet/Drugs, Sexuality/Suicide), you ask about his eating and exercise habits. He states that he used to be active in sports when in grade school. However he began college preparatory school at 7th grade, and since then has focused more on his studies. His primary source of exercise occurs three times a week as part of his physical education (PE) classes. Kelii notes, however, that after PE, he is hungry and eats more snacks.

M.T. Frank
Resident in Psychiatry, Boston University Medical Center

A. Guerrero, M. Piasecki (eds.), *Problem-Based Behavioral Science and Psychiatry*,
© Springer Science+Business Media, LLC 2008

*Lunch is typically fast food, and he snacks on candy bars, chips, and soda through-
out a typical day.*

*On physical exam, Kelii is 198 cm in height and weighs 118 kgs. You take a
moment and calculate that his body mass index (BMI) is approximately 30.*

*You recall that you are already treating Kelii's father and grandmother for Type-
II diabetes, and take several minutes to explain to the patient his multiple risk factors
for contracting this illness. You ask Kelii to come back to the clinic the next morning
in order to have blood drawn for labs, and you will call and speak with him about
the results when they come in.*

 **Please proceed with the problem-based
approach!**

At this point in the case, it is reasonable to suggest that the patient's lifestyle and
family history contribute to his obesity. Obesity and family history are also important risk factors for diabetes. While public health and primary care recommendations
regarding diet, exercise, and healthy body weight are commonplace, the diagnosis
of treatment non-adherence is premature in this case because specific behavioral
health prescriptions have not been made to Kelii regarding healthier habits.

Medical advances of the twentieth century are responsible for having brought
many formerly fatal, acute illnesses under control, and clinical attentions are
increasingly concerned with the prevention and treatment of chronic medical conditions, such as diabetes. It is within this environment that the modern prescriptions
for harm reduction, primary prevention, and behaviorally oriented health care have
flourished. Healthy habits are not solely the concern of older adults, however; the
bulk of existing research supports the conclusion that initiating and maintaining
healthy habits is of vital importance for young adults (Dubbert, Rappoport, &
Martin, 1987).

In addition, reviews of US mortality risk factors have concluded that more than
one-half of all deaths have direct behavioral health determinants, and behavioral
risk factors have been linked to many cancers, cardiovascular disease, lung and
liver disease, motor vehicle-related fatality and injury, and sexually transmitted disease, including acquired immunodeficiency syndrome (AIDS) (e.g., as reviewed by
Gochman, 1997).

The vignette at this point is an excellent opportunity to review the components
of a well-adolescent history, for which risk-assessment acronyms such as HEADSS
are commonly used.

Case Vignette 10.1.2 Continuation

A few days later, you review the results from Kelii's fasting labs:
  Afterwards you call the patient at home and arrange for a follow-up visit.

Sodium: 141 mEql/l	Bicarbonate: 24 mmol/l	Cholesterol (total): 245 mg/dl
BUN: 12 mg/dl	Glucose: 156 mg/dl	LDL: 170 mg/dl
Creatinine: 1.0 mg/dl	Glycosylated Hb: 7.0 %	Triglycerides: 239 mg/dl

When you enter the examination room where Kelii is waiting, you notice that he looks anxious. After reviewing the test results with him, you conclude "Kelii, you likely have Type-II diabetes and this means that you're going to have to make some changes in your lifestyle. Your current diet and exercise habits are for a big part of this illness, and so it's very important that you make healthier choices." You make mental note to schedule appointments for Kelii with the dietician and diabetes nurse educator before he leaves.

You inform Kelii that the diabetes nurse will show him how to use the glucose monitor, lancets, and test strips which you will prescribe for him today, and that you want him to monitor and record his blood sugars every morning for the next 4 weeks. You conclude your visit, and say to Kelii "Come back in one month and bring all your blood sugar records so I can see how you're doing. Do you have any questions at this time?" "...Nah, Doc," he replies and departs.

You next see Kelii 4 weeks later. You received word from the dietician and diabetes nurse educator that he never made his appointments, and you begin to wonder if Kelii is participating in his treatment. Kelii arrives on time for his appointment and you again note that he looks anxious. You ask about his success with the changes you prescribed last month. "Gee, Doc, I never thought I could make these changes, so I never tried. There's so much you wanted me to do. I just couldn't do it. Besides, I feel healthy! Why should I care about my sugar levels?"

 Please proceed with the problem-based approach!

This case illustrates how, for any given patient and with respect to any particular health behavior, non-adherence is a heterogeneous construct. For example, while Kelii did not perform blood glucose monitoring as requested, he succeeded in arriving on time for each of his appointments with you, but did not show up for his visits with the dietician or nurse educator. Non-compliance with diabetic self-care is extremely common. Although self-monitoring of blood glucose is a standard regimen component for adults with Type-II diabetes, compliance estimates range from 5 to 44 % (Kennedy, 2001) with lowest rates reported by patients who do not yet require medication (Harris, 2001). Concerning the nature of a given prescribed regimen, it is generally accepted that the more complex a prescription is perceived to be, the less likely it is that patients will be successfully adherent.

When assessing Kelii's risk for noncompliance, it is important to recall that examples of noncompliance often do not have an explicit intention to be noncompliant. For example, is a non-English speaking patient who cannot read the instructions on his pill bottle less compliant than the uninsured patient who chooses to feed his children instead of fill a prescription? How about the busy executive who misplaces his prescription versus the carefree adolescent who neglects to fill his prescription in first place? Each is an example of medication non-adherence, yet each scenario invites different anticipatory and corrective actions by the clinician who is intent on improving adherence.

Case Vignette 10.1.3 Conclusion

You feel yourself becoming frustrated as you contemplate how to proceed, when Kelii continues "You also keep referring to this 'Type-II diabetes' and I still don't know what you mean. Yeah, my Dad's also got it, but he sure as heck doesn't talk about it. How can I be sick with this disease if I don't feel sick?" You take a moment to let Kelii's words sink in, and begin to appreciate how you may have contributed to his noncompliance by failing to explain things in simpler terms, and by not assessing his thoughts and feelings more carefully.

When you are finished, you ask Kelii to repeat your explanation using his own words. Afterwards Kelii sighs deeply and jingles the change in his pocket. "I think I understand a little better, Doc, thanks. But I'm still not sure I can make all these changes you want – it's not cool!" You allow Kelii to discuss other perceived barriers to adherence and suggest several potential benefits of diet, exercise, and weight loss, including the possibility that his diabetes will resolve completely. As you conclude your visit, Kelii smiles and says "Well, Doc, I guess it's time I started taking better care of myself, and this diabetes might be just the swift kick in the pants that I need." As he leaves your office, you resolve to make compliance enhancement a higher priority with all your patients, and feel that Kelii wasn't the only one getting a swift kick in the pants today.

The vignette concludes with Kelii disclosing to his doctor the extent of his non-compliance with prescribed treatment and provides some insight into the particular factors at play. The principle diagnoses in this case are obesity, diabetes mellitus, and noncompliance with treatment.

For review, according to the DSM-IV, *noncompliance with treatment* is not considered a mental disorder, but rather is included with such entities as *malingering* and *partner/relationship problems*. The diagnosis of noncompliance with treatment can be used when the focus of clinical attention is non-adherence to important aspects of treatment for a mental disorder or general medical condition, and warrants independent clinical attention.

Common reasons for non-adherence are shown in Table 10.1.

Many theories have been used to explain and predict behavior change, perhaps the most popular within medical contexts is the *Stages of Change* model (e.g., DiClemente, 1993), which we discussed in Chap. 4, and the associated techniques of *Motivational Interviewing* (Miller & Rollnick, 2002). According to this model, Kelii starts out in *precontemplation*, where he does not recognize the problem or the need

Table 10.1 Common reasons for non-adherence

Reason	Examples
Discomfort resulting from treatment	Pricking finger with lancet
Cost of treatment	Time commitment, financial burden
Personal values, religious, cultural, or other beliefs about the advantages and disadvantages of the treatment	Alternate beliefs about what the treatment should be
Maladaptive personality traits or coping styles (please refer to Chap. 6)	Passivity, externalization
Presence of comorbid mental illness	Major depression, anxiety disorders
Doctor–patient variables	Inadequate instructions, physician does not elicit patient questions or concerns, low level of rapport

to change. When changes in diet and exercise are seriously considered, Kelii has entered the *contemplation* stage, which may be followed by *preparation*, in which he makes a commitment to try to change and takes the necessary steps to enter the *action* stage, in which he implements the plan for modifying his behavior. Finally, with successful change, Kelii enters a *maintenance* stage, in which he sustains his lifestyle modifications to avoid relapse and accommodates the new behavior. Stages of change are by no means sequential, and jumps can be made in both forward and backward directions. At the conclusion of the case, Kelii can be seen entering the *preparation* stage of behavior change, having moved forward from *precontemplation* at the start of the vignette.

As depicted in Table 10.2, with the construction of a bio-psycho-social formulation, it will be possible to target interventions to optimally manage all mechanisms leading to the principle clinical problem in this case: noncompliance with diabetes treatment.

Please take this opportunity to construct a bio-psycho-social formulation.

Additional Topics of Interest

- The role of public health departments and the promotion of healthy lifestyles
- The collection and evaluation of national health statistics (e.g., Morbidity and Mortality Weekly Report)
- Patient adherence within both general population and specific age groups
- Adherence within specific health domains (e.g., diet, exercise, seat belts, bicycle helmets, smoking cessation, substance abuse, chronic disease, obesity)
- Psychiatric conditions commonly associated with non-adherence (e.g., antisocial or avoidant personality disorders; affective, psychotic, or anxiety disorders; factitious disorder; malingering)
- America's "obesity epidemic", the populations most at risk for developing obesity, and the factors implicated in its etiology
- Type-II diabetes mellitus: risk factors, pathophysiology, and treatment approaches

Table 10.2 Bio-psycho-social case formulation

	Biological		Psychological		Social	
	Factor	Intervention	Factor	Intervention	Factor	Intervention
Predisposing factors	Genetic risk factors (e.g., family history of obesity)	–	Maladaptive personality traits (e.g., denial of illness)	Individual counseling; acceptance of personal responsibility	Modeling of noncompliant behaviors (e.g., family members are not good role models)	Family counseling; compliance enhancement targeted at specific family members
Precipitating factors	Medical condition requiring behavior change (e.g., diabetes)	Primary prevention of lifestyle-related medical conditions	Lack of behavior-specific self-efficacy	Individual counseling and building of required skill repertoires	Embarrassment regarding self-monitoring blood glucose in public	Individual counseling; use of less obtrusive monitoring equipment
Perpetuating factors	–	–	Avoidance of inconvenience associated with compliance	Individual counseling; time management strategies	Poor communication between patient and health care provider	Routine assessment of patient compliance with prescribed treatment; nonjudgmental orientation

Review Questions

1. Which of the following variables would not be expected to predict compliance with self-monitoring blood glucose (SMBG)?

   (a) Having promised someone that you will comply
   (b) Having successfully practiced SMBG in the past
   (c) High educational achievement
   (d) Absence of discomfort during testing

2. Behavior-specific self-efficacy refers to the belief that one is capable of performing the health behavior in question and that doing so will result in better health.

   (a) True
   (b) False

3. Which of the following preventive health behaviors would not be recommended to a single, sexually active 21-year-old woman?

   (a) Cervical cancer screening
   (b) Breast self-examination
   (c) Mammography
   (d) Bimanual pelvic examination

4. When a patient's health condition does not respond to your initial medical management, it is useful to inquire about compliance.

   (a) True
   (b) False

5. According to the principles of motivational interviewing, which of the following best describes a newly diagnosed diabetic in the "contemplation" stage of behavior change?

   (a) Actively following an 1800-calorie ADA diet and attending weekly diabetes support group
   (b) Struggling to resume dietary control after having overindulged during a 2-week vacation
   (c) Collecting information about alternative and complimentary diabetes treatment approaches
   (d) Angrily responding to a family member who reminds you that diabetes runs in the family and requests that you be evaluated for this disease

Answers

1. c, 2. a, 3. c, 4. a, 5. c

References

DiClemente, C. C. (1993). Changing addictive behaviors: A process perspective. *Current Directions in Psychological Science, 2,* 101–106.

Dubbert, P. M., Rappoport, N. B., & Martin, J. E. (1987). Exercise and cardiovascular disease. *Behavior Modification, 11,* 329–347.

Gochman, D. S. (Ed.). (1997). *Handbook of Health Behavior Research III: Demography, Development, and Diversity.* New York: Plenum Press.

Harris, M. I. (2001). Frequency of blood glucose monitoring in relation to glycemic control in patients with Type 2 diabetes. *Diabetes Care, 24,* 979–982.

Kennedy, L. (2001). Self-monitoring of blood glucose in Type 2 diabetes. *Diabetes Care, 24,* 977–978.

Miller, W. R., & Rollnick, S. (2002). *Motivational Interviewing.* New York: Guilford Press.

Chapter 11
Stress and Health

Michael K. Daines and Nikhil Majumdar

Psychological stress is an important contributor to medical problems. Many common health problems can be better managed when the role of stress is identified and managed.

At the end of this chapter, the reader will be able to

1. Provide a working definition of stress
2. Discuss the physiologic and pathophysiologic effects of stress
3. Describe common symptoms of stress
4. Discuss common medical conditions where stress causes or aggravates the illness
5. Discuss adaptive and maladaptive responses to stress

Case Vignette 11.1.1 Presenting Situation: David Rosenthal

You are called to the emergency room to provide a psychiatric evaluation of David Rosenthal. The chart describes him as a 43-year-old man who drove himself to the ER and reported to the ER physician the sudden onset of palpitations, profuse sweating, nausea and lightheadedness. He also has had tingling and numbness in his arms and hands. He felt that his chest was tight and it was hard to breathe. The symptoms started suddenly about 4 hours ago and reached peak intensity within about 5 minutes. He was in a business meeting at the time but didn't want to leave early "because it would have been too embarrassing." The symptoms gradually resolved after about an hour. He has had four similar episodes over the past 2 months and that he's becoming progressively worried that he "might drop dead the next time." His vital signs are: blood pressure 112/84, heart rate 96 and regular, respirations 14 and unlabored and temperature 37.2°C. An EKG report states "Non-specific ST segment and T-wave abnormalities. Clinical correlation required." Blood test results are pending.

M.K. Daines
Assistant Professor of Psychiatry, University of Nevada School of Medicine

A. Guerrero, M. Piasecki (eds.), *Problem-Based Behavioral Science and Psychiatry*,
© Springer Science+Business Media, LLC 2008

Please proceed with the problem-based approach!

A review of the DSM-IV-TR criteria for panic attacks and panic disorder indicates that he meets many, but not all, of the criteria. Mr. Rosenthal reports 7 of the 13 symptoms of a panic attack. Only four symptoms are required to meet the definition of a panic attack. He has had four such attacks over the last 2 months, which meets the severity and frequency criteria. He meets the criteria regarding persistent worry about the attacks. However, his condition does not satisfy one important criterion. The presence of a general medical condition has not been excluded. Additional information is required.

Case Vignette 11.1.2 Continuation

You introduce yourself, informing him that you are a third-year medical student assigned to the psychiatry service and that the ER doctor has requested a psychiatry consultation. Mr. Rosenthal erupts in anger. "Do you think I'm crazy? Do you think this is all in my head? Nobody has told me what my test results are. Nobody told me a psychiatrist was coming!"
How would you handle this situation?
This brief exchange demonstrates several valuable lessons.

1. There remains a significant stigma about seeing a mental health professional or having psychological symptoms (see Stigma and Medicine, Chap. 13).
2. When a physician requests a consultation, whether psychiatric or medical, the patient should be informed of the purpose and should give consent. (see The Physician–Patient Relationship, Chap. 8, and Ethics and Professionalism, Chap. 9).
3. Patients frequently do not acknowledge or understand the relationship between life stresses and physical symptoms.

Case Vignette 11.1.3 Continued

You acknowledge Mr. Rosenthal's anger. You validate his frustration about waiting for test results. "I can only imagine what it would be like to be in your shoes. I think I would want to be kept informed as much as possible. Would you like me to find out approximately how much longer it will take?" You make sure that you do not make promises or assurances that are outside your ability to keep. You assure him that the interview is voluntary and confidential. You inform him that life stresses can be important triggers for many illnesses. You offer to talk with him while awaiting the test results. Mr. Rosenthal becomes less defensive and replies, "Well, there has been a lot going on lately."

He has been married for 19 years and has two children, who are doing well socially and educationally. Mr. Rosenthal has a close relationship with his mother and his sisters. About a year ago, his father died of a heart attack. He was sad about this loss, but does not feel that he became depressed. Five months ago he received an important promotion and a pay raise. He is working longer hours, but he enjoys his work and likes most of the challenges. However, it does require that he give oral presentations to large groups of strangers which he finds quite anxiety provoking. His family has moved to a larger home, and he misses the friendships from his old neighborhood.

Recently Mr. Rosenthal has felt impatient and angry with his wife and children. He doesn't feel that they appreciate the sacrifices he has made to provide them with a high standard of living. He is not exercising as much as he did before the promotion. He has resumed smoking 8–10 cigarettes per day but drinks no more than two glasses of wine per week and has never used illegal drugs. He asks, "Do you think this has anything to do with my symptoms?" Before you can answer, the ER doctor enters the room and explains that his blood tests indicate that he has had a myocardial infarction.

 Please proceed with the problem-based approach!

There are multiple factors that are correlated with an increased risk of developing coronary artery disease (CAD). They include

- Abnormalities of lipoproteins
- Hypertension
- Family history of CAD
- Diabetes mellitus
- Smoking
- Psychosocial stress

When an individual has two or more of these risk factors, the increase in risk is greater than the sum of risk factors. A detailed review of the diagnosis and treatment of CAD or myocardial infarction (MI) is outside the scope of this chapter. However, the mechanisms by which some of these factors lead to CAD or MI are well described. Studying these mechanisms helps us to understand the role of the stress response in the development of CAD, MI and other diseases.

First, it is necessary to propose a working definition of stress. Common usage of the word stress combines the demands of life ("I'm under a lot of stress") with the physical and emotional reactions ("I'm feeling so much stress"). Usually there is a negative connotation to the word stress. For our discussion, we will refer to external demands as *stressors* and the combination of the physical and emotional effects as the stress response:

- Stressors can be physical, mental or emotional.
- Stressors and the stress response can be acute or chronic.
- A person's perception of a stressor dramatically affects the physiologic responses.
- Voluntary human behaviors can moderate or aggravate the effects of these responses.

Normally, the body is in a balanced state known as homeostasis. Though many processes are important in maintaining homeostasis, we will be primarily concerned with the autonomic nervous system (ANS) and the hypophyseal-pituitary-adrenal axis (HPA). The ANS is composed of two divisions: the sympathetic nervous system (SNS) and the parasympathetic nervous system (PNS). The SNS is sometimes referred to as "fight or flight." The PNS can be thought of as the "rest and digest" system. The SNS can be activated by consciously perceived stimuli or by reflexive unconscious response. In either case, activation stimulates sympathetic thoraco-lumbar spinal ganglia to release norepinephrine (NE) and neuro-peptide Y directly onto receptors in the heart, lungs and arterioles. This results in an increase in heart rate, blood pressure and cardiac output. The bronchi dilate allowing increased airflow. Perfusion of vascular beds in muscles increases. The pupils dilate allowing a better visual response. The animal becomes more alert and focused. The adrenal glands release the catecholamines epinephrine (EPI) and NE into the circulation, which sustains these effects. Glycogen that has been stored in the liver and muscles is metabolized to glucose providing immediate energy availability. This response evolved to allow organisms to escape from physical threats. Although much of modern stress is psychological rather than physical (deadlines, red lights) the physiological response is the same.

The HPA also responds to stressors. In response to stimuli perceived as stressful, the hypothalamus releases arginine vasopressin (AVP) and corticotropin releasing factor (CRF) from the peri-ventricular nuclei to the anterior pituitary. The anterior pituitary releases adrenocorticotropic hormone (ACTH), which stimulates the adrenal cortex to release cortisol and aldosterone. Cortisol mobilizes glucose and increases gluconeogenesis. Aldosterone and AVP causes the kidney to retain salt and water, thus increasing blood pressure and circulating volume.

Both the SNS and HPA axis are self-balancing. For example, cortisol and aldosterone act on receptors in the hippocampus, amygdala and hypothalamus to reduce the release of CRF. This keeps the activation of HPA from becoming too high or persisting too long.

Natural selection has favored the development of these "prepare and repair" systems to respond to acute threat or actual injury. When the threat has passed, homeostasis is restored. However, if a stressor is chronic and the activation of these systems persists, these same responses can be pathological.

If we look at the stress response in more detail, we find beneficial effects (+) of acute activation but adverse effects (−) of chronic activation:

- Cortisol reduces insulin release, insulin-dependent growth factor (IGDF) and insulin sensitivity:

  + Acutely provides immediate energy
  − Chronically contributes to development of diabetes mellitus, obesity and dyslipidemia

- Cortisol and norepinephrine increase inflammatory cytokines such as interleukin-6 (IL-6) and tissue necrosis factor alpha (TNF-a) and the acute phase reactant C-reactive protein (CRP):

  + Acutely activate cellular immunity to fight acute infection
  − Chronically cause inflammation in the arterial endothelium contributing to the development of atherosclerotic plaques, a risk factor for CAD
  − Chronically stimulate CRF release, perpetuating the stress response

- Norepinephrine and AVP constrict renal arterioles and promote sodium retention:

  + Preserves circulating volume and reduces the risk of hypovolemic shock in acute injury or bleeding
  − Contributes to the development of hypertension

Psychosocial stressors activate the stress response through both the SNS and HPA axis. The hormonal and immunologic responses to psychological stress can affect the onset and course of a variety of conditions including

- Diabetes mellitus
- Hypertension
- Inflammatory bowel disease
- Asthma
- Multiple sclerosis

In controlled experiments, it is possible to measure and reproduce the physiological responses to acute psychological stress. A group of volunteers is exposed to standardized triggers such as public speaking, mental arithmetic under time pressure or viewing frightening movies or photographs. Their physiological responses are compared to a control group with no exposures. The comparison reveals differences in hormonal secretion and the effects on pulse, blood pressure and blood glucose between the two groups.

Understanding the effects of chronic psychosocial stressors is more difficult because of multiple confounding variables. Some stressors such as death of a spouse or child, divorce or loss of employment are either present or absent. Other stressors such as job dissatisfaction or low social support have a range of severity. The duration of exposure to the stressor may also be difficult to measure. There may be multiple psychosocial stressors present in the study groups. It is intuitive that if one stressor is bad, two or more stressors are worse. The Recent Life Change

Questionnaire (RLCQ) developed by Holmes and Rahe is a widely used method that demonstrates temporal relationships between stressful events and illnesses and quantifies the additive effects of stress.

Chronic physiologic changes are also found with prolonged emotional or social stressors. For instance, working women with children have higher levels of NE than working women with no children. The risk for working mothers developing CAD increases linearly with the increased number of children. Work stress is characterized as high-demand work with low autonomy and low self-reported satisfaction. In one study, workers with this profile had higher than normal levels of fibrinogen, which can trigger clot formation in coronary arteries leading to MI. Negative emotions of depression, anxiety or hostility are associated with increased health risk. The inflammatory cytokine IL-6 and the acute phase reactant CRP are both persistently elevated in patients who exhibit these negative emotions prominently.

Lower socio-economic status (SES) is associated with higher risk and poorer outcome of CAD, DM, HTN and asthma. However, lower SES is also associated with many health-risk behaviors (smoking, alcohol or unhealthy diets). Low social support, divorce and low job satisfaction may be risk factors for low SES or may result from low SES.

Case Vignette 11.1.4 Continuation

Mr. Rosenthal is admitted to the intensive care unit and, after appropriate testing, undergoes coronary artery by-pass graft surgery. His hospital recovery is uncomplicated. You complete your psychiatry clerkship and have started your first rotation in the internal medicine clinic. By chance, he is scheduled for a follow-up visit with you. He has been participating in a cardiac rehabilitation program that includes dietary advice, smoking cessation education and progressive exercise. He tells you that he has not any of the symptoms that brought him to the ER. He doesn't have any pain. He feels that the cardiac rehabilitation program was initially good and he was feeling that his stamina had been increasing. For the last 2 weeks, however, he has lost interest in attending the program and has become pessimistic about returning to work. He has had difficulty sleeping. He looks sad. He has a large cold sore on his lip. He tells you in a slow, monotone voice, "I don't think it's worth it."

Please proceed with the problem-based approach!

Mr. Rosenthal's follow-up history suggests major depressive disorder, which is described in Chap. 22. In this chapter, we will continue our focus on the stress responses and its relation to depression, CAD morbidity and mortality and effects on the immune system.

Major depressive disorder and sub-clinical depression are part of a vicious cycle. Psychosocial stress activates the stress response, which may lead to depression. Depression has been shown to increase the risk of developing CAD and MI and to occur frequently in the post-MI period. Depression worsens the functional outcomes of patients who survive MI, e.g., return to work, satisfaction with relationships, overall sense of well-being and greater non-cardiac health concerns. These poor functional outcomes result in increased psychosocial stress.

As described above, stress activates pro-inflammatory cytokines, IL-6, TNF-alpha and CRP. The inflammatory response is necessary to fight infection and to repair damaged tissue. Inflammatory cytokines also cause behavioral changes that benefit healing and recovery. In animals, there is decreased motor activity, decreased novelty-seeking and decreased pursuit of reward. The same behaviors are seen in humans who give subjective explanations for these behaviors: fatigue, loss of motivation and loss of ability to experience pleasure (anhedonia). IL-6 activation in the CNS affects metabolism of serotonin, dopamine and norepinephrine in the hippocampus, amygdala and nucleus accumbens, portions of the limbic system that regulate emotion. This "let-down" feeling is beneficial for a short period of recovery, but if it persists may begin the vicious cycle of depression.

Case Vignette 11.1.5 Conclusion

During the follow-up visit, you determine that Mr. Rosenthal does not have suicidal ideation. He tells you that he thinks only "weak people" get depressed and that he has always been able to control his life before his MI. You discuss with him that depression is frequent after an MI and you provide a brief explanation about stress and health. Together you develop a treatment plan.

Please proceed with the problem-based approach!
STOP

Primary care physicians treat the majority of patients with depression. Your treatment plan might include a prescription for an antidepressant medication. Although the primary mechanism of action for the antidepressant effects is in the brain, some antidepressants have caused reductions of pro-inflammatory cytokines in humans and in laboratory animals.

It is important to pay attention to Mr. Rosenthal's coping strengths (please also refer to Chap. 6). Optimists expect that negative events are isolated occurrences that will eventually resolve and that these events could happen to anybody. Pessimists believe they are victims of repeated patterns of negative events that will persist and can be blamed on themselves or others. In a group of initially healthy men, those with optimistic interpretations of life events had half the number of MIs or

Table 11.1 Stress management techniques

Exercise	Aerobic, outdoor may be best
Social support	Family, friends, colleagues
Diversion	Sports, movies, artistic activities
Relaxation	Music, reading, yoga
Time management	Using planning tools
Diet	Avoid excessive caffeine, alcohol
Sleep	7 or more hours a night

cardiac deaths than pessimists. Optimism improves immune measures and reduces the intensity and duration of the stress response. Although optimistic and pessimistic dispositions are usually well-established traits by adulthood, it has been shown that people can learn to adopt an optimistic style. Psychological treatments that help patients to learn more optimistic thought patterns are known as cognitive behavioral therapies (CBT).

Individuals with positive coping strengths are less likely to engage in health-risk behaviors such as smoking or substance abuse and more likely to adhere to prescribed treatments of medication, diet and exercise. Humor and laughter are positive coping responses that have been shown to cause an immediate beneficial immune response in patients with rheumatoid arthritis and in healthy volunteers.

Stress management techniques can pro-actively allow for improvements in stress and coping before a medical problem occurs. Table 11.1 offers a summary of commonly employed stress management approaches. People with higher levels of social support appear to have more robust immune systems. Aerobic exercise programs may be as effective as antidepressant medications in some groups of depressed patients. Lifestyle changes can lead to dramatic improvements in well-being.

Conclusions

Psychosocial stressors activate physiologic responses in the autonomic nervous system, the hypophyseal-pituitary-adrenal hormonal system, the immune system and the clotting system to respond to stressors. These systems return to baseline levels when the stress has resolved. Extreme, cumulative or prolonged stressors can result in an excessive or prolonged stress response that may initiate, precipitate or perpetuate many serious illnesses. Patients can learn effective coping methods to improve health.

Review Questions

1. Stress responses are . . .

    (a) Always beneficial
    (b) Often beneficial chronically

    (c) Often beneficial acutely

    (d) Without benefit

2. Which of these is not an effect of chronic norepinephrine elevation?

    (a) Preservation of circulating volume and decreased risk of hypovolemic shock

    (b) Chronic corticotropin releasing factor release

    (c) Increased likelihood of developing hypertension

    (d) Increased likelihood of developing atherosclerotic plaques, a risk factor for CAD

3. Which of these is considered a safe antidepressant for a cardiac patient?

    (a) A tricyclic antidepressant

    (b) A monoamine oxidase inhibitor

    (c) A selective serotonin uptake inhibitor

    (d) None of the above

4. How is coping strength related to cardiac disease?

    (a) Optimists have more heart attacks and cardiac deaths than pessimists.

    (b) Optimists have fewer heart attacks and cardiac deaths than pessimists.

    (c) Pessimists and optimists have equal numbers of heart attacks and cardiac deaths.

Answers

1. c, 2. a, 3. c, 4. b

Bibliography

Holmes SD, Krantz DS, Rogers H, Gottdiener J, Contrada RJ. Mental stress and coronary artery disease: A multidisciplinary guide. Progress in Cardiovascular Disease, 2006; 49: 106–122.

Rahe RH, Veach TL, Tolles RL, Murakami K. The stress and coping inventory: An educational and research instrument. Stress Medicine, 2000; 16: 199–208.

Raison CL, Capuron L, Miller AH. Cytokines sing the blues: Inflammation and the pathogenesis of depression. Trends in Immunology, 2006; 27: 24–31.

VanItallie TB. Stress: A risk factor for serious illness. Metabolism, 2002; 51: 40–45.

Chapter 12
Health Care 101

David C. Fiore and Jason P. Crawford

> *Of all the forms of inequality, injustice in health care is the*
> *most shocking and inhumane.*
>
> Martin Luther King, Jr.

This chapter will give you an opportunity to explore some of the more interesting and important facets of the rapidly changing landscape of health care delivery. The cases highlight how Americans obtain and pay for their health care, how health care is financed, why the "system" is structured the way it is, and how "public health" fits into the system. We hope you'll be able to formulate your own opinions in regards to the relative advantages and disadvantages of health care delivery in the United States and how you believe health care may, or should, be delivered 5 or 10 years from today.

At the end of this chapter, the reader should be able to

1. Discuss the current organization, structure, and financing of the health care system in the United States
2. Articulate key strengths and weaknesses of our current health care system, including issues of quality, access, and cost
3. Describe the importance of "public health" and how public health differs from, yet complements, individual health care

As in the other chapters in this book, we will be using case vignettes as the vehicle for delving into these topics; but first, we would like to introduce the Baker family and provide some introductory information that will allow the reader to understand the health insurance situations that arise in the scenarios. Please note that this chapter modifies the PBL tables in order to best address the complex topic of health care financing.

> **Mrs. Betty Baker**: a 54-year-old graphic artist for Can-do advertising company who moved to the United States from Ottawa, Canada, when she was 28.
>
> **Mr. Bob Baker**: a 62-year-old human resources administrator for a mid-sized auto parts company who was born and raised outside of Detroit, Michigan.
>
> **Mr. Brian Baker**: a 19-year-old sophomore college student, son to Betty and Bob, currently an undeclared major, enjoying his early college years.

D.C. Fiore
Associate Professor, Family and Community Medicine, University of Nevada School of Medicine

A. Guerrero, M. Piasecki (eds.), *Problem-Based Behavioral Science and Psychiatry*,
© Springer Science+Business Media, LLC 2008

Ms. Bridget Baker-McGladrey: the 22-year-old daughter of Betty and Bob who is a healthy married woman who has completed 2 years of college but recently put it "on hold" when she became pregnant 6 months ago and decided to drop out to work at a local department store to save for her child's future.

Mr. Tom McGladrey: a 25-year-old male computer technician. He is employed in a "start-up" business of five employees. He is "buying in on the ground floor" by sweat equity, and the company has yet to show a profit. He's working at a fast-food restaurant part-time to supplement his meager income now that Bridget is pregnant. He has no current major medical issues.

Based on the character information above and your knowledge of health insurance options in the United States (see also Tables 12.1a and 12.1b), please fill in the below table and consider the potential sources of health insurance coverage each character may have out of the following list:

Self-pay (meaning "uninsured")
Private individual insurance
Employer-sponsored insurance
Medicaid
Medicare
State Children's Health Insurance Plan (S-CHIP)
CHAMPUS
Veterans Affairs
Canadian Health Act provincial insurance

Case Vignette 12.1.1 Presenting Situation: Betty Baker

During her annual physical, Betty Baker's primary care physician, Dr. Dulces, noticed a lump in her right breast and the mammogram confirmed a "suspicious lesion." Dr. Dulces referred Betty to the surgeon, Dr. Sherman, who confirms cancer with a biopsy and later performs a partial mastectomy. Dr. Dulces then refers Betty to Dr. Sung, a renowned oncologist, for chemotherapy. Unfortunately, Dr. Sung is not on Betty's employer-sponsored health maintenance organization (HMO) health insurance plan's list of contracted providers. So, she returns to Dr. Dulces, who now refers her instead to Dr. Walsh, who is indeed on her HMO plan's provider list.

Due to the stage and grade of her cancer, Dr. Walsh recommends initiation on a novel chemotherapy regimen only available through the University Hospital's Cancer Center. Betty discusses this with Dr. Dulces, who makes it clear that this is out of her area of expertise, but supports Betty's decision to opt for this treatment, even though the University Hospital is approximately 2 hours away. Unfortunately, she finds out that her HMO plan has refused coverage of the treatment as it is pending FDA approval and is still classified as "experimental" by the plan. After many calls to her insurance provider (and with much assistance from Dr. Dulces, who had tried to hide her frustration with the insurance company), Betty is "approved" for a consultation at the University, but no guarantee is made that the insurance company will pay for the treatment.

Table 12.1 Demographic information and potential health insurance coverage

a. Contents to be filled in by students

Person	Age	Employment status	Potential source of coverage	What else you need to know
Betty Baker				
Bob Baker				
Brian Baker				
Bridget Baker – McGladrey				
Tom McGladrey				

b. Populated table

Person	Age	Employment status	Potential source of coverage	What else you need to know
Betty Baker	54	Employed	Employer-sponsored (hers or husband's), self-pay	Size of the companies, what insurance plan they offer, how long she's been there
Bob Baker	58	Employed	Employer-sponsored, self-pay	As above, more about his injury and coverage rules at the VA
Brian Baker	19	Unemployed student	Private individual insurance, employer-sponsored (mother's or father's), self-pay	Student health plan availability and coverage, parental coverage of college-enrolled kids
Bridget Baker-McGladrey	21	Unemployed	Medicaid or S-CHIP, self-pay	Income level, Medicaid requirements (especially concerning pregnancy)
Tom McGladrey	23	Employed	self-pay, possibly on parent's insurance	Ability to cover adult children on parental plan
Kelly Zanjen	79	Retired	Canadian Health Insurance, private, self-pay	Availability of private insurance in Canada, coverage while in United States
Blake Baker	85	Retired	Medicare, VA, Medicaid, self-pay	Medicare coverage, VA

At her first visit in the University Oncology Center she meets other women with breast cancer and is startled to learn that some women were "approved" for treatment without any difficulty while others, like herself, have been stopped at almost every step. In addition to learning all she can about breast cancer, Betty is determined to learn more about the health care system: Why is she being "bounced around" from doctor to doctor? Why do some women have no problem getting their insurance company to pay for the University's Oncology Center treatment? Why is certain therapy only offered at major "centers" like the University?

 Please proceed with the problem-based approach!

Table 12.2 Betty Baker

	What are the facts?	What are your hypotheses?	What do you want to know next?	What specific information would you like to learn about?
Betty's medical condition				
What are Betty's options to receive care?				
How has the health care system impacted Betty's options?				
What options are available to Betty?				

Complete Table 12.2.

Like so many other Americans, Betty is confused by the complex nature of the US health care system's organization. The role of any health care system is to assure that the "right patient receives the right service at the right time and in the right place" (Bodenheimer, 2005; Rodwin, Kervasdoue and Kimberly, 1984). In order to accomplish this role, a number of organizational models evolved to provide defined levels of care within a health care system. In 1920, Lord Dawson published a report defining these levels of care: (1) *primary care* constitutes the overwhelming majority of health care encounters and refers to provision of preventive care and treatment of common health problems; (2) *secondary care* emphasizes specialty expertise and hospital-based services; and (3) *tertiary care* focuses on special investigation, treatment, and management of rare and complex diseases and disorders. (4) The term *quaternary care* has also more recently been coined to delineate highly advanced specialized care that is not widely available or used.

Overview of Health Insurance and Financing in the United States

The inevitability of illness throughout our lifetimes mandates the need for health care. The escalating costs of medical care outstrip other areas of the economy and make it difficult for most societies to finance health care. In an attempt to manage costs, the United States has tailored financing systems to fund health care. An essential component of most health care financing schemes is the availability of "health insurance" to provide a source of payment to providers of health care services. The use of health insurance allows the insured a partial shield against the high costs of health care while simultaneously providing funds to subsidize the health care costs of the actively ill. According to Bodenheimer (2005), health insurance allows the distribution of health care "more in accordance with human need rather than exclusively on the basis of ability to pay . . . funds are redistributed from the healthy to the sick, a subsidy that helps pay the costs of those unable to purchase services on their own."

Although the majority of health care financing and health insurance coverage worldwide rely heavily on public funding from governmental sources, the United States remains unique in its use of private funding for health care. According to 2006 US Census Bureau reporting, approximately 59.7 % of all non-elderly (less than 65) insured Americans are covered through employer-sponsored insurance, and privately funded employer-sponsored health insurance remains the dominant mode of our health insurance coverage (Denavas-Wait et al., 2007; Clemans-Cope et al., 2006).

The private health insurance model began in the 1930s. As health care costs quickly outstripped income potentials for the average US worker, health insurance allowed public access to the array of rapidly developing health care technologies and services. The private health insurance industry in the United States met even greater demand during World War II. The US wartime economy placed significant constraints on both workforce availability and salary increases, so non-salary-based "fringe" benefits became important for recruiting prospective employees. Health insurance coverage plans became very attractive to employees due to escalating health care costs. Federal government tax subsidies (equaling over $100 billion per year currently) provided significant tax shelter for employers and today are one of the cornerstones to the intimate link between employment status and health insurance coverage in the United States (Bodenheimer, 2005).

Significant gaps in health insurance coverage for the US population result from the reliance on private employer-sponsored health insurance plans. Those who cannot obtain employment, or who are employed by a business that does not offer health insurance, remained uninsured. The elderly, the permanently disabled, the poor, and children emerged as uninsured populations in the late 1950s (Bodenheimer, 2005).

The reaction to this uninsured population gap was the advent of Medicaid and Medicare, governmentally funded health insurance programs. As of 2006, these programs constitute 27.0 % of all health insurance coverage for the US population (Denavas-Wait et al., 2007). Medicare was enacted in 1965 in order to provide partial health insurance coverage for all persons 65 years or older and persons with permanent disabilities. The Medicaid program was developed to provide partial coverage for the poor, some persons with disabilities, children, pregnant women in need, and select elderly who also qualify for Medicare (the "dual eligible"). The State Children's Health Insurance Plan (S-CHIP) was enacted in 1997 to provide expanded coverage for children and adolescents below the 200 % federal poverty level (FPL). The military and Veterans Health Administration provide federally funded health insurance for the active, retired, and veteran populations of the US Armed Forces through programs such as the Comprehensive Health and Medical Plan for Uniformed Services (CHAMPUS), the Civilian Health and Medical Program of the Department of Veterans Affairs (CHAMPVA), and the Department of Veterans Affairs (VA). The VA system provides medical services to low-income veterans and those with permanent disabilities and is funded annually at the discretion of Congress.

The simplest models for health care delivery can be organized into two main subsets, the *regionalized model* and the *dispersed model*. The regionalized model emphasizes a strong base of primary care provision for all localities throughout the service area. Secondary and tertiary care is provided at more distinct district or regional locations, such as large urban centers, and services much larger subsets of the overall population within the health system. Access to higher levels of care originates at the primary care level. An example of this model is the English National Health Service (described in more detail later; Bodenheimer, 2005). The dispersed model of care places emphasis on provision of all levels of care throughout all localities of a service area. Though dispersed care models may intuitively seem the most advantageous to a population, the costs of health care delivery under this model are often prohibitive.

The high cost of health care delivery and organization prompted efforts to control the escalating costs of health care during the 1960s and 1970s. Betty's feelings of frustration and confusion regarding her own health care access and delivery stem from the development of such cost-containment strategies. The advent of the *health maintenance organization* (HMO) under the Nixon administration's HMO Act of 1973 and the *managed care* movement in the 1980s and 1990s had significant impact on the provision of health care within the United States. Unlike indemnity plans that offer reimbursement of health care expenses on a fee-for-service basis, HMOs and other types of managed care organizations (MCOs) use systems and techniques to control the use (and, ostensibly, the cost) of health care services (Ruth, 2005b). The ultimate goal of a managed care organization (MCO) is providing health care services to a defined population in a cost-efficient manner while maintaining the population's health.

Several forms of MCOs have developed over the last few decades. The most well known is the HMO. Members pay a fixed fee to access the HMO's network of contracted providers (who provide services to members at a discounted rate under contract with the HMO) to meet the member's health care needs. A primary care physician (PCP) provides preventive and routine health services as well as coordinates referrals for specialty care and advanced diagnostics and treatments. The emphasis for PCP is on prevention of disease, and medical care is generally directed by a set of approved guidelines within the HMO.

Health maintenance organizations can be further subdivided into a variety of models depending on how providers are contracted. *An Individual Practice Association* (IPA) is a group of independent providers who join together to contract with an HMO. In a *staff model HMO*, such as Kaiser Permanente, the HMO employs all providers and owns its own hospitals, clinics, and labs to provide services exclusively for HMO members. A *group model HMO* contracts with a single multispecialty group to provide services to members. In a *network model HMO*, the HMO contracts with a combination of groups, IPAs, and individual physicians (Baldor [1998]).

Two additional MCO models have developed during the 1990s to provide greater flexibility to their members. First, a *Point of Service* (POS) plan allows members to see providers outside of the contracted network but at a higher out-of-pocket expense to the member. Second, a *Preferred Provider Organization* (PPO) plan designates some providers as "preferred" and sets lower deductibles and co-payments for these physicians while still allowing members the option to use out-of-network physicians at higher out-of-pocket costs. Both POS and PPO plans differ from HMOs in that traditional HMO plans will not cover any of the costs for services of an out-of-network provider.

In Betty's case, her employer has contracted with an HMO that is restrictive to who can provide her services (i.e., the oncologists) and what services can be provided to her.

Health Care Costs Overview

Case Vignette 12.1.2 Conclusion

Through her research, Betty has learned that the innovations of health care in the past 30 years have vastly improved the prognosis for breast cancer. Depending on the stage of the cancer, 5-year survival ranges are over 50 %. Unfortunately, these advances did not come without a cost.

After reviewing some the bills related to her treatment, Betty wonders why the provision of health care is so expensive and where all of that insurance money goes to anyway. She simply cannot imagine how anyone could pay "out of pocket" for these huge bills. Betty concludes that the health care costs in the United States are spiraling out of control. Her oncologist prescribes a long-term medication for her breast cancer and she is cancer-free at 3-year follow-up.

Please proceed with the problem-based approach!

Please complete Table 12.3.

Betty is correct—the costs of health care in the United States are astronomical. National health expenditures rose at twice the rate of inflation from 2004 to 2005 reaching roughly $2 trillion. This accounts for 16 % of the gross domestic product (GDP) (Centers for Medicare and Medicaid Services (CMS), 2007b; National Coalition on Health Care (NCHC), 2007a; Organization for Economic and Co-operation Development (OECD), 2007). In other words, $1 of every $6 spent on US-made goods and services went to health care!

US per capita spending on health care has reached an unprecedented high worldwide of $6,700 (CMS, 2007b; NCHC, 2007a). The next closest countries to the US for expenditures on health care are Switzerland at 11.6 % of its GDP and Norway at $4,364 per capita (OECD, 2007). Unfortunately the health care costs in the United States continue to skyrocket. According to the Milliman Medical Index (MMI),

Table 12.3 Betty Baker

	What are the facts?	What are your hypotheses?	What do you want to know next?	What specific information would you like to learn about?
What are health care costs in the United States?				
Who pays this cost (individual, employers, government)?				
Where does the money go?				

the total costs of medical spending for a family of four in 2007 is estimated to be $14,500, an increase of 8.4 % over the 2006 MMI (Milliman Medical Index (MMI), 2007).

Where do these costs arise? At roughly 82 % of all health care cost, hospital and physician services account for the greatest majority of spending. Outpatient and inpatient hospital services increases at the most rapid rate of 9.0 and 9.8 %, respectively (MMI, 2007).

How does this impact out-of-pocket expenditures? The MMI estimates that the average family will spend $2,420 in out-of-pocket expenses through health insurance plan cost-sharing at the time of service (i.e., deductibles, co-payments), an increase of $210 over 2006 data (MMI, 2007). In addition, for the $14,500 annual premium for an insurance plan, the employee contributes 38 % ($3,171) via payroll deductions, while the employer contributes the remaining 62 % ($8,909). In combination, payroll deductions and out-of-pocket cost-sharing payments total $5,591 paid by the employee, an increase of over 100 % since 2000 (NCHC, 2007b).

Case Vignette 12.2.1 Presenting Situation: Bob Baker

After many years of uncontrolled hypertension, cigarette smoking, and hyperlipidemia, Bob suffered a large right-sided cerebrovascular accident 6 months ago. After an inpatient hospital stay, Bob spent 8 weeks at a rehabilitation center in order to adapt to the problems he had with moving his left arm and leg. He was unable to maintain his human resources position at the auto parts company and was forced into retirement due to disability. Bob purchased continuation coverage through his employer's Consolidated Omnibus Budget Reconciliation Act, or COBRA plan. He is increasingly concerned with expenses since his wife's diagnosis of breast cancer, since his COBRA plan's monthly premiums are significant. He is unsure whether he and his wife will be able to afford the premiums for the COBRA plans which now cover both of them and he wonders what alternatives he has. During one of his visits to Dr. Dulces, she informs him that he may qualify for Medicare due to his disability.

He replies that he thought Medicare was just for "old folks." He decides to explore this option in more detail on the Internet and effortlessly finds medicare.gov.

 Please proceed with the problem-based approach!

Please complete Table 12.4.

Medicare was developed as a tax-financed insurance program for all people aged 65 and older. It subsequently expanded to include people under 65 with permanent disabilities. The program is currently administered by the Centers for Medicare and Medicaid Services (CMS, http://www.cms.hhs.gov/), formerly known as the Health Care Financing Administration (HCFA), under the supervision of the Department of Health and Human Services (DHHS, http://www.hhs.gov/).

At age 65, a person is automatically enrolled in Medicare if he/she is eligible for Social Security (meaning the person or their spouse has paid into the Social Security System for 10 years) regardless of current income, retirement status, or medical history. A person under 65 with a permanent disability is eligible for Medicare coverage after receiving Social Security disability benefits for 24 months, though persons with chronic kidney disease often have the 2-year waiting period waived (Bodenheimer, 2005; Henry J. Kaiser Family Foundation (KFF, 2006b). As of 2006, Medicare provides coverage for 13.6 % of all insured Americans, equating to nearly 43 million persons (Denavas-Wait et al., 2007; KFF, 2006b). In 2006, total Medicare benefit spending equaled $342 billion, accounting for 14 % of the federal budget (CMS, 2007b; KFF, 2006b).

Medicare is subdivided into four parts. *Medicare Part A* provides payment for inpatient hospital, skilled nursing facility, home health, and hospice care. *Medicare Part B*, the Supplementary Medical Insurance Trust Fund, pays for physician services, both outpatient and preventive, and some medical equipment and home health costs and requires beneficiary premiums. This standard monthly premium for 2007

Table 12.4 Bob Baker

	What are the facts?	What are your hypotheses?	What do you want to know next?	What specific information would you like to learn about?
Who does Medicare cover?				
About what Medicare covers				
How is Medicare financed?				
What are the challenges Medicare is facing?				

equaled $93.50 but may be as high as $161.40 depending on household income levels (CMS, 2007b). *Medicare Part C*, or the Medicare Advantage program, allows managed care companies to administer Medicare benefits. *Medicare Part D*, begun in 2006, provides a partial outpatient prescription drug benefit to beneficiaries. It requires a beneficiary premium of about $25 per month.

Medicare is by no means a comprehensive health insurance program. In general, Medicare covers only 45 % of total health care costs for beneficiaries due to cost-sharing measures such as annual deductibles, monthly premiums, and coverage exemptions that require out-of-pocket spending for the beneficiary. Therefore, many Medicare recipients purchase supplemental private health insurance coverage, known as "Medigap," to lower annual out-of-pocket expenses (KFF, 2006b; Ruth, 2005a). Additionally, over 7 million Medicare beneficiaries are dually eligible for state-based Medicaid coverages to help fund their Medicare premiums, deductibles, and non-Medicare-covered health expenses such as long-term care services (KFF, 2006b).

As the US population ages, and with a decline in the ratio of workers to beneficiaries, Medicare currently faces a "funding warning." As Medicare spending increases to meet the health care needs of the aging "baby boomer" generation, the Medicare Part A Trust Fund reserves are projected to be exhausted by 2018 (KFF, 2006b).

The Consolidated Omnibus Budget Reconciliation Act (COBRA) of 1996 requires that employers with 20 or more employees offer employees and their families a temporary extension of health coverage (known as "continuation coverage") under their sponsored health plan when coverage under the plan would otherwise end. COBRA may be purchased at the time of voluntary or involuntary termination, reduction in work hours (thereby disqualifying employee for benefits), divorce or separation from covered employee, or death of covered employee. In general, COBRA plans provide no employer sponsorship of the premium payments, therefore the employee bears the entire cost for coverage.

Case Vignette 12.3.1 Presenting Situation: Bridget McGladrey

Bridget and Tom began their relationship about 2 years ago. They recently learned that she was about 12 weeks pregnant and quickly had the wedding they had been planning for the following summer. Bridget dropped out of college last year and has been working at a local department store that offers health insurance benefits only after employment for 6 months. She is currently uninsured. Money has been "tight" considering Tom's business has only just opened and his income has been very low. Bridget is very concerned about how she can afford prenatal care for her pregnancy and care for the new baby. She has been contemplating her options and was told by a friend at work that she may qualify for the state-based Medicaid program. She is unfamiliar with Medicaid and gets on the Internet to find out if she will qualify.

Please proceed with the problem-based approach!

Please complete Table 12.5.

The Medicaid program serves as the nation's major public health insurance program for low-income people. Medicaid, unlike Medicare, is a state-based program funded jointly by the state and federal governments. Like Medicare, CMS provides federal supervision over Medicaid programs.

The federal government creates minimum eligibility guidelines and allows the state authority to optionally extend Medicaid eligibility beyond these minimums. To be eligible for Medicaid coverage, a person must meet financial criteria and fall within one of three eligibility groups: *categorically needy, medically needy,* and *special groups* (CMS, 2005). These groups include children and newborns, pregnant women, people with disabilities, certain subpopulations with specific medical conditions, low-income workers, and dual eligible Medicare beneficiaries. As of 2006, 12.9 % (45.7 million) of all insured Americans received benefits through state-based Medicaid programs (Denavas-Wait et al., 2007; CMS, 2006).

Medicaid services vary by the state. Federally mandated coverages include the inpatient and outpatient hospital treatment, professional services (physicians, dentists, midwifes, and nurse practitioners), laboratory and x-ray, nursing home and home health care for those 21 and older, family planning, pregnancy-related, well-newborn, and well-child care, and rural health clinic/federally qualified health center services. Optional services determined by state authority include prescription drugs, clinic services, prosthetic devices, hearing aids, intermediate care facilities, and other elder services.

Medicaid remains the major source of coverage for low-income individuals who need mental health services and substance abuse treatment and is accountable for

Table 12.5 Bridget and Tom

	What are the facts?	What are your hypotheses?	What do you want to know next?	What specific information would you like to learn about?
What are the origins of the Medicaid program?				
How is Medicaid funded?				
Who does Medicaid cover?				
What does Medicaid cover?				

44 % of public mental health spending (Substance Abuse and Mental Health Services Administration (SAMHSA), 2005).

Medicaid spending accounts for, on average, 22 % of state budgets (CMS, 2007b; NCHC, 2007b). This places Medicaid spending second only to education as the states' highest governmental expense. On average, the federal government finances 57 % of all Medicaid programs (KFF, 2006a). The largest proportion of expenditures is attributable to the dual eligible elderly and disabled, accounting for 70 % of Medicaid spending. Medicaid payments for nursing home care, a service not covered by Medicare, remains the most costly at 44 % of all expenditures (KFF, 2006a).

Case Vignette 12.3.2 Continuation

Bridget has completed 6 months of employment at the department store, but has had to reduce her time to 20 hours per week, so she still does not qualify for health insurance. Her prenatal care is covered by Medicaid, but she had to call many doctors to find one who would accept her insurance. Bridget wonders if Medicaid will still cover her and little Tommy once he's born, if they qualify for her employer-sponsored insurance. Her friend at work told her the insurance plan "stinks" and Bridget is unsure about how to proceed.

 Please proceed with the problem-based approach!

Complete Table 12.6.

A third governmental-sponsored program, the State Children's Health Insurance Plan (S-CHIP) aims to address the growing problem of uninsured children nationwide by increasing coverage for children less than 19 years whose family income

Table 12.6 Bridget and Tom

	What are the facts?	What are your hypotheses?	What do you want to know next?	What specific information would you like to learn about?
What are Bridget's options?				
How does the government provide care to children?				
What are employer-sponsored insurance opportunities for part-time workers?				

is below 200 % of the federal poverty level (FPL) (set at $41,300 for a family of four in 2007) (CMS, 2007a). This group is referred to as "targeted low-income children" and is comprised of children whose families earn too much to be eligible for Medicaid but not enough to purchase private insurance. Enrollees in the state-based S-CHIP programs cannot be eligible for Medicaid or private insurance (Ruth, 2005b).

Like Medicaid, S-CHIP provides federally mandated minimums. Within these federal guidelines, each state can design a program of eligibility, enrollment, payment, benefits, and operation/administration. The coverage must include those stipulated by the federal guidelines for Medicaid, specifically targeting well-newborn/well-child care, immunizations, and emergency services.

The federal and state governments, similar to Medicaid, jointly fund the S-CHIP programs. The federal government allocates funds to each state via an annual capped block grant that matches (up to 85 % of) the respective state's annual contribution to the program. The total federal and state S-CHIP expenditures for 2006 were $5.4 billion and $2.4 billion, respectively, for a total governmental expenditure of $7.8 billion (Center for Children and Families, 2007; KFF, 2007a). Continued federal support for S-CHIP will be voted on by Congress during the 2007–2008 session.

Case Vignette 12.3.3 Continuation

Since Bridget spends a lot of time in the waiting room at the Maternity Clinic she has made friends with some of the other women there. Her best new friend, Juanita Juarez, shocked Bridget with stories of how much difficulty her family (some of whom are undocumented immigrants) has in getting health care. Juanita claims her niece died of pneumonia because she could not see a doctor soon enough and her parents were too afraid of deportation to go to the ER. When Bridget shares this with Tom, he scoffs that this could not be true in the United States, because everyone, regardless of insurance status, can go to the ER anytime they want for "free" care.

 Please proceed with the problem-based approach!

Complete Table 12.7.

The US Census Bureau indicates a steady rise in the uninsured US population over the last decade. According to 2006 data one in six Americans lack coverage (Denavas-Wait et al., 2007). In addition to the uninsured population, an estimated additional 30–40 million are considered "underinsured" due to coverage restrictions, financial barriers, and/or lack of access to care (Bodenheimer, 2005).

Table 12.7 Health Access

What are the facts about access to health care and the uninsured?	What are your hypotheses?	What do you want to know next?	What specific information would you like to learn about?
How many Americans are uninsured?			
Who are the Uninsured?			
Why are they uninsured?			
What are some medical and financial consequences of being uninsured?			
What are some recent proposals to address this problem?			

Who are the uninsured? Currently 80% of uninsured Americans come from low-income working families—70% with one or more full-time workers and 11% with part-time workers (Denavas-Wait et al., 2007; KFF, 2006c). The elderly and children have more access to health care coverage via the Medicare, Medicaid, and/or S-CHIP programs, leaving non-elderly adults to constitute 80% of the uninsured population. Eighty percent of the uninsured are native or naturalized US citizens, although non-citizens have a higher population uninsured rate (40–50%) compared to the US average due to income and eligibility factors (KFF, 2006c; KFF, 2007b). Uninsured rates vary by racial/ethnic group and are presented in decreasing order: Hispanics (34.1%), American Indian/Alaskan Native (29.9%), Native Hawaiian/other Pacific Islanders (21.8%), Black (20.5%), Asian (15.5%), and White (14.9%) (KFF, 2006c; KFF, 2007b). The largest concentrations of the uninsured are found in the South (19.0%) and the West (17.9%). California, Texas, Florida, and New York represent the states with the highest percentage of uninsured population (Denavas-Wait et al., 2007).

Why are the uninsured uninsured? Contrary to popular belief, only 7% of those who are uninsured state that they "do not need health insurance" (KFF, 2006c). Most of the uninsured (53.3%) cited "cost" as the number one reason for their lack of health insurance (Centers for Disease Control and Prevention (CDC), 2006). With insurance premiums increasing by 143% since 2000 compared to a mere 20% increase in wages over the same time period, low-income working families are no longer able to afford the premium payments.

The second and third most common reasons for lack of health insurance are reported to be "lost job or change in employment" (26.9%) and "employer did not offer or insurance company refused" (14.1%) (CDC, 2006). Since the economic recession of 2001, employment opportunities have shifted from full-time, high-wage jobs to part-time, low-wage jobs, many of which offer no employer-sponsored insurance plans. Additionally, companies previously offering employer-sponsored plans began to drop coverages or shift more of the premium contributions to employees due to the rapid inflation of insurance premium costs. The poor and near poor are hardest hit by these shifts in employment opportunities and costs, further increasing these populations' uninsured rates.

How does lack of insurance affect the health care for the individual? The uninsured have a much greater probability of not having a regular source of care, with over 20% (versus 3% of the insured) reporting emergency rooms as their usual source of care (KFF, 2006c). For uninsured people, the out of pocket costs of health care lead to postponement of needed care and preventive health measures. This leads to delays in diagnoses and presentations at later stages in disease often mandating higher acuity and more expensive care. In fact, in 2004, per capita costs for the uninsured are almost twice as high as the insured (KFF, 2006c). Additionally, lack of financial resources often leads to non-adherence with prescription medications and recommended follow-up. These barriers to health care for the uninsured lead to an estimated 10–15% reduction in health overall and projected 18,000 potentially preventable deaths per year in the 25 to 64-year-old age group (Institute of Medicine (IOM), 2006).

Insurance coverage status has a significant impact on mental health as well as physical health. The majority of insurance plans do not provide as comparable coverage for mental health services as medical and surgical benefits. Less than one-half of people with diagnosable mental disorders receive treatment during their lifetime. The Mental Health Parity Act of 1996 was passed in an attempt to close the gap between mental health and medical service coverage by prohibiting insurance companies from paying less for mental health care than for general medical care. Although Medicare and Medicaid provide mental health coverage, significant out-of-pocket expenses and coverage gaps lead to a high uninsured/underinsured rate in this population.

In the United States, there is no such thing as "free" care for the uninsured; 35 % of all uncompensated care is paid for out-of-pocket by the uninsured (KFF, 2006c). Americans are divided on whether or not health care is a "right." Approximately 50 % of Americans believe that the government should insure all Americans (Rasmussen Report, 2007). However, others have noted that health care is not a right delineated in the Constitution (unlike access to legal council). Many countries and international bodies do recognize health care as a right (http://www.nesri.org/fact_sheets_pubs/Right %20to %20Health %20Care.pdf).

Case Vignette 12.4.1 Presenting Situation: Brian Baker

Brian has recently returned to school after summer vacation for his sophomore year. Due to the recent financial constraints from his mother and father's illnesses, at the start of the new college year, they decided not to purchase him the school's optional student health plan. After a sexual encounter at a fraternity party, Brian develops a greenish penile discharge. He is very concerned but is hesitant to visit the student health clinic due to the anticipated expense of the visit. After an embarrassing disclosure to his roommate regarding his current condition, the roommate recommends that he go to the local public health department's STD clinic. Brian did not even know there was a public health department or what "public health" is. He calls the student health center to get directions.

 Please proceed with the problem-based approach!

Please complete Table 12.8.

Defining "public health" as a whole can be an elusive task. In a theoretical sense, public health is the "fulfillment of society's interest in assuring the conditions in which people can be healthy" (IOM, 1988). Public health focuses on promoting,

Table 12.8 Brian Baker

What are the functions of a "health department?	Why did this structure develop?	What do you want to know next?	What specific information would you like to learn about?
Questions (what is public health, roles, levels)			

protecting, and improving a population's health status. Public health relies upon a multitude of disciplines from biology and medicine to statistics and epidemiology to achieve these goals.

The primary federal agency for public health matters in the United States is the Department of Health and Human Services (DHHS, www.hhs.gov). With a 2007 budget of $698 billion, DHHS represents almost one-quarter of all federal outlays and contains 11 operating divisions. Within DHHS, the US Public Health Service (USPHS) serves as the federal focal point for public health concerns. Eight agencies are found within USPHS:

1. *Substance Abuse and Mental Health Services Administration* (SAMHSA, http://www.samhsa.gov/)—enhances the quality of substance abuse prevention, addiction treatment, and mental health services in the United States
2. *National Institutes of Health* (NIH, www.nih.gov)—currently the world's premier medical research organization
3. *Centers for Disease Control and Prevention* (CDC, www.cdc.gov)—provides a myriad of disease control and prevention services as well as health statistics and surveillance
4. *Food and Drug Administration* (FDA, www.fda.gov)—conducts safety and efficacy research of pharmaceuticals, medical devices, biological products
5. *Indian Health Service* (IHS, www.ihs.gov)—administers health services to American Indians and Alaskan Natives
6. *Health Resources and Services Administration* (HRSA, www.hrsa.gov)—the nation's "access" agency to health care for the low income, the uninsured, and community health centers, contains 6 bureaus and 12 offices.
7. *Agency for Healthcare Research and Quality* (AHRQ, http://www.ahrq.gov/)—evidence-based information on health care outcomes and quality of care, 2007 budget of $319 million
8. *Agency for Toxic Substance and Disease Registry* (ATSDR, http://www.atsdr.cdc.gov/index.html)—research, education, and prevention efforts regarding hazardous substance exposure

The US Public Health Service Commissioned Corps (http://www.usphs.gov/) also resides within DHHS and is led by the Surgeon General, known as "America's chief health educator" (www.surgeongeneral.gov). Several other federal agencies also provide some public health-related responsibilities for the United States including the Environmental Protection Agency and the Departments of Homeland Security, Education, Agriculture, Defense, Transportation, and Veterans Affairs.

The US Constitution places the States as the primary fulcrum for protecting the health of their populations and a large amount of responsibility for public health planning, program implementation, health promotion and education, and evaluation occurs at the state level. Though each state (and territory of the United States) contains a state-based public health agency, their organization and mandated responsibilities vary based upon state-specific laws and regulations. Quite often federal statutes mandate the states' responsibilities for public health, such as the Clean Air Act, Clean Water Act, and the Occupational Safety and Health Act (OSHA). The Association of State and Territorial Health Officials (ASTHO, http://www.astho.org/) reports the following to be largely state health agency responsibilities: women, infants, and children (WIC) program administration; oversight of public health laboratories; maintenance of vital statistics; tobacco prevention and control; food safety; health facility regulation; and environmental health (ASTHO, 2002).

Case Vignette 12.4.2 Conclusion

Brian skips his morning classes and finds the Public Health Department. He is evaluated and treated for gonorrhea. The nurse throws a handful of condoms into the bag with the penicillin. Another health department official asks him the name of his sexual partner. He sheepishly replies that he has no idea.

As our nation continues to spend more on health care (now exceeding 16% of GDP) and as we face the aging of the "baby boomer" population it is becoming apparent to even the most optimistic American that our health care system is soon going to reach the breaking point. The Americans have been citing health care as a top priority for them during each election cycle in recent history. The time for action cannot wait much longer, or we will not be improving a challenged system, but rather picking up the pieces of a destroyed system. With the information gained in working through this chapter, it is our hope that the reader will join in the health care policy debate and help shape the future of health care for all of us in the United States.

Review Questions

1. Approximately what percent of non-elderly insured Americans receive their insurance through an employer-sponsored plan?

    (a) 10%
    (b) 30%
    (c) 60%
    (d) 90%

2. Approximately what percent of the United States GNP is spent on health care?

    (a) 6%
    (b) 16%

(c) 32%
(d) 66%

3. Approximately how much do Americans spend on health care per capita?

(a) $600
(b) $1,500
(c) $3,600
(d) $6,700

4. Please match the type of insurance coverage with the most appropriate description.

(a) Medicare
(b) Medicaid
(c) Private insurance

1.Federally funded and is designed to cover the elderly and people with certain long-term disabilities
2.Federally and state funded, designed to cover primarily the poor
3.Primarily employer-based, "fee for service," and "HMO" models exist

Answers

1. c, 2. b, 3. d, 4. a–1, b–2, c–3

References

Association of State and Territorial Health Officials. *2002 Salary Survey of State and Territorial Health Officials.* 2002. http://www.astho.org/tcmplates/display_pub.php?pub_id=128.
Baldor R. *Managed Care Made Simple,* 2nd ed. Blackwell. 1998.
Bodenheimer TS and K Grumbach. *Understanding Health Policy: A Clinical Approach*, 4th ed. McGraw-Hill/Appleton & Lange. 2005.
Center for Children and Families. Georgetown University Health Policy Institute. *Federal SCHIP Expenditures by State, 1998–2007.* 2007. http://ccf.georgetown.edu/.
Centers for Disease Control and Prevention. *QuickStats:* "Reasons for No Health Insurance Among Uninsured Person Aged <65 Years." *Morbidity and Mortality Weekly Report (MMWR)* 55 (49): 1331. 2006.
Centers for Medicare and Medicaid Services. *Medicaid at a Glance, 2005.* Publication #CMS-11024-05. 2005. www.cms.hhs.gov/MedicaidEligibility/downloads/POV07ALL.pdf.
Centers for Medicare and Medicaid Services. *2006 Medicaid Managed Care Enrollment Report Summary Statistics as of June 30, 2006.* 2006. http://www.cms.hhs.gov/ MedicaidDataSources-GenInfo/Downloads/mmcer06.pdf.
Centers for Medicare and Medicaid Services. *2007 Poverty Guidelines.* 2007a. www.cms.hhs.gov/ MedicaidEligibility/downloads/POV07ALL.pdf.
Centers for Medicare and Medicaid Services. Statistics home Page. 2007b. http://www.cms. hhs.gov/NationalHealthExpendData/02_NationalHealthAccountsHistorical.asp#TopOfPage.

Clemans-Cope L, B Garrett, and C Hoffman. *Changes in Employee's Health Insurance Coverage, 2001–2005.* #7570. Kaiser Commission on Medicaid and the Uninsured. 2006. www.kff.org.

DeNavas-Wait C, BD Proctor, and J Smith. US Census Bureau, Current Population Reports, P60-233. *Income, Poverty and Health Insurance Coverage in the United States: 2006.* US Government Printing Office, Washington, DC. 2007.

Institute of Medicine. *The Future of Public Health.* National Academy Press. 1988.

Institute of Medicine. *Care Without Coverage, Too Little, Too Late.* National Academy Press. 2006.

Milliman Medical Index. 2007. http://www.milliman.com/expertise/healthcare/products-tools/mmi/pdfs/milliman-medical-index-2007.pdf.

National Coalition on Health Care. *Facts on Health Care Costs.* 2007a. http://www.nchc.org/facts/cost.shtml.

National Coalition on Health Care. *The Impact of Rising Health Care Costs on the Economy, Effects on the State Budgets.* 2007b. http://www.nchc.org/facts/Economy/effects_on_state_governments.pdf.

Organization for Economic and Co-operation Development. *OECD Health Data 2007: Statistics and Indicators for 30 Countries.* 2007. http://www.oecd.org/document/30/0,3343, en_2825_495642_12968734_1_1_1_1,00.html.

Rasmussen Report 10/11/07, accessed on 10/23/07 at http://www.rasmussenreports.com/public_content/politics/free_health_care_not_if_it_means_switching_insurance_coverage.

Rodwin VG, J Kervasdoue, and J Kimberly. *The End of an Illusion: The Future of Health Policy in Western Industrialized Nations.* University of California Press. 1984.

Ruth E. *Health Care Financing and Reimbursement.* 2005a. http://www.amsa.org/uhc/2005_healthcare_financing.pdf.

Ruth E. *Health Insurance in America.* 2005b. http://www.amsa.org/uhc/2005_health_insurance.pdf.

Substance Abuse and Mental Health Services Administration. *National Expenditures for Mental health Services and Substance Abuse Treatment, 1991–2001.* DHHS Pub# SMA 05-3999. 2005.

The Henry J. Kaiser Family Foundation. *Dual Eligibles: Medicaid's Role in Filling Medicare's Gaps.* 2004. www.kff.org.

The Henry J. Kaiser Family Foundation. *Medicaid Program at a Glance.* 2006a. www.kff.org.

The Henry J. Kaiser Family Foundation. *Medicare at a Glance Fact Sheet.* 2006b. www.kff.org.

The Henry J. Kaiser Family Foundation. *The Uninsured: A Primer, Key Facts About Americans Without Health Insurance.* 2006c. www.kff.org.

The Henry J. Kaiser Family Foundation. *State Health Facts, 2007.* 2007a. http://www.statehealthfacts.org.

The Henry J. Kaiser Family Foundation. *Myths About the Uninsured.* 2007b. www.kff.org.

Chapter 13
Stigma and Medicine

Barbara Kohlenberg, Melanie Watkins and Lindsay Fletcher

In everyday medicine, stigma impacts the care that people receive. Felt stigma is a term that describes feelings, such as shame, that interfere with asking for help. Enacted stigma is when health care providers treat people differently because of judgments they have made about that person's background or behavior. In this chapter we take a slightly different approach to problem-based learning. We present cases that target responses from the reader, and we invite the reader to consider those responses as the cases unfold. In addition, our PBL tables have a different format from most chapters in this book. Our tables invite further exploration of the reader's thoughts, feelings and behaviors.

At the end of this chapter, the reader will be able to

1. Describe the effects of enacted stigma on the provision of health care
2. Discuss the effects of self-stigma, or "shame" on seeking and receiving health care
3. Describe how enacted and self-stigmas interact to produce faulty assessment, treatment and outcome in medical care
4. Discuss how health care providers might reduce the effects of stigma in health care

Case Vignette 13.1.1 Presenting Situation: LaNita Michaelson

LaNita is a 32-year-old African American woman who is pregnant with her fourth child. She presents to the emergency department at approximately 27 weeks gestation. She is unsure about her last menstrual period; therefore the gestational age of the fetus is estimated by an ultrasound performed at her last visit to the emergency department. She was diagnosed with HIV 2 months prior to her pregnancy. Her CD4 count is 325 and she is not currently on anti-retroviral therapy. She has a history of non-compliance and her prenatal care has been sporadic. She is in subsidized housing and has three children in foster care.

B. Kohlenberg
Associate Professor of Psychiatry, University of Nevada School of Medicine

A. Guerrero, M. Piasecki (eds.), *Problem-Based Behavioral Science and Psychiatry*,

LaNita has been experiencing sharp right-sided abdominal pain for approximately 2 days. The pain comes and goes and she has felt feverish. In addition, she has had nausea, vomiting and decreased appetite. She reports good fetal movement. There is no vaginal bleeding or discharge.

You are the ER physician assigned to LaNita. You have been working long hours and you are halfway through a 14-hour shift.

 Please proceed with the problem-based approach!

Visualize this patient and notice what emotional reactions come up in you. Be honest and write down what first comes to mind without censoring your responses. Please proceed with the problem-based approach. In this case, your thoughts, feelings and behavior will be explored. Table 13.1 is modified from Chiles and Strosahl (2004).

Physicians may find it difficult to come up with positive and compassionate responses to LaNita, and it may be easier to generate negative, judgmental responses. Similarly, few physicians would be proud of their difficulties in these areas and may, in fact, feel that their responses are justified. Given the combination of being exhausted and asked to provide health care for a woman who seems negligent of her own HIV status, her children and her pregnancy, it could be very difficult to generate positive, compassionate responses while providing health care. Situations like LaNita's, which highlight the contrast between the way the physician is supposed to think, feel and act and the way he/she actually thinks, feels and behaves, give rise to critical, self-evaluative thinking and lead to burnout (Falk, 2001).

Table 13.1 LaNita-Physician response (adapted from Chiles and Strosahl, 2004)

Dimension of response	My response	How I feel about my own response?
What is your primary *positive* emotional response?		
What is your primary *negative* emotional response?		
What aspects of this person's situation and behavior elicit the most *negative* or *judgmental* response from you?		
What aspects of this person's situation and behavior elicit the most *positive* or *compassionate* response from you?		
What is the biggest barrier you would encounter continuing to interact with this person?		

Case Vignette 13.1.2 Continuation

During her previous visits to the county hospital, emergency room employees became frustrated with LaNita. She missed follow-up prenatal appointments and she continued to use the emergency department for routine care. She reported concern that the pregnancy clinic staff "won't take me seriously."

LaNita approaches the admission staff, who know her by name from her visit 3 weeks prior. You hear the staff say reprovingly: "You will have to wait your turn, LaNita. Did you even see your obstetrician at the clinic?"

Please proceed with the problem-based approach!

Stigma

Stigma is a term with highly social, political and personal implications. The term stigma traces to the notion of a physical mark placed on slaves to easily identify and separate them from the general culture. Today, people are not marked physically, yet they are stigmatized when they belong to certain categories considered abnormal or unconventional (Falk, 2001). Stigma is from a label or stereotype that links a person to unfavorable characteristics. Global health initiatives are targeting stigma because of its effects on the response of nations, communities, families and individuals to illness (Keusch, 2006).

Enacted stigma describes what happens when a person or group is shunned, denied protection under the law or dehumanized. In health care, targets of enacted stigma have included but are not limited to patients with epilepsy, certain infectious diseases (e.g., Hansen's disease and HIV/AIDS), obesity, substance abuse, mental illness and physical disabilities. Gender, race, religion, age and socio-economic status also stigmatize patients in the health care system inasmuch as prejudice exists, resulting in health care disparity and poor outcomes in the stigmatized group (3). There is something about the patient and the group they belong to that makes the physician feel frustrated, afraid, incompetent or uncomfortable in some way. In part, to help avoid these unpleasant thoughts and feelings, physicians tend to find reasons to discount and to not fully engage with the needs of the patient, who may, in turn, not receive effective health care. Stigma can curtail opportunities for people in these and other categories. For example, stigmatized people face restricted access to resources and opportunities (e.g., housing, jobs, effective health care). In its most overt and egregious form, stigma results in discrimination and abuse.

Self-stigma occurs when a person believes the enacted stigma focused on them. Self-stigma refers to the internalized effects of stigma upon the stigmatized person. This could include low self-esteem, isolation and hopelessness. A stigmatized person may deprive themself of dignity. Self-stigma may also result in people avoiding health care, not seeking help when needed and not following through with medical instructions because they believe that they are not deserving of help.

In every patient encounter, the physician brings biases about certain groups or categories of people based on their own experience. For example, a physician might negatively stigmatize a patient seeking pain medication if the physician himself/herself has a history of a substance use disorder. In such an example, the patient might be inappropriately categorized as an addict, user or drug seeker and denied treatment for pain. At the other end of the continuum, physicians may have a positive feeling about a patient, who may then not receive the care appropriate for his/her illness. For example, physicians are likely to assume adherence to medical regimens in patients with whom they are well acquainted, an assumption that may be false (Miller et al., 2002). They may think, "I know this patient really well, and I'm sure they are taking their medications." The provider may not fully engage with the evaluation of the patient. Often, clinical judgments are based on outward features of a patient, previous actions or membership in a certain group. This bias may result in suboptimal care because the details of the patient's medical problems are not assessed. At both ends of the continuum, enacted- and self-stigmatization describe how a physician judges a person and how that person responds, all leading to a distance between the patient's needs and his/her treatment.

LaNita belongs to many different groups, each of which has associations with prejudice and stigma. She is a single pregnant woman, is African American, is HIV positive, has children in foster care and has a history of non-compliance with prenatal care. Each of these attributes can give rise to enacted- and self-stigma, a process resulting in social isolation and rejection (Jones et al., 1984), clearly impacting health care. In LaNita's case, the physician might engage in negative enacted stigma, which might result in the following behaviors:

1. Failure to elicit LaNita's concerns
2. Inadequate time spent educating and treating her because of her past failure and her predicted failure to follow through in the future
3. Blame toward LaNita for her poor health
4. Rationalization for not optimally engaging with this patient, followed by feelings of guilt, defeat and burnout

Case Vignette 13.1.3 Conclusion

LaNita becomes upset with staff and begins to raise her voice. She is hungry, tired and in pain. She shouts, "I've been working at a new job and my boss won't let me off for my appointments." She has been trying to get "back on track" to be able to create a good life for her new baby and to try to re-establish a relationship with her other children. She feels frustrated and ashamed. She bursts into tears and resolutely mutters to herself, "I'm out of here." She leaves the clinic before being seen by clinic staff.

Table 13.2 LaNita-Patient response (adapted from Chiles and Strosahl, 2004)

Dimension of response	LaNita's response	Positive and negative effects on LaNita
What is her primary *positive* emotional response?		
What is her primary *negative* emotional response?		
What aspects of this situation and staff behavior elicit the most *negative* or *judgmental* response from her?		
What aspects of this situation and staff behavior could elicit the most *positive* or *compassionate* response from her?		
What is the biggest barrier she would encounter in continuing to try to receive treatment?		

Now imagine that you are LaNita, with her history and current situation. (See Table 13.2.)

> *What might be LaNita's reactions at this point?*
> *Does this additional information change your perceptions about LaNita? If so, how?*
> *What are your emotional responses?*
> *How might your emotional responses be different if LaNita were white/HIV negative/middle class?*

LaNita may feel a great deal of shame about her present situation. She may, in fact, have avoided health care just because of her own shame around her condition (Lazare, 1997). She may be afraid about pregnancy and her HIV status, and her avoidance of health care may be related to her attempts to not think about her own precarious health. After all, if she does not see a doctor, perhaps she can forget that she is, in fact, ill. Perhaps she can ignore her pregnancy and the addition of new responsibilities. Also, she may be accurately afraid of coming in for help from past experiences of being stigmatized by health care providers. In this situation, both enacted stigma and felt stigma are interacting to produce a very poor health care outcome.

How might the physician improve this situation?

First, it is important to note it is not possible to completely eliminate judgmental thoughts and feelings from one's mind. Indeed, we are trained on many levels to make judgments of our patients in an attempt to evaluate and help them. These judgments include features of personality and risk factors for poor compliance and prognosis. When these judgments cause us to under-evaluate a patient, to treat them condescendingly or harshly or to withhold our best intentions, we begin the downward spiral of stigma. It is not possible to be without judgment but it is possible to decide not to allow one's actions toward patients to reflect these judgments.

Physicians may strive to provide excellent health care even when their thoughts and feelings are inviting them to take short cuts that do not serve the patient's health care needs.

To be more effective, think about how you might engage less with the judgmental thoughts and feelings you identified with this case, and focus on how to provide respectful, effective health care. In daily life there are many examples where we behave effectively even when our thoughts and feelings dictate otherwise, e.g., going to work even when tired or depressed. It is possible to provide effective health care even when you feel discouraged and defeated by the patients themselves.

Sample Dialogue

Here is an example of how one doctor might avoid stigmatizing LaNita or another patient:

Physician: It is great you came in. I am glad you are here. You look really tired. Was it hard to get here?

Patient: I'm so tired. The buses were all late and I had to borrow money for the fare. I'm not feeling good at all and I am worried about my baby . . .

Physician: I'm glad you care so much. We want to help. I notice this is your fourth visit to the ER. It must be hard, but did you have chance to make it to your obstetrician appointment since we last saw you? Is there something that can be done to help make it easier for you to attend your outpatient appointments? I wonder if there is a way to get you some bus passes . . . would that help?

Please use Table 13.3 to identify other strategies to elicit the most positive and cooperative responses.

In caring for a patient with felt stigma and shame, it could help to be empathic and to invite the patient to share what he/she may feel and to discuss how important it is to seek health care anyway. Much the way you have to learn to behave as a competent physician in spite of judgmental feelings, the patient must also take care of his/her body even when he/she is feeling ashamed. For example: "LaNita, I know how hard it must be to come in here. I know that many times, people who have had problems like this feel embarrassed and feel some shame. I am so glad that you are in here today; even though it is hard, and I am going to try really hard to have this visit go well for you."

Table 13.3 Strategies to elicit the most positive and cooperative responses in Case Vignette 13.1

How might you, as her physician, elicit the most *positive* and cooperative response from her?

Case Vignette 13.2.1 Presenting Situation: Mary Kormitte

Mary is a 23-year-old woman who presents to the emergency department on a Friday evening. Her chief complaint is suicidal ideation that has worsened over the past few days. Mary reports to the medical assistant that her boyfriend of 6 months has left her because she is "too much" for him. She is also "a mess" because she is in her second year of medical school and exams are coming up. She is tearful and distraught. When the medical assistant tries to console her, Mary replies, "Look, I just want to see the doctor, okay?"

On exam, Mary is a thin, anxious appearing young woman. She has superficial lacerations on her left forearm. Her mood is irritable and labile. Her vital signs are within normal limits, except for an elevated pulse of 115. When the ER physician opens the door, Mary recognizes him as her attending from her second year physical examination and diagnosis course. She is immediately embarrassed. He begins by telling her, "Mary, I see that you have been diagnosed with bipolar disorder and also that you have been to the emergency department four times this year. Looks like you haven't been taking your medication according to the refill log. It will be hard for you to progress in your career if you go on like this."

Mary is reluctant to discuss what brought her in. She feels numb and detached. She raises her voice, "You don't know what you are talking about. You have no idea. I just want it over!" The physician looks at the computer and notices that Mary also has a diagnosis of borderline personality disorder. He sighs and says, "I see you have been cutting. Why would you do something like that to yourself?"

 Please proceed with the problem-based approach!

Here a complex set of issues emerge. This patient is clearly in distress. She is also a medical student. You are the attending physician in the emergency room. What is your response to the patient? Please use Table 13.4 to organize your thoughts.

Mary is falling into the category of having mental illness: she may have bipolar disorder, borderline personality disorder, and is also currently suicidal. She is also cutting on her arm. These problems are very difficult for anyone, including physicians, to deal with. These types of mental health issues are highly stigmatized in our culture. People with mental illness are often severely judged, feared and given suboptimal health care. Mary's dysfunctional behavior may be particularly difficult to accept because she is a medical student and may evoke particular responses on the part of the physician. In the area of substance abuse, enacted stigma is particularly severe as it tends to evoke even greater negative social attitudes.

Table 13.4 Responses to Case Vignette 13.2

Dimension of response	My response	How I feel about my own response. Include both positive and negative feelings
What is your primary *positive* emotional response?		
What is your primary *negative* emotional response?		
What aspects of this person's situation and behavior elicit the most *negative* or *judgmental* response from you?		
What aspects of this person's situation and behavior elicit the most *positive* or *compassionate* response from you?		
What is the biggest barrier you would encounter continuing to interact with this person?		

Case Vignette 13.2.2 Conclusion

Mary is distraught. She doesn't want to tell the attending that she is feeling hopeless because her boyfriend broke up with her. She fears he will not take her seriously. The attending's pager beeps.

"I have some really acute patients to take care of, Mary. What do you need right now?"

Mary can't pinpoint what she needs. She does know that she feels intense anxiety about her relationship and her studies. She is suddenly unsure that she can trust the attending to maintain confidentiality.

"Nothing! I have nothing. I need nothing! I'll go home deal with it."

 Please proceed with the problem-based approach!

When physician judgments result in enacted stigma, the following may occur:

1. Referral to psychiatry immediately, without any discussion with Mary
2. Minimization of the problems because of her medical student status, e.g., "You will feel better after finals . . ."
3. Blame toward the patient for their poor health. "You didn't take your meds . . ."
4. Temporary feelings of justification in not having engaged with this patient; followed by feelings of defeat and burnout

When physician judgments do not lead to enacted stigma, the following might occur:

1. Quality time spent with the patient; genuine engagement with her and under-standing of her problems; development of a thoughtful, collaborative referral if indicated
2. Connection with her medical student status; empathy toward the demands; encouragement to take care of herself
3. Assessment of her problems with adherence to medications, including an assess-ment of side effects, costs and benefits, and alternative treatment regimens
4. Consultation from trusted colleagues about your own feelings about treating someone who is so distressed and yet may share a profession with you

Now imagine you are Mary. She is embarrassed, overwhelmed and anxious about how she might be perceived and how best to cope with her feelings. Take a few minutes to consider how you would feel in the encounter described. Please use Table 13.5 to organize your thoughts.

Does this additional information change your perceptions about Mary? If so, how?

How might your reactions be different if Mary were African American, poor, uneducated, HIV positive?

In this case, it is likely that Mary feels tremendous felt stigma or shame. Seeking treatment from the same people who teach and evaluate her is likely very difficult. She may, in fact, have avoided seeking help earlier due to her own shame around her condition. Mary is also at risk for avoiding seeking help in the future if she were to leave the ER feeling that she did not receive good care or that her career is now in danger. In addition, her suicide risk is high: a problem that would greatly affect other medical school students in her class and reflect poorly on the school and community.

Table 13.5 Mary's feelings in Case Vignette 13.2

Dimension of response	Mary's response	Positive and negative effects on Mary
What might she have felt prior to entering the emergency room that felt positive to her?		
What might she have felt prior to entering the emergency room that felt negative to her?		
What is her primary *positive* emotional response?		
What is her primary *negative* emotional response?		
What aspects of this situation and staff behavior elicit the most *negative* or *judgmental* response from her?		
What aspects of this situation and staff behavior elicit the most *positive* or *compassionate* response from her?		
What is the biggest barrier she would encounter in continuing to try to receive treatment?		

Table 13.6 Strategies to elicit the most positive and cooperative responses in Case Vignette 13.2

How might staff/you elicit the most *positive* and cooperative response from her?

To be more effective with Mary, think about how you might engage less with your judgmental thoughts and feelings and focus more on the provision of respectful, effective health care. Please use Table 13.6 to organize your thoughts. It is possible to provide effective health care even when you feel judgmental and defeated. Learning these skills will help you teach them to Mary. Empathize with how she may be feeling under these conditions and reinforce her willingness to seek help when needed. Connect with Mary's value of taking care of herself and thus succeeding in her medical career.

Sample Dialogue

Please consider the following as one possible way to avoid stigmatizing Mary or another patient:

Physician: Mary, I understand you may feel uncomfortable because we know each other from the medical school. Coming in when you need help even when you could feel some awkwardness is very admirable and a good step in taking care of yourself. I will do my best to keep what we discuss here between the two of us.

Patient: Thank you. I'm so upset. My boyfriend just broke up with me. I think it is because I have bipolar disorder. I'm scared. I'm scared to be alone. And exams are coming. I can't focus or concentrate. I can't do what I need to do.

Physician: It's hard to focus when you are trying to sort out feelings. I am wondering if you are having feelings about harming yourself.

Patient: I've had those thoughts. That's probably what scares me the most. I have been cutting. It takes away the pain for a while and then it becomes unbearable all over again.

Physician: It must be hard for you to share this with me. You sound worried about your thoughts and feelings. I am concerned about you and want to make sure that you get the help you need. What is important is that you get help when you need it so that you can pursue your goals and stay healthy.

Conclusion

Avoiding the effects of stigma may well be the most difficult aspect of providing equal health care to all people. This may be the case because doing so requires the disciplined efforts of all health care personnel to monitor their feelings and thoughts and to control their actions. Within groups, one person has the power to promote a culture of tolerance and compassion. Consider an internal medicine resident asking the staff psychiatrist to help him understand a patient with borderline personality disorder: "She has brought me to my wit's end...I can't stand her...I feel terrible." For one minute, the psychiatrist sits with the resident, validates his feelings, commends him for recognizing the problem in himself and then states simply that this patient's emotional progress became retarded ever since she was raped at home as a teenager. "And so she still sees the world as a young teenager in many ways, even though she is well educated and physically very capable." The resident and the patient will benefit because the resident sought help to manage his feelings of frustration and burn out, and a senior colleague took time to think the problem through.

Review Questions

1. Why do you think enacted stigma causes others to feel shame? What kind of verbal and non-verbal signals have you seen people use to send this demeaning signal to others?
2. Why should a patient's self-imposed stigma burden a physician who is adequately treating the patient otherwise?
3. What specific personal goals can you make, to reduce the demoralizing and debilitating effects of stigma your working environment?
4. When is shame a positive emotion? When is shame a negative emotion? When have you felt stigma in your life? How can you ward off the ill effects of this stigma?

Bibliography

Chiles, J., Strosahl, K. (2004). *Clinical Manual for Assessment and Treatment of Suicidal Behavior.* American Psychiatric Publishing, Washington, DC.

Falk, G. (2001). *Stigma. How We Treat Outsiders.* Prometheus Books, New York.

Jones, E., Farina, A., Hastorf, A., Markus, H., Miller, D. T., Scott, R. (1984). *Social Stigma: The Psychology of Marked Relationships.* Freeman, New York.

Keusch, G. (2006). *www.thelancet.com* 367, Feb 11, 2006.

Lazare, A. (1997). Shame, humiliation, and stigma in the medical interview. In M. Lansky and A. Morrison (Eds), *The Widening Scope of Shame* (pp. 383–396). The Analytic Press, New Jersey.

Miller, L. G., Liu, H., Hays, R. D., Golin, C. E., Keith Beck, C., Asch, S. M., Ma, Y., Kaplan, A. H., Wenger, N. S. (2002). How well do clinicians estimate patients' adherence to combination antiretroviral therapy? *Journal of General Internal Medicine* 17 (1), 1–11. doi:10.1046/j.1525-1497.2002.09004.x.

Wailoo, K. (2006). *www.thelancet.com* 367, Feb 11, 2006.

Chapter 14
Culture, Ethnicity, and Medicine

Anthony P.S. Guerrero

Culture is a part of who we are and how we manage our health and illnesses. During training, most physicians are confronted with people who represent cultures and values that are remarkably different from their own background. This chapter offers information on approaching cultural differences.

At the end of this chapter, the reader will be able to

1. Discuss the definitions of culture and culturally competent care
2. Discuss ethnic factors that can impact on the epidemiology and presentation of common medical illnesses
3. Approach situations in which culture may impact upon help-seeking behavior and treatment adherence

Case Vignette 14.1.1 Pinky

"Pinky" is a 7-year-old female brought by her mother to the pediatrician for symptoms of acute gastroenteritis. The mother recently immigrated to the United States and speaks English as a second language. While the physician and patient share the same ethnic background, the physician was born and raised in the United States.

Mother: So what does my daughter have?
Physician: It seems that your daughter may have a stomach flu, and that's why she's having the stomach ache and diarrhea.
Mother: What medicine does she need?
Physician: Actually, she doesn't need medicine at this time. Because it's a virus, there's no antibiotic that can treat this. She needs to drink a lot of fluids, though.
Mother: Is this normal, then?
Physician: Not necessarily "normal," but certainly, this is "common."

A.P.S. Guerrero
Associate Professor of Psychiatry and Pediatrics, Associate Chair for Education and Training, Department of Psychiatry University of Hawai'i John A. Burns School of Medicine

A. Guerrero, M. Piasecki (eds.), *Problem-Based Behavioral Science and Psychiatry*,
© Springer Science+Business Media, LLC 2008

Mother: So she just needs to drink more? (almost crying)
Physician: I think that's what would help her the most.
Mother: (silence, definitely crying at this point)
Physician: I'm sorry to see that you're crying. Can you tell me what you're thinking?
Mother: Nothing, really . . .

Please proceed with the problem-based approach!

Basic Principles and Definitions

Whether or not we believe that a patient is from a "culture" different from our own, it is important to recognize that in every patient encounter, we bring with us a set of assumptions and styles of communication that undoubtedly affect the care the patient receives. In the above case, in which the parent seems confused and upset over what would ordinarily be a routine explanation for a benign acute illness, any of the following may have occurred:

- Physician's failure to elicit (or recognize the need to elicit) what the parent is most worried about and/or what the parent feels the child needs most at this time (e.g., medication)
- A language barrier, in which terms such as "virus" or "not normal but common" do not necessarily provide the intended reassurance
- Physician's assumption that asking directly "what are you thinking" is the most effective way to elicit concerns or questions
- Parent's fear that she will not be able to satisfactorily explain the child's illness to the decision-maker or authoritative figure in the family (who was unable to make this visit)

Case Vignette 14.1.2 Conclusion

Concerned and perplexed, you consult with your front office receptionist, who is able to speak in the native language with the mother. As it turns out, Pinky's mother is concerned that her own mother (child's grandmother) will be upset if the child does not go home with a medication. The mother seemed relieved as further explanation was given while the grandmother was on the telephone.

Traditionally, culture has been defined along the lines of values, beliefs, and/or practices shared by populations of people. Obviously, culture is not the same as "ethnicity" or "race," as there can be many different types of "culture" (e.g., the medical culture) that have nothing to do with race—which is not even universally accepted as a valid concept.

Lewis-Fernandez and Kleinman (1995) have defined culture as the *"processes that emerge out of the patterns of everyday social life—taken-for-granted common sense, historically determined ways of being and doing, preferred forms of ordinary interpersonal interaction, socially elaborated bodily states."* We will use this definition for the purposes of this chapter.

Adaptiveness of Diversity

We believe that culture—like anything else for which "differences" among people exist—is best understood as something that must have been adaptive. In order to provide optimal care for a diverse patient group, this principle is important to consider, in terms of both medical/biological issues and social/cultural issues.

Case Vignette 14.2.1 Presenting Situations

You are a busy pediatrician at a community health center in a large west-coast city. The following are vignettes from your practice:

Junior, a 3-day-old Filipino-Caucasian male infant comes to your office for a routine post-hospitalization check. He is feeding both breast milk and formula. He is jaundiced to the mid-trunk. Mother is O+, and baby is also O+, Coombs' negative. You wonder how much you should be concerned about the jaundice, since it does not appear that there are obvious risk factors.

John-boy, a 7-year-old Pacific Islander boy, comes in with a stuffy nose, headache, fever, and a history of ill contacts. His throat was mildly sore in the beginning but not now. On exam, his throat is minimally red, without exudates or adenopathy. You wonder whether you should obtain other studies. Although this is not a well-child check (and therefore only his weight is measured and not his height or BMI), you notice that he is significantly overweight.

Lisa, a 17-year-old Japanese female, comes in with nausea, vomiting, and headache. She was recently started on escitalopram by her psychiatrist, who was concerned that there may be other causes of her physical symptoms, since the starting dose given of the medication was very small.

 Please proceed with the problem-based approach!

Culturally competent care implies not only integrating awareness of cultural dynamics (as illustrated in the first case) into the patient care encounter, but also considering biologically mediated differences—whether they correspond to ethnicity, gender, or other classification—that may impact upon medical care. While it is likely true that there is little biological reality behind the entire concept of "race," it is undeniably true that there are populational differences (even within "races") in disease prevalence, drug metabolism, and dietary practices. Similar to how "cultural" differences must have had an adaptive function, such biological differences are also likely a product of evolution and adaptation to environment. Some examples are summarized in Table 14.1.

Case Vignette 14.2.2 Conclusion

Regarding Junior, your newborn patient, you astutely ask further details about the infant's ethnicity and learn that the mother identifies herself as pure Filipino. You also inquire about any family history of any blood problems or dietary restrictions, and you learn that there is a maternal male cousin who was jaundiced as an infant and who needed to avoid certain foods and medications. You therefore order (in addition to your usual tests) a test for glucose-6-phosphate dehydrogenase and monitor the child very carefully over the next few days.

Table 14.1 Potential adaptiveness of certain genotypes associated with certain illnesses and other conditions

Phenotype	Higher prevalence in	*Possible* evolutionary adaptive role of associated genotype
Cystic fibrosis	Caucasians	Protection against cholera (Bertranpetit, Calafell, 1996)
Thalassemia	Southeast Asians, Mediterranean peoples	Protection against malaria (Kwiatkowski, 2005)
Glucose-6-phosphate dehydrogenase deficiency	Southeast Asians, Mediterranean and African peoples	Protection against malaria (Kwiatkowski, 2005)
Obesity, diabetes mellitus, metabolic syndrome, in the context of Western diets	Pacific Islanders, other indigenous peoples	Energy conservation during prolonged periods of limited food access (Chukwuma and Tuomilehto, 1998)
Lactose *tolerance* (rather than intolerance)	Caucasians	Ability to have dairy products as part of diet
Aldehyde dehydrogenase *non*deficiency	Non-Asians	Ability to have fermented drinks as part of diet
Rheumatic fever	Polynesians (Kurahara et al., 2002)	Immunogenetic factors that may otherwise confer protection against other rheumatological illnesses and possibly infections
Cytochrome P450 2C19 ultra-metabolizer	North Africans, Middle Easterners (De Leon et al., 2006)	Role in detoxification

Regarding John-boy, the 7-year-old boy, you appropriately query whether or not existing practice guidelines for the evaluation of possible streptococcal pharyngitis are truly applicable to your population. You decide to obtain a throat culture, which proves to be positive for group A beta-hemolytic streptococcus. You also provide the patient and parent counseling on diet and activity, attempting to be sensitive to: the family's indigenous dietary preferences, the role of other family members in the child's care, and other realities (e.g., expense of healthier meals, access to safe recreational areas) related to their socioeconomic status. Finally, given the prevalence of childhood obesity in your practice, you decide to implement new clinic protocols to adequately screen for and manage obesity. (Please also refer to Chap. 27: Eating Disorders).

Regarding Lisa, your 17-year-old patient, you conduct a history and physical examination and conclude that an adverse reaction to the escitalopram is the most likely cause of her symptoms. You research the drug metabolism of escitalopram and discover that it is metabolized by cytochrome P450 2C19 and that 10–25 % of East Asians are, in fact, cytochrome P450 2C19-poor metabolizers (De Leon et al., 2006). You communicate with her psychiatrist, who eventually is able to successfully treat her using an alternate medication. (The author predicts that, in the future, pharmacogenomic testing may become more widely used in these clinical situations).

While a discussion of all diseases that vary in prevalence by ethnicity is beyond the scope of this textbook, we advocate that culturally competent physicians should be of the mindset that certain conditions may affect certain ethnic groups more than others presumably because of evolutionarily adaptation and not because any ethnic group is inferior or superior to the other.

Reducing Health Disparities

We also advocate that culturally competent physicians should consider social and environmental factors that may lead to health disparities among cultural and ethnic groups.

Case Vignette 14.3.1 Presenting Situation

You are a family physician who is seeing Sammy, a 22-year-old Pacific Islander male with a history of a seizure disorder. According to his record, Sammy has a past history of methamphetamine abuse. A previous CT scan done in the emergency room showed an area of ischemic infarction, presumed secondary to the methamphetamine abuse. There is a long history of "noncompliance" and subtherapeutic levels of his anticonvulsant medications. Before you enter the room, your colleagues tell you . . . "Oh, he only comes back whenever he needs a disability form signed." You begin to wonder how you will address issues of compliance in this patient.

Please proceed with the problem-based approach!

As suggested in Chap. 10, apparent "noncompliance" should be viewed as a clinical finding that has its own set of differential possibilities. The case above illustrates possible causes for "noncompliance" that should be considered by the culturally competent clinician, in particular:

- Is the regimen too costly for the patient?
- Does the patient metabolize a medication in an unexpected way (leading to too many side effects or inadequate response)?
- Does the patient have alternative beliefs about the illness, including etiology and treatment?
- Does the patient have adequate social support or access to resources?
- Does the patient have an interfering psychiatric illness, the symptoms of which are under-reported because of the stigma of mental illness?
- Are there language barriers that prevent adequate explanations from being given?
- Did the clinician fail to involve key family members who are important in the patient's care?

Case Vignette 14.3.2 Continuation

Sammy insists, with a somewhat bland affect, that he has been taking the medications. He is able to repeat (again with a bland affect) that he has a "seizure problem" and that the medications are "for the seizures."

He denies any other medical or psychiatric illnesses. He adamantly denies any further substance abuse, and his girlfriend confirms this. He says that it's "all in the past" and that he now associates with "good people." Although he denies any history of depression, he admits to not being quite as talkative as he used to be. He denies any use of herbal medications or visits to a traditional healer for his condition.

He lives with his girlfriend and her extended family. He is a first-generation immigrant to the United States. English is a second language for him; however, he is able to converse fluently and appears to understand most of the explanations given. He denies that there is anyone else who is significantly involved in making decisions about his treatment or in implementing treatment recommendations. He does, however, rely on his girlfriend for transportation, as he does not feel comfortable driving given the history of his seizure disorder. He is on government-supported health insurance, which completely covers the cost of his medications. He denies any unusual stressors in his life other than his illness.

Please proceed with the problem-based approach!

There are numerous examples of health disparities in medicine, which are likely explained by complex interactions between biological, social, and environmental factors. Prominent examples, according to the CDC, are summarized in Table 14.2 (CDC Office of Minority Health).

It is also important to minimize cultural barriers and stigma (see Chap. 13) that may occur on the individual clinician level.

Case Vignette 14.3.3 Conclusion

You refer Sammy to a psychiatrist for possible depression. Because of subtle cognitive findings and the history of a neurological disorder, the psychiatrist suggests a follow-up neuroimaging study, which actually shows a brain tumor in an anatomic location that fully explains the seizures experienced by the patient, as well as the apparent poor judgment and blunted affect. Following radiation treatment of the brain tumor, his affect appears to brighten, and he no longer has issues of noncompliance.

In summary, when approaching the issue of health disparities, the culturally competent clinician should be mindful that (1) a patient may be at risk for certain illnesses as a consequence of living in a biological/psychological/social environment different from what he/she may be initially adapted to (e.g., a dark-skinned person being at risk for vitamin D deficiency in a polar latitude or a light-skinned person being at risk for skin cancer in an equatorial latitude) and (2) cultural differences

Table 14.2 Disparities in prevalence of illness by ethnicity

Condition	Higher in
Infant mortality	African Americans, Native Americans, Puerto Ricans
Mortality from cervical cancer	African Americans
Mortality from breast cancer	Caucasian Americans
Death from cardiovascular disease	African Americans
Diabetes mellitus	Native Americans and Alaska Natives
AIDS	African Americans and Hispanics
Underimmunization for influenza and pneumococcus in the elderly	Hispanics and African Americans
Depression and substance abuse	Native Americans and Alaska Natives
Hepatitis B	Asians and Pacific Islanders
Syphilis	African Americans
Tuberculosis	Asians and Pacific Islanders

between the clinician and the patient may prevent optimal diagnosis and treatment of illness (as illustrated in Case Vignette 14.1). We close with the following case.

Case Vignette 14.4.1 Presenting Situation

You are a supervising physician in a pediatric clinic. Your resident raises the concern that Julius, a mixed Asian/Pacific Islander toddler, seen for a well-child check, has on his back several marks that might suggest abuse. Your resident states, "This almost feels like a board review question...where they're sort of checking our so-called cultural competence. I thought about coining and cupping as indigenous healing practices, but these marks don't look like they come from coins or cups. I also thought about Mongolian spots, and these definitely don't look like them. I really think these were inflicted by a hand. I hate to stereotype, but I've heard from other families that corporal punishment is standard discipline in certain cultures."

You and the resident examine the patient together, and you confirm that this is likely a case of child abuse, probably inflicted by the stepfather. You inform the mother, who becomes tearful, that you will need to involve child protective services.

You commend the resident for identifying a case of child abuse, which is likely under-identified in primary care practice. (See Chap. 7.) You encourage the resident to critically appraise the notion that child abuse could ever be a culturally acceptable or adaptively advantageous practice. You discuss the principle of "acculturative stress" and help the resident to elicit the further history that this child's family, in immigrating to the United States, lost the strong extended family and community network that they otherwise would have had in their native countries, experienced significant financial stress, and became exposed to substances of abuse that would have been relatively absent in their traditional culture. Your resident is grateful for your instruction and plans to integrate knowledge of these issues into a comprehensive, "bio-psycho-social-cultural-spiritual" (see Chap. 1) treatment plan to prevent further child abuse, should this child ever return to the mother's care.

Review Question

1. Which of the following could be called "effective habits" of the culturally competent clinician?

   (a) Evaluating one's own style of communication with patients
   (b) Asking patients how they understand their condition and its treatment
   (c) Knowledge about ethnic differences in risk for certain conditions and response to treatment
   (d) Advocacy for improving access to care and reducing health disparities
   (e) All of the above

Answer

1. e

References

Bertranpetit J, Calafell F. Genetic and geographical variability in cystic fibrosis: evolutionary considerations. Ciba Found Symp 1996;197:97–114; discussion 114–8.

CDC Office of Minority Health. Eliminating racial & ethnic health disparities. http://www.cdc.gov/omh/AboutUs/disparities.htm (accessed 09/22/2007).

Chukwuma C Sr, Tuomilehto J. The 'thrifty' hypotheses: clinical and epidemiological significance for non-insulin-dependent diabetes mellitus and cardiovascular disease risk factors. J Cardiovasc Risk 1998;5(1):11–23.

De Leon J, Armstrong SC, Cozza KL. Clinical guidelines for psychiatrists for the use of pharmacogenetic testing for CYP450 2D6 and CYP450 2C19. Psychosomatics 2006;47:75–85.

Kurahara D, Tokuda A, Grandinetti A, Najita J, Ho C, Yamamoto K, Reddy DV, Macpherson K, Iwamuro M, Yamaga K. Ethnic differences in risk for pediatric rheumatic illness in a culturally diverse population. J Rheumatol 2002;29(2):379–83.

Kwiatkowski DP. How malaria has affected the human genome and what human genetics can teach us about malaria. Am J Hum Genet 2005;77(2):171–92. Epub 07/06/2005.

Lewis-Fernandez R, Kleinman A. Cultural psychiatry. Theoretical, clinical, and research issues. Psychiatr Clin North Am 1995;18(3):433–48. Review.

Chapter 15
Quantitative Measures in Healthcare

M. Anand Samtani, Earl S. Hishinuma, and Deborah A. Goebert

Medical students often ask themselves, "Why should I learn statistics for my future medical practice?" Statistical techniques are used in just about every discipline and profession as tools to organize and analyze data. In medicine, it is essential to have a basic understanding of statistics to:

1. Critically understand and interpret studies in medical literature
2. Properly conduct well-designed studies on human participants
3. Make informed and sound decisions about existing and new medications in one's clinical practice

Source: Appleton (1990, p. 1013)

At the end of this chapter, the reader will be able to:

1. Discuss fundamental concepts of statistical measurement
2. Discuss fundamental concepts of study design
3. Describe fundamental concepts of hypothesis testing and statistical inference
4. Interpret medical literature with basic statistical concepts

The primary goal of this chapter is to provide the student with a fundamental knowledge of the statistical tools relevant to clinical practice and clinical research. This chapter assumes some basic knowledge of quantitative measurements. A supplemental glossary (Appendix) is provided at the end of the chapter.

Case Vignette 15.1.1 Melinda

Melinda, a fourth-year medical student, presents a patient at the state mental hospital at the weekly case conference. This patient had been diagnosed with bipolar disorder with psychotic features, has been on a certain atypical antipsychotic (with supposedly fewer extra pyramidal side effects) for several years, and is now

M.A. Samtani
Statistician, Department of Psychiatry, University of Hawai'i John A. Burns School of Medicine

A. Guerrero, M. Piasecki (eds.), *Problem-Based Behavioral Science and Psychiatry*,
© Springer Science+Business Media, LLC 2008

exhibiting Parkinson-like symptoms. After discussion at morning report, Melinda is asked to present an article on drug-related movement disorders.

One week later, Melinda presents an article titled "Assessment of drug-related movement disorders in schizophrenia," published in Advances in Psychiatric Treatment (Gervin & Barnes, 2000). She recounts the case she presented the previous week. She discusses the link between long-term use of antipsychotic drugs and movement disorders commonly found in Parkinsonism. Following her presentation, the attending psychiatrist (who is well-known for successfully mentoring students and residents in clinical research) proposes that she investigate the topic further by conducting her own research project on movement disorders in patients treated with this particular antipsychotic at their facility.

The attending psychiatrist explains that before Melinda can embark on her project, she has to consider several key elements in selecting a study design and analyzing the collected data.

 Please proceed with the problem-based approach!

Learning Issues

In this section, we break down Melinda's project into 15 discrete steps. Her chances of success are significantly increased if she is able to think through each of the 15 steps and get help with research design and data analysis **before** she starts her project.

(1) Identify the research question:

    (a) What is the primary research question of your study?

    (b) Write down your research hypothesis (i.e., your proposed theory to answer your research question).

    (c) Identify other goals/objectives of your study.

(2) Conduct a literature review:

    (a) Are there similar studies that have been conducted?

    (b) What new idea or information can you contribute?

(3) Select the appropriate study design:

    (a) Decide on the type of study.

    After the research question has been defined, selecting the right type of study is essential to the success of the project. The aim and research question(s) of your study must fit the study design.

There are many ways to categorize study designs. Here, studies are classified under two main headings: observational and experimental. Experimental studies involve indirect and/or direct intervention by the investigator(s) during the data collection process, whereas observational studies require no intervention in the collection process. Many experimental studies require informed consent from the participants.

In general, experimental studies are considered more rigorous than other studies because these studies are prospective in nature (i.e., current and future data are collected vs. past data in a retrospective study) and there is more control over the participants and treatment(s). However, experimental studies usually require more protocols, IRB oversight, and expenses. Table 15.1 describes the types of studies:

1. Observational studies: These studies involve no intervention with the participants/ patients and treatments used in the study. Many study designs fall under this heading. They include: cohort, case–control, cross-sectional, case series, and community surveys.
2. Experimental studies: These studies involve intervention (e.g., treatment) on the part of the investigator(s). Studies under this heading include: clinical trials and community intervention trials.
   Please refer to Table 15.1 for a summary of the different study designs.

(4) Select tools for measurement (scales, types of measurement).
   It is important to know what type of data you have before selecting a statistical test for analysis. Data can be categorized into four levels, known as scales or types of measurement (see Table 15.2). The type of measurement will determine the statistical test employed. Since nominal and ordinal data are considered discrete (or categorical) data, non-parametric tests would be needed to analyze the data. This is because non-parametric tests do not assume a normal distribution. For interval and ratio scale data, parametric tests may be used for analysis.

   Parametric statistical tests assume that the data approximate a normal distribution (interval and ratio data), whereas non-parametric tests are less restrictive, assuming no particular distribution of the data (nominal and ordinal). With multiple data types in an analysis (i.e., discrete and continuous), non-parametric tests are applied. However, when possible, parametric tests should be employed as they have more explanatory power.

(5) Instruments and diagnostic tests.
   How consistent and accurate are your instruments? You should assess the validity and reliability of your instruments (e.g., surveys). These two concepts and how to test for them are discussed in the next case. If your study requires the use of a screening test for a particular disease, testing the accuracy of the results is crucial. Simple calculations are used to produce the sensitivity and specificity of these tests.

   Sensitivity refers to the probability that a positive result on a screening test truly indicates that the patient does have a certain disease or condition for which he or she is tested. It is the probability of a true positive.

Table 15.1 Study designs

Type of study	Experimental/ observational	Analytical/ descriptive	Retrospective/ prospective	Description/examples	Advantages	Disadvantages
Case–control	Observational	Analytical	Retrospective	<ul><li>Often used to study rare diseases</li><li>Examines the outcome to determine the possible risk factors</li><li>Case group: participants with disease</li><li>Control group: participants without the disease</li><li>Odds ratio often used in analysis</li></ul>	<ul><li>Economical</li><li>Data can be analyzed relatively quickly (Kuzma, 1992)</li></ul>	
Cohort	Observational	Analytical	Prospective; it can also be retrospective	<ul><li>As a prospective study: data are collected over a determined period of time</li><li>The influence of the selected risk factors on the outcome is examined in the group exposed to vs. the group not exposed to the risk factors</li></ul>	<ul><li>Better control over sample selection and data collected</li><li>Prospective study design reduces bias</li></ul>	<ul><li>More costly and time-intensive</li></ul>
Cross-sectional	Observational	Descriptive	Retrospective/ prospective	<ul><li>Examines relationship of variables at a specific point in time. It is a snapshot view of what is happening</li><li>Often used to assess prevalence</li><li>Example: a political poll</li></ul>		
Case series	Observational	Descriptive	Retrospective/ prospective	<ul><li>A descriptive study of a group with common attributes, experiences, etc.</li><li>Also used to determine the association between exposure to a particular factor and outcome</li><li>Data may include personal background and diagnoses</li></ul>		

Table 15.1 (continued)

Type of study	Experimental/ observational	Analytical/ descriptive	Retrospective/ prospective	Description/examples	Advantages	Disadvantages
Community surveys	Observational	Descriptive	Prospective	▪ A study designed (e.g., questionnaires and surveys) to provide a basic understanding of a selected community (e.g., demographic, concerns, opinions)		
Clinical trails	Experimental	Analytical	Prospective	▪ Apply intervention (e.g., therapy, new drugs, procedure) to one of the groups studied to determine its effects against a control group (receiving a placebo intervention or the standard treatment) ▪ Often single or double-blinded measures (in which either the patient or both the patient and the administrator do not know whether what is being administered is a placebo or active treatment) ▪ Example: testing whether a new drug is more effective than the current drug for a particular disease	▪ Offers more robust data (reduces bias) and is considered the "gold standard" in research	▪ More time and capital-intensive
Community intervention trials	Experimental	Analytical	Prospective	▪ Experiments are done at the community rather than the individual level (as with clinical trials) ▪ Requires significant coordination with community leaders (e.g., community advocates and tribal and religious leaders)		

Table 15.2 Scales of measurement

Type of data	Examples	Discrete/ continuous	Characteristics	Type of statistical test
Nominal	Gender, ethnicities, religion	Discrete	▪ Membership ▪ May be assigned numeric value; however, these values have no true meaning	Non-parametric
Ordinal	Educational level (e.g., elementary, graduate to professional education), Likert scale (agreement scale)	Discrete/ continuous*	▪ Membership ▪ Values are in some ranking order ▪ Spacing between values are NOT equivalent	Non-parametric
Interval	Temperature (i.e., Celsius and Fahrenheit), a severity of pain scale (e.g., 0–10)	Continuous	▪ Membership ▪ Values are in some ranking order ▪ Equivalent intervals ▪ Arbitrary zero point	Parametric
Ratio	Age, length, weight, height, screening tests (e.g., prostate-specific antigen [PSA] levels)	Continuous	▪ Membership ▪ Values are in some ranking order ▪ Equivalent intervals ▪ Absolute zero	Parametric

* As a general rule, ordinal data may be treated as continuous data if there are many ranks (similar to an interval scale). Nonetheless, some researchers disagree with this rule, arguing that ordinal data are only discrete (or categorical)

On the other hand, **Specificity** refers to the probability that a negative result on a screening test truly indicates that the patient does not have a certain disease or condition for which he or she is tested. It is the probability of a true negative. Providing accurate results is important as lack of treatment (if the result is a false negative result) could result in harm to the patient's health.

Tables 15.3, 15.4, and 15.5 apply this to an example: detecting Parkinson's disease.

For predictive values, if the test is negative, the negative predictive value, the probability of Parkinson's disease is TN/(FN + TN). It is the probability that a negative test result is a true negative. If the test is positive, the positive predictive value, the probability of Parkinson's disease is TP/(TP + FP). It is the probability that a positive test result is a true positive (Table 15.5).

False positive rate (α) is the relative frequency of a positive test result of a certain disease when in fact the patient does not have the disease. Using Table 15.3,

Table 15.3 Sensitivity and specificity

	Parkinson's disease		
	Present	Absent	
Test positive	(TP) 85	(FP) 7,100	(TP + FP) 7,185
Test negative	(FN) 15	(TN) 92,800	(FN + TN) 92,815
	(TP + FN) 100	(FP + TN) 99,900	(TP + FP + FN + TN) 100,000

TP = true positives; FP = false positives; FN = false negatives; TN = true negatives

Table 15.4 Sensitivity and specificity

Sensitivity	Specificity
TP / TP + FN	TN / (FP + TN)
85/100 = 85 %	92,800/99,900 = 93 %

Table 15.5 Predictive values

Positive predictive value	Negative predictive value
TP / TP + FP	TN / (FN + TN)
85/7,185 = 1 %	92,800/92,815 = 99.98 %

the calculation is $FP/(FP + TN) = 7,100/99,900 = 7\%$ (or 1–specificity). False negative rate (β) is the relative frequency of a negative test result when in fact the patient does have the disease. The calculation for this rate is $FN/(TP + FN) = 15/100 = 15\%$ (or 1–sensitivity).

(6) Sampling.

Selecting an appropriate and feasible sampling technique and sample size are essential in providing data for a more robust analysis with minimal bias (good representation of the population studying). **Simple random sampling** is when a sample of the population is randomly selected, making sure each observation has an equal chance of being picked. **Stratified sampling** is when there are several different groups within the population and each one needs to be represented equally. For each group, the simple random sampling technique is applied to generate the sample. **Self-selection sampling** is when the sample is based on convenience of data collection or some other factor determined by the investigator (e.g., the selection of a set of schools or programs in which consent could be easily obtained). This technique could result in bias in the data. **Systematic sampling or assignment** is when a list of the population is available, the first observation is randomly selected, then every

nth observation (decided by the investigator) is selected until the determined sample size has been reached.

(7) Significance level and statistical errors.

Hypothesis testing involves comparing empirically observed sample findings with theoretically expected findings—expected if the null hypothesis (Ho) is true. This comparison allows one to compute the probability that the observed outcomes could have been due to chance or random error.

   Significance level is the alpha or significance level that is set by the researcher, generally at 5 %. It is the level at which the test results are determined to be statistically significant. The significance level is also

- The probability at which the null hypothesis (Ho) would be rejected.
- The level or probability selected by the researcher that determines the probability of committing a Type I error.
- See Table 15.6.

   Type I error is rejecting a true null hypothesis. A researcher can mistakenly reject the null hypothesis when in reality it is true (not false). It is giving "false affirmation" to the results of a study (Vogt, 2005). This, in turn, generates a false positive. The objective of minimizing Type I error is to have a small probability claiming something is true when in reality it is not true (e.g., statistically significant difference between two drugs, when there is no difference). It is inversely related to a Type II error.

   Type II error is failing to reject a false null hypothesis (accepting a false null hypothesis). It is failing to reject (mistakenly accepting) the null hypothesis when in reality it is false. It is giving "false denial" (Vogt, 2005) to the results of a study (e.g., no significant difference between two drugs, when there is a difference). This, in turn, generates a false negative.

   Statistical power is the probability of rejecting a truly false null hypothesis. In other words, it is the probability that statistically significant differences will be found in a study. It is the inverse of the probability of a Type II error (e.g., if power = 80 %, then probability of a Type II error = 20 %). A general rule is that statistical power of 80 % or higher is acceptable.

Table 15.6 Type I and Type II errors

	Reject the null hypothesis	Do not reject the null hypothesis
Null hypothesis is true	**Type I error** Alpha	Correctly determining there is no difference 1-alpha
Null hypothesis is false	**Power** Correctly determining that there is a difference 1-beta	**Type II error** Beta

(8) Establish protocols for study (the actual steps necessary on how you conduct your study):

  (a) Determine how your participants will be selected.
  (b) Are signed consent and/or assent forms needed? If yes, develop a plan to collect and store the confidential data.
  (c) Train the project members/administrators on collecting data (e.g., interviews, IQ tests).

 (9) Run the study on a test group (i.e., a pilot study).
(10) Develop a codebook of all variables and possible values collected.
(11) Conduct the study (collect primary data).
(12) Clean/recode the data (making appropriate notes in the codebook).
(13) Analyze the data:

  (a) Revisit the hypothesis stated.
  (b) Descriptive and inferential analysis:

    (1) Run basic frequencies and correlations of the study variables.

A correlation (r) is the statistical relationship between two variables. This numerical relationship is often referred to as a bivariate distribution. It tests whether or not there is an association between the variables. The values range from -1 to $+1$. A value of -1 indicates a perfect negative or inverse relationship. A value of $+1$ indicates a perfect positive or direct relationship. A value of 0 indicates no relationship, except in the case of a curvilinear relationship (other techniques need to be employed to determine the association).

There are different ways to calculate the correlation coefficient depending on the type of variable being used (i.e., ordinal, interval, or ratio). If the scale of measurement for the variables is ordinal (i.e., a ranking order with no uniform intervals or absolute zero), then Spearman's rho or Kendall's tau may be applied. The most common and widely used correlation coefficient is Pearson's product–moment (Pearson's r). Pearson's r carries certain assumptions and distribution requirements. It is this statistic that measures the degree of the linear relationship (i.e., strength and direction of the association) between variables.

    (2) Choose the appropriate statistical test (see Fig. 15.1). For this chapter, the focus is on basic statistical tests.
    (3) Review results: Is there a statistically significant difference between the null hypothesis and your research hypothesis?

(14) Write your paper.
(15) Submit the paper for presentation and publication.

Choosing a test

1. Scale?

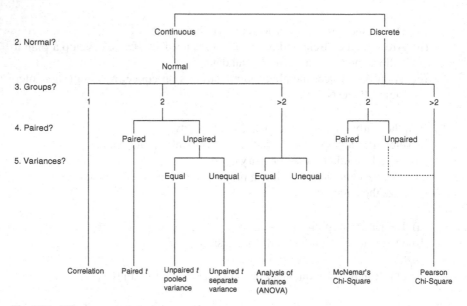

Fig. 15.1 Selecting a statistical test
Source: Garb (1996). Understanding medical research: A practitioner's guide. Boston: Little, Brown. Figure 15-3, p. 184.
Note: See supplemental glossary for explanations of statistical tests.

Case Vignette 15.1.2 Conclusion

Following considerable thought to her study design options, Melinda selects a case–control study to evaluate the relationship between long-term use of antipsychotic drugs and movement disorders commonly found in Parkinsonism. A randomized clinical trial with case and control groups would be the ideal. However, that option requires a significant amount of time and capital.

After receiving permission from the hospital, she conducts 100 chart reviews (retrospective data) of patients with and without the Parkinsonism symptoms. The Pearson correlation was applied to test for an association. The result was 0.7, confirming a reportable and direct relationship. The next step is to apply a randomized controlled trial to determine whether or not a significant causal relationship exists. Melinda noted that this study may provide useful insight into further studies (i.e., experimental) and assist in successfully applying for grants that would provide the funding for a more involved data collection.

Case Vignette 15.2.1 Shyla Sing

Shyla Sing is a 12-year-old girl who was brought to the primary care clinic by her mother. Mrs. Sing explains to the medical psychologist and the first-year resident who is shadowing that day that though Shyla appears to be physically fine, she is worried about her child's mental development. Some of Mrs. Sing's concerns include Shyla's difficulty in interacting with her peers. Also, Shyla is extremely shy and refuses to separate from her mother.

Please proceed with the problem-based approach!

Case Vignette 15.2.2 Continuation

Shyla's physical examination revealed no abnormalities and suggested that she is a normal 12-year-old girl. Furthermore, the results of standard laboratory tests did not reveal any medical problems.

Mrs. Sing explains that for the past 2 years, Shyla has had "erratic behavior." Examples include simple dialog resulting in major tantrums. Mrs. Sing may ask for a spoon from the kitchen drawer, and Shyla would suddenly start to cry. When Mrs. Sing approaches her, Shyla would often yell out, "Get away from me. You do not care whether I live or die!" At times, she would escalate the situation by throwing utensils and/or hitting her mother. This type of behavior usually occurs when she is alone with her mother.

Furthermore, Shyla's academic performance has shown a decline over the past 2 years. Her parents have met with the school principal on three occasions during the time period to discuss her failing to near-failing grades in her classes. After meeting with the principal, the parents, mainly the mother, would talk with the Shyla about improving her grades. Sometimes it would result in a "shouting match." Usually, within a month, Shyla's grades would show a steady improvement. This would last for 3–4 months and then decline again.

Since there is an array of possible diagnoses related to the patient's behavior, the behavioral health consultant suggests conducting a structured interview with the patient. The Diagnostic Interview Schedule for Children (DISC) was brought up as a possibility. The resident was not very familiar with this instrument. Therefore, he decides to investigate its application for this particular case.

Please proceed with the problem-based approach!

There are advantages of employing the DISC scoring algorithms for mental health diagnoses. It has been reviewed and approved by the National Institute of

Mental Health (NIMH). Also, since the DISC is a highly structured interview, the administration of the computerized version requires no clinical and little hands-on training.

In terms of the instrument's **reliability** and **validity**, the DISC has been widely used since 1983. Since that time, there have been many inquiries and reviews as to its reliability (e.g., tests and retests). Although there may be some detractors, the DISC appears to have a history of reliable and valid results.

Reliability is concerned with the consistency of a measurement or instrument over multiple applications. With a survey or questionnaire, it is the consistency of the results over time with the same individual or the consistency within a set of items administered at the same time. While reliability is focused on the consistency of the instrument, **validity** is concerned with its accuracy. Does the instrument measure what it is expected to measure? A test could be reliable or consistent over time. However, it might not be an accurate or valid measure. This term can be further categorized into internal and external validities.

A common metaphor used to describe the relation between these two concepts is a dartboard or target. The objective is to hit the center (i.e., the bull's eye) of the board. One possibility may involve a tight grouping of darts on the periphery of the board. The results would be considered very reliable but not valid or accurate (i.e., totally missing the center). The ideal case is for all the darts to hit the bull's eye. This result would be both reliable and valid.

There are many types of reliability. For this chapter, two types are discussed: **internal reliability** (or internal consistency) and **inter-rater reliability**. Internal reliability assesses the consistency (correlation) among the responses from the items (e.g., questions) within the same instrument (e.g., test, survey). Inter-rater reliability assesses the consistency of the raters' or observers' assessment of the same event.

One popular measure of internal reliability is Cronbach's alpha. It is a reliability coefficient, ranging from 0 to 1 (values close to 1 are considered to reflect a high reliability). Values of 0.7–0.8 are regarded as satisfactory; however, clinical applications require higher values (Bland & Altman, 1997).[1]

A way to gauge for inter-rater reliability is **Cohen's kappa**. Its values range from 0 to 1. Values less than 0.4 are considered to be "poor," 0.4–0.6 are "moderate," 0.6–0.8 are "substantial," and above 0.8 are "almost perfect."[2]

Internal validity is the extent to which the observed results demonstrate a causal relationship between the variables (dependent and independent) examined. In other words, to what extent do the studied independent or explanatory variables cause a variation (one way or another) in the dependent or outcome variable? It is the degree to which valid conclusions can be drawn about the causal effects of one variable on another (Vogt, 2005). **External validity** is the ability to apply the test results outside the study or generalize them to another or larger group.

---

[1] For the calculations of Cronbach's alpha, see Campbell and Machin (1999, pp. 174–175).

[2] For the calculations of Cohen's kappa, see Campbell and Machin (1999, p. 175).

Case Vignette 15.2.3 Conclusion

Before committing to the DISC as a diagnostic tool, the resident further examines its reliability and validity. For internal consistency, the calculated Cronbach's alpha was 0.89. This is more than satisfactory. For inter-rater reliability, the calculated Cohen's kappa was 0.72, considered substantial.

Finally, for external validity, the resident gains permission to review past medical charts from different clinics where the DISC was used. He then compares DISC results with physicians' diagnoses. For the most part, the outcomes were consistent. The resident continued to evaluate its validity by comparing a small group of at-risk patients (potential for suicidal thoughts or actions based on DISC results) with their follow-up appointments. His investigation validates the DISC results as many of these patients later admit to have had suicidal thoughts and some have attempted to act on it.

In the end, the resident decides to administer the structured interview with the patient. After running the computerized version and reviewing the results with the DSM-IV, the resident felt better equipped to diagnose the patient. Shyla was diagnosed with depression and anxiety disorder. Six months later with the behavioral treatment and medication, she showed significant and consistent improvement in her behavior.

Case Vignette 15.3.1 Nate

As an assignment for his next journal club, Nate, a second-year medical student, was asked to present on the essential elements in critically understanding a journal article. He selected an article from a reputable, peer-reviewed journal on a meta-analysis done on an existing oral hypoglycemic medication (Drug X) that has been on the market for 10 years.[3]

In his presentation, Nate notes that the authors of the study applied a meta-analysis to examine retrospective data from 40 of 104 relevant studies in which Drug X was used. They proposed that Drug X is potentially harmful because it increases the incidence of cardiac events (i.e., myocardial infarction). Literature searches were conducted using various public and private databases. Inclusion criteria for the meta-analysis included studies that had a randomized control group not receiving Drug X, studies that were conducted for least a period of 20 weeks, and studies with outcome data for cardiovascular events.

The average age of the participants was approximately 53 years. Of 13,100 patients on Drug X, 95 experienced a cardiovascular event. Of 12,700 patients not on Drug X, 70 experienced a cardiovascular event. When comparing the treatment group to the control group, the odds ratio for a cardiovascular event was 1.32 (at

---

[3] This fictitious case is loosely based on facts and findings from an article published in the *New England Journal of Medicine* (Nissen & Wolski, 2007).

the 95 % confidence interval [CI], 1.04–1.85; p=0.04). The authors concluded that Drug X is associated with a significant increase in the risk of a cardiovascular event.

Please proceed with the problem-based approach!

It is important that consumers of research literature be critical of the method, analysis, and results of any study. Most journal articles offer current and relevant information on research topics of interest. It is the responsibility of health care professionals to be informed and properly evaluate and interpret published studies in order to provide the best clinical care for their patients.

Case Vignette 15.3.2 Continuation

After reading the article a few times, Nate made a list of questions to critically examine the methods and results of the published study.

The list includes:

(1) Have you critically examined the methods to determine the validity of the study? How was the sample selected (e.g., simple random sample, stratified sampling)?

(2) Pretend that you were conducting the study yourself (see the previous case for the checklist of designing a study). Would you do it differently? If yes, how would you change it? Would your changes significantly impact the results of the published study?

(3) What do the results mean?

(4) Can the findings be applied in a practical sense (e.g., in my practice)? If yes, how can I apply them?

Additional questions for meta-analysis include:

(5) When dealing with multiple studies, you have to deal with multiple study designs, sampling, data collection techniques, and protocols. Were the values from different studies placed on a standard or common scale?

(6) How were the data combined into one data set? Do you have access to the original data sets? Did any of the studies in the meta-analysis use the same data set (partial or complete)? This would entail double-counting.

(7) Were the studies with opposing or negative results reported?

Please proceed with the problem-based approach!

STOP

Learning Issues

A **meta-analysis** is conducted by gathering data from multiple journal articles to increase its sample size. The data, from various secondary sources, are compiled and considered as one large data set in the analysis. Each study included in the meta-analysis is considered a unit of measurement.

Criteria for an Acceptable Meta-analysis

1. The study objectives were clearly identified.
2. Inclusion criteria of articles in general and specific data to be accepted were established before selection.
3. An active effort was made to find and include all relevant articles.
4. An assessment of publication bias was made.
5. Specific data used were identified.
6. Assessment of article comparability (e.g., controls, circumstances) was made.
7. The meta-analysis was reported in enough detail to allow replication.

Source: Riffenburgh (2006, p. 163).

Relative risk is a risk ratio comparing the probability of developing a disease in two groups: the incidence of those exposed to a specific risk factor (e.g., smoking and alcohol consumption) and the incidence of those not exposed to the risk factor. It is often applied in prospective data analysis (e.g., cohort studies and clinical trials), where the two groups are selected at the beginning of the study. Consequently, this ratio is not used in case–control studies (retrospective data analysis with a focus on the outcome first). The following example of relative risk examines the influence of alcohol on liver disease (see Table 15.7). The exposure group included men who drank the alcohol equivalent of 50 or more beers a week. The group not exposed to significant alcohol consumption drank the alcohol equivalent of 1–8 beers a week (social drinking).

Based on the calculated relative risk, a man who drank heavily was approximately 1.5 times more likely to develop a liver disease than a man who drank socially.

The **odds ratio** is the ratio of two probabilities: the probability that an event will occur (a/c for simplicity, the data in Table 15.7 are used) and the probability that an event will not occur (b/d). It is often used in the analysis of retrospective cases (e.g., case-control studies of rare diseases).

Table 15.7 Example of relative risk

		Liver disease		
		Present	Absent	Totals
Exposure to alcohol	Yes	(a)	(b)	(a + b)
	(50 or more)	70	150	220
	No	(c)	(d)	(c + d)
	(1–8)	250	950	1200

The relative risk is calculated by the following formula:

$$\frac{a/(a+b)}{c/(c+d)} \rightarrow \frac{70/(70+150)}{250/(250+950)} \rightarrow \frac{0.318}{0.208} \rightarrow 1.53$$

The odds ratio is calculated by the following formula:

$$\frac{a/c}{b/d} \rightarrow \frac{70/250}{150/950} \rightarrow \frac{0.280}{0.158} \rightarrow 1.77$$

While the odds ratio is often used as an estimate for relative risk, we can see by applying the same example from Table 15.7 that, the odds ratio is different from the relative risk. A man who drank heavily was approximately 1.8 times more likely to develop a liver disease than a man who drank socially. As the ratios move away from 1, the difference become more apparent.

Case Vignette 15.3.3 Conclusion

Nate applies the critical questions to examine the validity of the authors' claims. Based on the data, methods, and analysis, it is difficult to say with confidence that the association between Drug X and cardiac events is truly noteworthy. Specific reasons include:

(1) Methods: The retrospective data come from other multiple sources. Moreover, the authors did not have access to the original source data. This is a considerable limitation.

(2) Methods: It appears that most of these studies were not designed to study cardiac outcomes.

(3) Analysis: The actual number of cases with cardiac outcomes was relatively small given the sample size. For participants on Drug X, 95 of 13,100 patients experienced a cardiovascular event. For participants not on Drug X, 70 of 12,700 patients experienced a cardiovascular event.

(4) Analysis: Although statistically significant (p = 0.04), the odds ratio of 1.32 appears to be low. Nonetheless, to test whether this ratio is relatively high or low, a comparative analysis with other similar drug(s) should be conducted.

Ideally, a randomized clinical trial (prospective analysis) should be conducted to properly examine whether a significant causal relationship exist. In the end, it is up to an informed practitioner to decide how to interpret and apply the findings of this article and other journal articles in his/her practice.

Review Questions

1. Study designs:

A group of clinician-researchers hypothesized that household crowding may be an important risk factor for pediatric obsessive–compulsive disorder (via increased risk for streptococcal pharyngitis). The researchers chose to analyze a database that was derived from one-time surveys of youth attending community high schools that agreed to participate in the study. The surveys included questions on the number of people in the household and structured interview questions to assess for symptoms of obsessive–compulsive disorder. While all students at the high schools were approached for potential participation in the surveys, the only students included in the study were those for whom there was both youth and parental consent. Which of the following statements pertaining to the study design is FALSE:

(a) The study would involve retrospective data analysis.
(b) This is a cohort study design.
(c) This is a cross-sectional study design.
(d) Self-selection sampling was done.
(e) None of the above.

2. Sensitivity, specificity, predictive values:

Based on the following data on Blood Test A used to diagnosis Lyme disease, calculate (a) the sensitivity and specificity of the screening test and (b) the positive and negative predictive values.

Lyme Disease

	Present	Absent
Blood Test A Positive	240	12,300
Blood Test A Negative	60	107,400

3. Correlations:

If both samples in Case 1 and Case 2 are representative, which case would you rather have?

Case	r	r^2	N	Significance
1	high(0.90)	0.81	6	No
2	low (0.10)	0.01	4000	Yes

Answers

1. Study designs:
   Answer: (b).
2. Sensitivity, Specificity, Predicative Values:

Disease

	Present	Absent	
Test Positive	(TP) 240	(FP) 12,300	(TP + FP) 12,540
Test Negative	(FN) 60	(TN) 107,400	(FN + TN) 107,460
	(TP + FN) 300	(FP + TN) 119,700	(TP + FP + FN + TN) 120,000

TP = True Positives   FP = False Positives
FN = False Negatives   TN = True Negatives

Sensitivity	Specificity
TP / TP + FN	TN / FP + TN
240/300 = 80 %	107,400/119,700 = 90 %

Positive Predictive Value	Negative Predictive Value
TP / TP + FP	TN / FN + TN
240/12,540 = 2 %	107,400/107,460 = 99.94 %

3. Correlations:

Depending on the purpose of the study, Case 1 or Case 2 could be valid answers.

For Case 1, the Pearson r or correlation coefficient is very high (0.9). However, the sample size is very small ($N = 6$). Also, the results show that it is not statistically significant. Nonetheless, if one is conducting a pilot study and wants to illustrate a very strong effect, Case 1 is the better option.

For Case 2, the correlation coefficient (0.10) appears to be very low. However, the sample size is large, and the correlation is statistically significant. For large sample sizes, the r can be low and still reach statistical significance. Accordingly, if one wants to illustrate a statistically significant relationship regardless of a very small effect, then Case 2 is the better option.

Appendix: Populated problem-based tables for the case vignettes

Case Vignette 15.1

What are the facts?	What are your hypotheses?	What do you want to know next?	What specific information would you like to learn about?
▪ There appears to be a link between long-term use of antipsychotic drugs and movement disorders commonly found in Parkinsonism	▪ There is a relationship between long-term use of this particular atypical antipsychotic drug and movement disorders commonly found in Parkinsonism ▪ A significant portion of the variation in occurrence of this movement disorder can be explained by the long-term use of this drug	▪ Have observational or experimental studies been conducted on this topic?	▪ How to select and conduct a study? ▪ Study designs ▪ Scales of measurement for data collection ▪ Types of sampling techniques ▪ Sensitivity and specificity tests ▪ How to analyze data (e.g., basic statistical tests used to analyze data)

Case Vignette 15.2

What are the facts?	What are your hypotheses?	What do you want to know next?	What specific information would you like to learn about?
▪ 12-year-old girl ▪ Mother worried about mental development ▪ Difficulty interacting with peers ▪ Shy	▪ Possible anxiety disorder ▪ Normal separation anxiety or temperamental variation ▪ Depression ▪ Child abuse	▪ Physical appearance (e.g., any bruises, residual marks, etc.) ▪ Cognitive awareness of environment ▪ Home environment	▪ What are the normal developmental milestones at this age? ▪ Other ways to approach and communicate with this girl ▪ Available diagnostic tools/instruments ▪ Reliability ▪ Validity

Case Vignette 15.2 (Continued)

What are the facts?	What are your hypotheses?	What do you want to know next?	What specific information would you like to learn about?
▪ Refuses to separate from mother	▪ Posttraumatic stress disorder ▪ Nutritional deficiency ▪ Possible endocrine disorder (hypothyroidism) ▪ Mother is overly concerned	▪ School performance ▪ Parents' disposition (temperament) ▪ Possible substance use ▪ Possible parental substance use	

Case Vignette 15.3

What are the facts?	What are your hypotheses?	What do you want to know next?	What specific information would you like to learn about?
▪ The journal article purports that through the use of meta-analysis, Drug X is associated with a significant increase in the risk of a cardiovascular event	▪ That the study has many limitations and should be treated with cautious reception	▪ Of the 64 relevant studies not selected, how many claimed no significant relationship between Drug X and cardiac events	▪ Meta-analysis ▪ Relative risk ▪ Odds ratio

Bibliography

Appleton, D. R. (1990). What statistics should we teach medical undergraduates and graduates? *Statistics in Medicine, 9,* 1013–1021.

Bakeman, R., & Robinson, B. F. (2005). Understanding statistics in the behavioral sciences. Mahwah, NJ: Lawrence Erlbaum.

Bell, F. D. (1995). Basic biostatistics: Concepts for the health sciences: The almost no math stats book. Dubuque, IA: Wm. C. Brown.

Bland, J. M., & Altman, D. G. (1997) Cronbach's alpha. *British Medical Journal, 314,* 572.

Bowers, D. (1996). Statistics from scratch: An introduction for health care professionals. West Sussex: Wiley.

Campbell, M. J., & Machin, D. (1999). Medical statistics: A commonsense approach (3rd ed.). West Sussex: Wiley.

Carvounis, C. P. (2000). Handbook of biostatistics: A review and text. New York: Parthenon.

Dawson-Saunders, B., & Trapp, R. G. (1990). Basic and clinical biostatistics. Norwalk, CT: Appleton & Lange.

Diagnostic Interview Schedule for Children brochure. http://www.promotementalhealth.org/downloads/DISC %20Brochure.pdf. Accessed 10/18/07.

Garb, J. L. (1996). Understanding medical research: A practitioner's guide. Boston: Little, Brown.

Gervin, M., & Barnes, T. R. E. (2000). Assessment of drug-related movement disorders in schizophrenia. Advances in Psychiatric Treatment, 6, 332–343.

Greenhalgh, T. (1997). Statistics for the non-statistician. 1. Different types of data need different statistical tests. British Medical Journal, 315, 364–366.

Greenhalgh, T. (1997). How to read a paper: Statistics for the non-statistician. II: "Significant" relations and their pitfalls. British Medical Journal, 315, 422–425.

Harris, M. B. (1995). Basic statistics for behavioral science research. Needham Heights, MA: Allyn & Bacon.

Huck, S. W. (2000). Reading statistics and research. New York: Longman.

Kerlinger, F. N., & Lee, H. B. (2000). Foundations of behavioral research. Orlando, FL: Harcourt College Publishers.

Kuzma, J. W. (1992). Basic statistics for the health sciences. Mountain View, CA: Mayfield.

Lang, T. A., & Secic, M. (1997). How to report statistics in medicine: Annotated guidelines for authors, editors, and reviewers. Philadelphia, PA: American College of Physicians.

Matthews, D. E., & Farewell, V. T. (1996). Using and understanding medical statistics. Basel: Karger.

National Institute of Mental Health (NIMH) Diagnostic Interview Schedule for Children Version IV (NIMH DISC-IV): description, differences from previous versions, and reliability of some common diagnoses.

National Institute of Mental Health Diagnostic Interview Schedule for Children (NIMH-DISC). http://chipts.ucla.edu/assessment/pdf/assessments/disc_for_the_web.pdf.Accessed 10/18/07

Nissen, S. E., & Wolski, K. (2007). Effect of rosiglitazone on the risk of myocardial infarction and death from cardiovascular causes. New England Journal of Medicine, 356, 2457–2471. http://content.nejm.org/cgi/content/full/NEJMoa072761. Accessed 10/13/07.

Pedhazur, E. J. (1997). Multiple regression in behavioral research: Explanation and prediction. Orlando, FL: Harcourt Brace College Publishers.

Petrie, A., & Sabin, C. (2005). Medical statistics at a glance. Oxford: Blackwell.

Riffenburgh, R. H. (2006). Statistics in medicine. Burlington, MA: Elsevier.

Shaffer, D., Fisher, P., Lucas, C. P., Dulcan, M. K., & Schwab-Stone, M. E. (2000). Journal of the American Academy of Child and Adolescent Psychiatry, 39(1), 28–38.

Vogt, W. P. (2005). Dictionary of statistics & methodology: A nontechnical guide for the social sciences. Thousand Oaks, CA: Sage.

Chapter 16
Death, Dying, and End-of-Life Care

Lori Murayama-Sung and Iqbal Ahmed

All physicians face end-of-life issues during their training and many continue to work in specialties where life and death are part of their daily duties. This chapter addresses a key challenge for physicians who work with older and critically ill patients.

At the end of this chapter, the reader will be able to

1. Understand psychological issues surrounding end of life, including stages of grief, psychiatric illness, and psychosocial/spiritual needs
2. Understand what the standard of care is with regards to euthanasia and physician-assisted suicide
3. Discuss sensitive issues with patients including diagnosing death, organ donation, and how to address families at the time of death
4. Understand what palliative care is and when to refer someone to hospice

Case Vignette 16.1.1 Presenting Situation: Kim

Mr. Kim is a 63-year old Chinese man who is admitted for pleuritic chest pain and dyspnea. He has no known medical or psychiatric history except for an 80 pack-year smoking history. He had not sought medical treatment in years but finally decided to seek treatment at the urging of his second wife.

After you perform a full work-up, you gently break the bad news to him that he has end-stage lung cancer. You explain to him that his prognosis is poor and that the recommended treatment at this time would be palliative chemotherapy.

Mr. Kim barely says a word during this discussion, but you brush this off because he seems "all right" at the time. Later, however, you become concerned that he may be suffering from depression because the nursing staff has witnessed him crying frequently in his room. He also has been barely touching his food.

L. Murayama-Sung
Chief Resident, General Psychiatry Program
University of Hawai'i John A. Burns School of Medicine

A. Guerrero, M. Piasecki (eds.), *Problem-Based Behavioral Science and Psychiatry*,
© Springer Science+Business Media, LLC 2008

You decide to address these issues; however, before you do, you try to recall the recent grand rounds on "stages of grief." You also think about how you will need to differentiate between depression that needs treatment and an adjustment reaction that will dissipate with time.

Please proceed with the problem-based approach!

Kubler-Ross's stages of grief provide a model for the different emotional and cognitive stages that people experience when they are faced with loss. Not everyone progresses through these stages in this particular order and some people skip stages. Table 16.1 describes the stages and offers examples for each of them.

In addition to recognizing stages of grief, you need to determine if Mr. Kim meets the criteria for a normal grief reaction (preparatory grief) versus a major depressive episode (Table 16.2). While people can have symptoms similar to those seen in depression, during acute grief the intensity and duration of symptoms appear less. Grief also does not typically have symptoms of extreme guilt or suicidal thoughts. See Chapter 8, Physician–patient relationship for information on breaking bad news.

Case Vignette 16.1.2 Continuation

Mr. Kim tells you that for months, he knew that something was "not right" with his body but delayed seeking treatment because of concerns that it could be something bad. He explains that when you initially told him he had end-stage cancer, he felt numb and was in disbelief. However, after a few days, his situation has started to sink in.

Mr. Kim admits to feeling sad and anxious with regards to his cancer. He denies actual thoughts of wanting to hurt himself at this time. He also denies any feelings of hopelessness or worthlessness. He does admit to recent weight loss, decreased energy, and some difficulty sleeping due to lower back pain secondary to compression fractures from bony metastasis.

Please proceed with the problem-based approach!

At this point, it seems most likely that Mr. Kim may be suffering from a grief reaction. However, in addition to assessing for grief and depression, it is also important to assess for other psychiatric conditions such as anxiety disorders, mood and anxiety disorders secondary to a general medical condition, and delirium.

Table 16.1 Stages of grief (Kubler-Ross, 1969)

Stage	Example
Denial	Mr. Kim is in disbelief that he has lung cancer
Anger	Mr. Kim gets angry at himself or his physicians for not recognizing his illness earlier. He also gets angry with God because he feels his situation is unjust
Bargaining	Mr. Kim tries to make deals with God or with himself such as "If my cancer remits, I promise I won't smoke anymore"
Depression	Mr. Kim starts to feel sad or despondent
Acceptance	Mr. Kim realizes that he has cancer, starts to cope with the realities of having cancer, and starts to focus on the treatment and his day-to-day relationships

Table 16.2 Determining the differences between grief and depression (Block, 2000; Periyakoil and Hallenbeck, 2002)

Bereavement/grief	Depression
Occurs in most terminally ill patients	Occurs in 1–53 % of terminally ill patients
Grief/sadness relapses and remits and is triggered by loss/illness	The patient feels overwhelmed in all aspects of life. Depression is constant
The patient may still find pleasure in things	The patient does not enjoy anything
Somatic symptoms are present, including minor changes in sleep, appetite, concentration, and energy level	Somatic symptoms can be more severe, including severe sleep disturbances, significant weight loss
The patient may experience minor guilt. The patient maintains a sense of hope, but what is hoped for may shift with time	Severe guilt, worthlessness, hopelessness, and helplessness
The patient may have thoughts of a quick, pain-free, dignified death, but this is different from an active desire for death	Severe and persistent suicidal ideations
Able to look forward to things in the future	No positive outlook for future
The patient may have illusions about the deceased person	Overt psychotic symptoms: hallucinations and delusions
The patient tries to go back to a normal routine	Failure to go back to routine
Grooming and hygiene are good	Poor hygiene and grooming
Severe symptoms dissipate in < 2 months	Severe symptoms persisting beyond 2 months
	If left unaddressed, can have a direct impact on medical illness and care
Treatment includes increased support with loved ones, support groups, regular contact with physicians, counseling	Treatment can include antidepressants, stimulants, antipsychotics, and ECT
Medications, primarily to help with short-term issues such as sleep	

Case Vignette 16.1.3 Continuation

When discussing his medical issues, Mr. Kim describes his fear about what will happen to his body and his ability to function as he approaches death. He remembers watching his father die from gastric cancer and is worried that he will experience the same amount of pain. He states that if the pain became unbearable, he would want you to put him out of his misery like those people in the television special he saw on Dr. Jack Kevorkian. Mr. Kim tells you how important it is for him

*to have a dignified death. You pause to think about what other goals patients may
have at the end of life.*

 **Please proceed with the problem-based
approach!**

Although Mr. Kim brings up end-of-life issues on his own, for many patients,
these discussions are often avoided for various reasons including the following
(Larson and Tobin, 2000):

- Patient barriers: The patient may be scared, confused, unaware of the seriousness,
  or too embarrassed to approach the topic. Cultural or family factors may impede
  discussions as well.
- Physician barriers: The physician may feel too nervous to deliver bad news or
  may not feel adequately trained in delivering this type of news.
- Systems barriers: With multiple physicians treating the patient, it may be unclear
  who is responsible for bringing up this discussion.

In order to improve these end-of-life discussions, Balaban [2000] created a four-
step approach described below:

- Initiate end-of-life discussion:

  - Provide a supportive/sympathetic environment for the patient and his/her fam-
    ily by listening and encouraging open discussions.
  - Designate a surrogate decision maker.
  - Elicit the patient's general ideas about end-of-life care.

- Clarify prognosis:

  - Be frank yet compassionate about their prognosis.
  - It may be necessary to repeat explanations.
  - Clarify the patient's understanding.
  - Avoid medical jargon.

- Identify goals at the end of life:

  - See Table 16.3.
  - Discuss goals in terms of medical care.

- Create a treatment plan:

  - Help patients understand their medical options including where they will
    receive their care and about pain management.
  - Provide recommendations in terms of treatment.
  - Identify the patient's preferences with regard to resuscitation.
  - Discuss palliative care if appropriate.

Table 16.3 Common treatment goals at the end of life (Block, 2000; Larson and Tobin, 2000)

Goals	Ways to approach these topics
1. Maintain sense of identity and operate as independently as possible within the limits of illness and prognosis.	"What barriers prevent you from feeling comfortable and in control as you deal with your illness?" "How would you like your loved ones to remember you?" End-of-life discussions including treatment options can provide sense of control
2. To avoid/limit pain and suffering	"Is pain or the possibility of pain/suffering a concern for you?" Do not say: "There is not much that can be done for you" Instead say: "I believe there is much that can be done to manage your pain, provide you comfort, and assist you in living every day to its fullest"
3. Maintain/enhance important relationships and resolve conflicts with others	"Are there people in your life you want to get closer to or make up with?" "How do you want to tell your loved ones good bye?" Encourage families to share emotions and memories, and collect memorabilia
4. Pursue remaining dreams and setting goals	"When you think about your future, what is of greatest importance to you?" "Are there unresolved issues that you need to take care of and bring closure to?" Help patients come up with goals such as attending their son's wedding or going to a grandchild's graduation
5. Finding meaning in life and death	Patients often question what type of legacy they have left behind. Allowing patients to share memories, words of wisdom
6. Preparation for death: being able to hand over control to family and loved ones	"In what ways can you help your family prepare for and cope with your death?" Organize end-of-life plans (living wills, funeral arrangements) Having a frank conversation with the patients about their prognosis and what happens as they are about to die can be helpful Telling the patients that you will be there until the end can be reassuring to patients

During this case, Mr. Kim brought up his goal of having a "good death." End-of-life conversations should include finding out from patients what their goals are even if faced with a terminal illness. Some common goals that people have at the end of life and ways to phrase these conversations are provided in Table 16.3.

Pain Management in Palliative Care

Another issue that Mr. Kim was trying to ask is "Will my pain be addressed?" This is an important concern for many end-of-life patients that is often incompletely addressed as evident by the SUPPORT study (The SUPPORT Principal Investigators, 1995).

When evaluating pain for palliative care patients, the physician must assess etiology, quality, severity, timing, and relieving/exacerbating factors. Principles for pain management (particularly with cancer patients) include the following (World Health Organization, 1986; Jacox et al., 1994):

- Mild to moderate pain: nonopioid analgesics (NSAIDs, aspirin, acetaminophen) +/− adjunctive agents.
- Moderate to severe pain: addition of opioid analgesics, to provide additive analgesic effects.

  − Moderate pain: opioids like codeine or hydrocodone.
  − Moderate to severe pain: use higher potency opioids like morphine, methadone (long half-life), or fentanyl (short half-life).

- When prescribing for patients with chronic pain, it is better to have scheduled rather than PRN analgesics to decrease break-through pain.
- Other adjunctive agents can be used for various types of pain. Medications such as tricyclic antidepressants or gabapentin can be used in neuropathic pain.
- Behavioral techniques such as relaxation techniques, biofeedback, or cognitive restructuring can be used as well.
- Physical methods, such as heat/cold and acupuncture, may be tried.
- Treat co-morbid psychiatric conditions, which can increase the patient's subjective experience of pain.

Physician-Assisted Suicide and Euthanasia

Euthanasia is when the physician actively participates with intentionally ending a patient's life. It is illegal and considered a criminal act in all states but some countries like the Netherlands have regulated systems for it (Van der Heide, 2007).

Physician-assisted suicide (PAS) is when the physician provides the patient with medications, interventions, or information that the patient will use to commit suicide. While this is currently legal in Oregon, many medical organizations such as the American Medical Association have made statements against these practices (American Medical Association, 2005; Emanuel, 2002).

Many Americans support euthanasia and PAS for those in severe pain (Emanuel, 2002). Pain, however, does not appear to be the main reason why people request these interventions. Psychosocial and existential factors appear to play more of a role. According to a systematic review performed by Hudson et al. [2006], depression/hopelessness, burdening others, loss of autonomy, physical symptoms, anxiety about the future, and existential worries were common themes behind these requests.

If Mr. Kim were to bring up the topic of PAS/euthanasia, it would be important to consider the following:

- How serious is the request? → Was Mr. Kim just reacting to his current situation or was he actually seeking information or assistance?
- What is the underlying reason for wanting PAS/euthanasia? → Mr. Kim discussed his concerns about unaddressed pain.

- Do not assume that a decision is final. Studies have shown that depression and hopelessness have strongly been associated with requests for euthanasia or PAS and that such requests can dissipate with time (Chochinov et al., 1995; Emanuel, 2002).
- Assess for psychiatric symptoms and even consider a psychiatric consultation → is depression contributing to Mr. Kim's request?
- Find out about the patient's support system.
- Educate the patient that alternatives such as treatment withdrawal, aggressive management of pain (even if it may shorten the patient's life), and withholding fluids or nutrition are legal and is not considered PAS.

Case Vignette 16.1.4 Continuation

Over the next 2 weeks, Mr. Kim appears to have accepted his prognosis. You initiate a discussion about his end-of-life goals. He reflects on all the things he would still like to accomplish, especially since he has only been married to his wife for 2 years. He describes the plans they had to travel to Europe when he retired at 65. He also tells you that he has not spoken to his three adult children for several years after a bitter divorce from their mother and how he would like to reconcile with them. He worries about his wife, who also has multiple medical problems, and asks you if his death could possibly impact her health. You ask Mr. Kim whether faith or religion is an important part of his life. He says that he has not attended church in years but would like to speak with the hospital chaplain.

 Please proceed with the problem-based approach!

Impact of Death on the Surviving Spouse

Studies have shown that the loss of a spouse can significantly impact the physical and psychological health of the survivor. Rates of hospitalizations and mortality increase (Greenblatt, 1978) with higher rates from accidental, alcohol-related causes, and violent means and moderate increases from lung cancer and ischemic heart disease (Martikainen and Valkonen, 1996).

Spirituality and Religion at the End of Life

Physicians are often uncomfortable asking about faith, but as Mr. Kim has shown, spirituality can play an important role for the terminally ill. Research has shown that only 10 % of physicians discuss spirituality with their patients despite 65–95 %

of patients wanting this addressed (Puchalski, 2002). Thus, simply asking "Is your faith important to you in this illness?" can open up the discussion (Larson and Tobin, 2000).

Religion or spirituality can be the way that people explore the meaning of their death and cope with their dying process. Studies have shown that spiritual well-being can help with cognitive symptoms of depression in elderly medical inpatients (Koenig et al., 1995). It can also be a protective factor against despair experienced at the end of life (Puchalski, 2002).

Discussions about faith are important because many religions have certain beliefs about end-of-life care. Finding out the patient's religious background and specific needs during the dying process can show commitment to caring for the patient as a whole. For example, some religions want their religious leaders present at the time of death (Roman Catholics have last rites) or have special requests for the care of the body before and after the patient's death. Certain religions, such as Islam and Judaism, also have traditions that can impact autopsy or organ donation (Kahn et al., 2003)

Case Vignette 16.1.5 Continuation

Mr. Kim then asks you about hospice and about the process of organ donation because the social worker came in earlier asking if he would like more information. As you glance over his chart, you notice that his code status has not been addressed, therefore you ask him about his resuscitation wishes.

Hospice/Palliative Care

Mr. Kim asks you about hospice, but before this topic can be discussed further, the general principle of palliative care should be discussed. The goals of palliative care are to enhance quality of life and relieve pain and suffering for patients with advanced disease (Morrison and Meier, 2004). It is a multidisciplinary approach that addresses psychosocial as well as spiritual issues and offers support to patients and families. Palliative care may be offered alongside other medical treatments. It aims to neither quicken nor delay death.

In order to qualify for hospice, a patient must be deemed to be terminally ill with a life expectancy of 6 months or less (Morrison and Meier, 2004). The patient and their family's goals must be directed at symptom relief rather than curative treatments aimed at prolonging life.

Organ Donation

In this vignette, Mr. Kim asks about the process of organ donation and the criteria for it. Most sources for organs are brain-dead donors with intact circulation (Hauptman and O'Connon, 1987).

Previously, the criteria for organ donation were strict with potential donors being under 50 with limited co-morbid conditions. Today, there is no national standard in terms of absolute or relative contraindications. Transplant centers each have their own criteria, often on a case-by-case basis because of the few absolute contraindications. Patients and their families may need to understand the concept of brain death and the process of organ donation in order to decide what is best for them.

Case Vignette 16.1.6 Continuation

After discussing his code status with you, Mr. Kim decides that he does not want life-sustaining measures if there is no hope for recovery or if he is unable to interact with his family. He names his wife as his Durable Power of Attorney (DPOA) in case he becomes incapacitated and is unable to make medical decisions for himself.

Several days later, Mr. Kim's respiratory function rapidly deteriorates. He becomes increasingly hypoxic and less responsive. Sensing the gravity of his situation, you gather his family members, including his estranged children.

Because of his previously stated wishes, you prepare to deliver comfort care to minimize his feelings of dyspnea as well as his bony pain. There is conflict, however, among the newly arrived family members. They are pushing for intubation despite the patient's wishes. You are frustrated by Mr. Kim's children who demand aggressive treatment against his stated wishes.

End-of-Life Discussions with Family Members

The conflict between Mr. Kim's and his family's wishes is a common theme seen in the hospital. Here are some ways to address this issue (Balaban, 2000; Weissman, 2004):

- Understand that acceptance of the patient's prognosis occurs differently for different people. Often times it is more difficult for families to accept the patient's impending death than it is for the patient.
- Go over clinical information with the patient and his/her family in a manner that is simple and jargon-free.
- Allow the patient and his/her family time to express their feelings and ask questions.
- Sometimes families want "everything done" despite the patient having a poor prognosis. In these cases, it is important to uncover the underlying motivation. Assessing the family dynamics can provide insight into unresolved issues or conflicts. Occasionally, families may not realize the futility of treatment; therefore, prognosis should be discussed.
- If these discussions are unable to progress, the ethics committee or legal counsel can help.

Case Vignette 16.1.7 Continuation

You arrange a family meeting to ascertain the family's understanding of Mr. Kim's condition and overall prognosis. His children repeatedly ask, "Why can't we use machines to help him breathe so we can keep him alive until he recovers?" They also ask why he is unresponsive and whether he is brain dead. You explain to them the difference between coma and brain death.

Diagnosing Death

Mr. Kim's family brings up a topic that can often be confusing for families. Table 16.4 helps to distinguish between persistent vegetative state (PVS), coma, and brain death. While there are differences in opinion with what to do with patients in a PVS, if a patient is diagnosed as being brain dead, they are considered legally dead. Once a person is considered legally dead, organ donation can commence and life support can be disconnected.

Case Vignette 16.1.8 Conclusion

Soon after the family meeting, there is a call from Mr. Kim's nurse saying that he is increasingly tachycardic and tachypneic. Family members at the bedside are distressed by his breathing pattern and are asking for measures to make him comfortable. "He looks like he's drowning. Can't you do something?" After you give him morphine to make him feel better, he eventually becomes more hypoxic with agonal breathing, progressing to complete unresponsiveness and asystole.

Table 16.4 Differentiating between various states of conscious (Multi-Society Task Force on PVS, 1994)

Persistent vegetative state	Coma	Brain death
The patient is awake and has sleep/wake cycles but is unaware of himself/herself and his/her surroundings	Sustained unconsciousness Can progress to consciousness, PVS, or death	Irreversibly comatose Legally dead; therefore, life support is futile
Hypothalamic and brain-stem autonomic functioning is intact but there are no purposeful responses to stimuli	Due to dysfunction in the ascending reticular activating system (which can be damaged at the site of the brain stem or both cerebral hemispheres). The patient is unable to be aroused, and this status lasts longer than 1 h	Absence of all brain functions including the brain stem, reflexes, and cranial nerves

As you are performing the "death pronouncement," you can hear the family sob-bing at the bedside. You then turn to them and say "I'm very sorry. When you are ready, we can meet in the family room where we can talk and I can answer any questions you may have."

Please proceed with the problem-based approach!

How to Address the Family at the Time of Death (Jurkovich et al. 2000; Williams et al., 2000)

Addressing Mr. Kim's death with his family is difficult, but here are some ways to improve these conversations with families:

- Meet the family in a private area. Identify their relationships to the deceased.
- Families like to be told in a sympathetic and unrushed manner what happened. Use the patient's name rather than "the patient." Advise them if an autopsy is required.
- Allow the family to ask questions and express their feelings.
- Allow them time to view the deceased, and prepare them if there are any medical devices left or if the body has been altered physically.
- Assist the family with what to do next (e.g., how to make funeral arrangements, when they can go home).
- Offer to request a visit from a pastoral counselor.
- Give handouts about the grieving process.

Review Questions

1. Which of the following is more likely a sign of depression rather than attributable to a grief reaction?

    a. Difficulty sleeping for several days
    b. Minor guilt
    c. Feelings of worthlessness

2. What are the stages of grief?
3. What are the three goals people commonly have at the end of life?
4. What is a typical pharmacologic approach to treating cancer patients with mod-erate to severe pain?

5. What are the goals of palliative care?
6. True/False:

   a. Euthanasia is legal in the USA.
   b. Physician-assisted suicide is illegal in all states.

7. Is a patient in a persistent vegetative state considered brain dead?

References

American Medical Association. E-2.211 Physician-assisted suicide. Last updated 2005. http://www.ama-assn.org/ama/pub/category/8459.html. Accessed 11/1/07.

Balaban RB. A physician's guide to talking about end-of-life care. Journal of General Internal Medicine 2000; 3: 195–200.

Block SD. Assessing and managing depression in the terminally ill patient. Annals of Internal Medicine 2000; 132: 209–218.

Cancer pain relief. Geneva: World Health Organization, 1986.

Chochinov HM, Wilson KG, Enns M, Mowchun N, Lander S, Levitt M, and Clinch JJ. Desire for death in the terminally ill. American Journal of Psychiatry 1995; 152: 1185–1191.

Emanuel EJ. Euthanasia and physician-assisted suicide. Archives of Internal Medicine 2002; 162: 142–152.

Greenblatt M. The grieving spouse. American Journal of Psychiatry 1978; 135: 43–47.

Hauptman PJ and O'Connon KJ. Procurement and allocation of solid organs for transplantation. New England Journal of Medicine 1987; 333(6): 422–431.

Hudson PL, Kristjanson LJ, Ashby M, Kelly B, Schofield P, Hudson R, Aranda S, O'Connor M, and Street A. Desire for hastened death in patients with advanced disease and the evidence based of clinical guidelines: a systematic review. Palliative Medicine 2006; 20; 693–701.

Jacox A, Carr DB, and Payne R. New clinical-practice guidelines for the management of pain in patients with cancer. New England Journal of Medicine 1994; 330: 651–655.

Jurkovich GJ, Pierce B, Pananen L, and Rivara FP. Giving bad new: the family perspective. The Journal of Trauma: Injury, Infection, and Critical Care 2000; 48: 865–870.

Kahn MJ, Lazarus CJ, and Owens DP. Journal of Clinical Oncology 2003; 21(15): 3000–3002.

Koenig HG, Cohen HJ, Blazer DG, Kudler HS, Krishnan KR, and Sibert TE. Religious coping and cognitive symptoms of depression in elderly medical patients. Psychosomatics 1995; 36(4): 369–375.

Kubler-Ross E. On death and dying. New York: Macmillan, 1969.

Larson DG and Tobin DR. End of life conversations. Journal of the American Medical Association 2000; 284(12): 1573–1578.

Martikainen P and Valkonen T. Mortality after the death of a spouse: rates and causes of death in a large Finnish cohort. American Journal of Public Health 1996; 86(8): 1087–1093.

Morrison RS and Meier ED. Palliative care. New England Journal of Medicine 2004; 350(25): 2582–2590.

Multi-Society Task Force on PVS. Medical aspects of the persistent vegetative state—first of two parts. New England Journal of Medicine 1994; 330; 1499–1508.

Periyakoil VS and Hallenbeck J. Identifying and managing preparatory grief and depression at the end of life. American Family Physician 2002; 65(5): 883–890, 897–898.

Puchalski CM. Spirituality and end-of-life care: a time for listening and caring. Journal of Palliative Medicine 2002; 5(2): 289–294.

The SUPPORT Principal Investigators. A controlled trial to improve care for seriously ill hospitalized patients. The study to understand prognoses and preferences for outcomes and risks of treatments (SUPPORT). Journal of the American Medical Association 1995; 274(2): 1591–1598.

Van der Heide A, Onwuteaka-Philipsen BD, Rurup ML, Buiting HM, Van Delden JJM, Hanssen-de Wolf JE, Jansses AGJM, Pasman HRW, Rietjens JAC, Prins CJM, Deerenberg IM, Geveres JKM, Van der Maas PJ, and Van der Wal G. End-of-life practices in the Netherlands under the Euthanasia Act. New England Journal of Medicine 2007; 356: 1957–1965.

Weissman DE. Decision making at a time of crisis near the end of life. Journal of the American Medical Association 2004; 292(14): 1738–1743.

Williams G, O'Brien DL, Laughton KJ, and Jelin GA. Improving services to bereaved relatives in the emergency department: making healthcare more human. Medical Journal of Australia 2000; 173: 480–483.

Part IV
Behavioral Neuroscience and Clinical Psychiatry

Chapter 17
Basic Principles of Evaluation: Interviewing, Mental Status Examination, Differential Diagnosis, and Treatment Planning

Anthony P.S. Guerrero, Daniel A. Alicata, and Nathanael W. Cardon

This chapter helps bring everything you are learning full circle as we discuss the actual patient encounter. We compare and contrast the psychiatric evaluation to that of general medicine and describe what is expected in your psychiatric clerkship as you examine, diagnose, and develop a treatment plan. This chapter provides the context for applying the principles of psychiatry.

At the end of this chapter, the reader will be able to

1. Discuss the basic structural components of a psychiatric interview, including history and mental status examination
2. Discuss the basic principles to guide the process of an effective interview, including establishing and maintaining rapport, prioritizing safety, and efficiently gathering data sufficient to yield a differential diagnosis
3. Discuss the process of differential diagnosis according to the DSM-IV-TR
4. Discuss the process of bio-psycho-social-cultural-spiritual formulation and treatment planning

Case Vignette 17.1.1 Dan, Tony, and Melissa

Dan, Tony, and Melissa are second-year medical students who are starting their "brain and behavior" clinical skills preceptorship. They are quite apprehensive about performing their first interview, because they believe that "everything is totally different when it comes to 'psych'."

Students often worry that the basic history and examination skills they learned on other clinical services will not work in psychiatric settings. In reality, the entire assessment and treatment planning process learned in other parts of medicine are completely relevant to psychiatry, with a few relevant adaptations, as shown in Table 17.1.

A.P.S. Guerrero
Associate Professor of Psychiatry and Pediatrics, Associate Chair for Education and Training, Department of Psychiatry, University of Hawai'i John A. Burns School of Medicine

A. Guerrero, M. Piasecki (eds.), *Problem-Based Behavioral Science and Psychiatry*,
© Springer Science+Business Media, LLC 2008

Table 17.1 Components of the psychiatric assessment

Traditional "medical exam" component	Psychiatric assessment component
Identifying data	Same
Source and reliability	Same
Chief complaint	Same
History of the present illness, with attention to "pertinent positives" and "pertinent negatives"	Same—with attention to the psychiatric review of systems and the different psychiatric and general medical conditions that should be "ruled in" and "ruled out"
Past medical history	Same *plus* a specific past psychiatric history
Family history	Same—with attention to psychiatric conditions
Social history	Same—often more lengthy because of the role of social factors in psychiatric illness
Review of systems	Same—because general medical conditions (detectable in the review of systems) can often explain psychiatric symptoms
Physical examination	Same—with more emphasis on the neurological exam and the MSE as a detailed branch step of the physical examination
	Mental status examination (described further below)
Problem list and assessment of each problem	Psychiatric formulation and differential diagnosis, based on the DSM-IV-TR
Plan, with additional information/diagnostic testing, specific treatments, and patient education	Same

Case Vignette 17.1.2 Continuation

The three students feel less anxious, knowing that they can apply the skills that they have already learned. They successfully meet the requirements of the preceptorship.

The three students are now third-year medical students new to the psychiatry clerkship. They each are about to do their first patient interview for the clerkship. Dan, who received positive recognition in his previous clerkships for his patience and his excellent bedside manner, states: "All I need to do is listen, and I think the patient will tell me what I need to know in 30 minutes (which is the time allotted to the interview)." Tony, who was recognized in his previous clerkships for his high exam scores, states: "I think I have everything figured out: all I need to do is ask the patient everything in this master template that I made, and everything will be fine." Finally, Melissa, who was recognized in her previous clerkships for her overall stellar performance, states: "I've never had a problem interviewing patients. I just need to get Honors in this clerkship because I want to go into a competitive specialty."

Following their first interview, the three students are flustered. In a de-briefing meeting with their clinical supervisor, Dan states: "I couldn't get a word in during the interview. All I was able to find out was that this patient is married and that he is a Christian. I was totally lost during the rest of the interview, and I didn't want to interrupt him because it seemed like he would get mad." Tony states: "Even though I kept telling the patient how important it was to answer all of my questions, all he could do was give one-word answers, look quickly from one side of the room to the next, and then ask to go back to his room ... which he did anyway after only 15 minutes. I ran out of time and we didn't even get to why he overdosed." Melissa states: "Because my patient kept crying so much, I didn't get a chance to test all of that important stuff for psychiatry, like ask about rolling stones gathering no moss and what to do with a stamped envelope."

Their supervisor, hoping to help their subsequent interviews with these patients to go smoother, encourages them to think of the interview as an opportunity to apply the problem-based approach. "What do you mean?" they ask. The preceptor encourages them to proceed with a modification of the familiar problem-based approach.

Although this is not the typical problem-based learning scenario, use of a modified PBL table may be helpful in guiding the process of the interview, as shown in Table 17.2.

 Please proceed with the problem-based approach!

Table 17.2 Modified PBL table for Case Vignette 17.1.2

What are the observations about the process of the interview?	What are the hypotheses about why the interview is going this way?	What might I need to ask about and/or do next?
(for Dan) Difficult to interrupt patient "I'm lost"	Bipolar mania Schizophrenia Methamphetamine intoxication	Summarize, ask clarifying questions Do one's best to elicit relevant history
(for Tony) One-word answers Looking quickly from one side of the room to the next Wants to go back to room	Suspicion about the interview process Irritability from depression	Ask about and try to optimize patient's comfort Re-orient patient to purpose and context of interview Do one's best to elicit relevant history
(for Melissa) Crying so much	Depression Grief	Recognize patient's emotions and provide empathic comments as appropriate

While the structural elements of the psychiatric interview are essentially identical to elements of the general medical interview, a distinguishing characteristic of psychiatric interviewing is the likelihood that the very illness that one is trying to assess (such as the primary mood or psychotic disorder that Dan's patient above likely was demonstrating symptoms of) may impact the very *process* of the interview. Whenever something unexpected happens in an interview (ranging from intense tearfulness, to a request to leave the interview early, to an unusual question being asked of the interviewer), the most appropriate next step is often to use this occurrence as an opportunity to gather more information about what might be happening. For example: "I notice that you're really wanting to go back to your room . . . We'll be done in a few minutes, but I wonder if you could tell me what you're thinking right now or if there's anything we could do to help you feel more comfortable right now."

Even though it is easy to remember what the structural elements of an interview should be, students often feel challenged in getting through a "complete interview" in a time-limited period—which often needs to be done in real-life situations. We suggest that, during a time-limited interview, students should establish the following priorities:

1. *Attempt to establish and maintain rapport through*

   - Unconditional positive regard for the patient and attentiveness to patient comfort. This can be conveyed through a friendly demeanor and supportive and empathic statements ("That must have been a tough time for you").
   - Adequate preparation for the interview (explaining the context).
   - Appropriate use of open-ended (yet context-appropriate) questions, such as "What happened that led to your hospitalization?" or "Could you tell me more about that?" or "What's your understanding of what the medications are being prescribed for?"
   - Responsiveness to the patient's emotions and other potential barriers to effective rapport. For example, Tony observed irritation in his interview, and Melissa observed overwhelming sadness during her patient interview but neither responded to the patient's mood state. Failure to address such barriers may interfere with subsequent data-gathering and may be more time-costly in the long run.

2. *Assess safety, specifically*

   - Suicidality and thoughts of violence toward others: current ideations as well as previous dangerousness, command hallucinations, acute stressors, mood symptoms; and (if a recent attempt had been made), degree of premeditation (including suicide notes and other preparatory acts), method of discovery, perception of lethality, and what the patient perceives as having changed since the attempt. (Apparently, Tony did not prioritize this in his interview).
   - Abuse and being victimized (particularly for minors and dependent adults).

- Serious psychotic symptoms that impair reality testing and would interfere with a patient's ability to meet basic needs.
- Serious general medical conditions.
- Substance intoxication and/or withdrawal (which could be life-threatening).

3. *Attempt to elicit history and examination findings to at least establish a differential diagnosis* (not necessarily the definitive diagnosis—which may be unrealistic to determine in a short period of time):

- Pertinent positives and pertinent negatives, based on criteria from the *Diagnostic and Statistical Manual of Mental Disorders*, currently in its fourth edition, text revision (DSM-IV-TR).
- To the degree possible, review of the key areas of history and psychiatric review of systems.

Another distinguishing characteristic of the psychiatric interview is the need to thoughtfully perform a mental status examination (MSE). While it may initially seem (as it probably did to Melissa) that the mental status examination is an academic exercise with little relevance to the rest of medicine, each of the elements has practical clinical relevance and represents an indirect assessment of neurological functions. Detailed descriptions of observations are more clinically relevant than clinical jargon. A good MSE will "paint a picture" of the patient at the time of the exam. The components of the MSE are summarized in Table 17.3.

Following the psychiatric interview and mental status examination is the bio-psycho-social-cultural-spiritual formulation (discussed in Chap. 1) and a differential diagnosis according to the DSM-IV-TR, which describes diagnostic assessment according to the following five axes:

Axis I Major psychiatric conditions (all psychiatric conditions other than personality disorders and mental retardation; includes substance use disorders)
Axis II Personality disorders and mental retardation
Axis III General medical conditions
Axis IV Stressors (e.g., primary support group, occupational, educational, legal, other social)
Axis V Global assessment of functioning: current and in the past year (on a scale of 0–100; examples: 70 = mild impairment, 60 = moderate impairment, 50 = severe impairment, 40 = impairment of reality testing, 20 and below = acute dangerousness)

It may sometimes seem that the checklist approach used by the DSM-IV-TR for diagnosing psychiatric disorders is "cookbook" medicine because there is no "gold standard" along the lines of a definitive blood test or histopathological finding. However, it should be noted that other medical conditions, such as rheumatologic disorders and disorders affecting multiple systems, are diagnosed and very effectively treated through a similar approach.

Table 17.3 Components of the mental status examination

Mental status examination component	How assessed	Sample descriptive terms	Part(s) of the brain being tested or neurobiologic mechanisms	Examples of practical clinical relevance
General appearance	Observation	Well developed, well nourished, thin, overweight, good/poor hygiene, no obvious deformities, etc.	Multiple	Patients whose illness affects ability to care for self may have significant findings on general appearance
Eye contact	Observation	Good, adequate, fair, poor, etc.	Multiple	May be decreased as a result of depression or distraction from hallucinations, etc.
Cooperation with interview	Observation	Cooperative with interview, guarded, etc.	Multiple	Several conditions can impact upon rapport
Motor activity	Observation; sometimes formal testing for abnormal motor movements, tremor, and/or rigidity	Psychomotor agitation or retardation (or none), abnormal motor movements (or none), tremor and/or rigidity present (or not)	Basal ganglia, motor cortex, other areas	Major depression may cause psychomotor retardation, while mania may case psychomotor agitation. Antipsychotic medications may cause abnormal motor movements, tremor, and/or rigidity
Speech	Observation	Normal or increased or decreased rate and/or volume and/or amount; normal (or not) clarity	Multiple areas, including speech centers	Mood disorders and/or substance intoxication may affect the rate, volume, and/or amount of speech. Neurological conditions (that may also cause psychiatric symptoms) may affect clarity of speech
Mood—expressed emotional state	Direct questioning about how the patient has been feeling; rate mood from 1 to 10, 10 = best possible	Euthymic, depressed, anxious, expansive, irritable	Hypothalamus, limbic system, other parts	Mood disorders and/or substances may affect patient's reported mood and observed affect

Table 17.3 (continued)

Mental status examination component	How assessed	Sample descriptive terms	Part(s) of the brain being tested or neurobiologic mechanisms	Examples of practical clinical relevance
Affect—observed emotional state	Observation	Mood-congruency (mood-congruent, mood-incongruent) Range (broad, restricted, flat) Lability (labile or not) Overall quality (neutral, depressed, anxious, euphoric, irritable)		
Thought process	Observation	Linear (remains on topic) and goal-directed, circumstantial (goes off topic but eventually returns to the original topic), tangential (goes off topic without ever returning to the original topic), flight of ideas (without production of a coherent thought), word salad (in which even the individual words may not coherently link together)	Inappropriate mesolimbic dopamine release, poor cortical filtering; other areas	Primary psychotic disorders such as schizophrenia and/or substances may affect thought processes
Thought content	Observation, some direct questions	Delusions (present or not, with specific examples); paranoid ideations (present or not, with specific examples); future orientation; etc.		Primary psychotic disorders such as schizophrenia and/or substances may affect result in delusions; depression with suicidal ideations may lead to a patient not having a future orientation

Table 17.3 (continued)

Mental status examination component	How assessed	Sample descriptive terms	Part(s) of the brain being tested or neurobiologic mechanisms	Examples of practical clinical relevance
Perceptions	Direct questions, with some observation for distractibility of other evidence of response to internal stimuli	Auditory and visual hallucinations (present or not); appearance (or not) of seeming to respond to hallucinations; other hallucinations (e.g., tactile, olfactory, etc.) also important to note if present	See above, relevant sensory cortices (auditory, visual, etc.)	Primary psychotic disorders such as schizophrenia, substances, and/or delirium may result in hallucinations
Alertness	Observation	Alert, drowsy, stuporous, comatose	Reticular activating system	Delirium may cause fluctuations in level of alertness
Orientation	Direct questions, with some observation	Oriented (or not) to person, place, time (date, month, year), situation	Often depends on alertness and memory	Delirium may cause disorientation. Other memory-impairing conditions such as dementia may cause disorientation
Concentration	Direct questions, with some observation	Able (or not) to perform serial 7's ("take the number 100, subtract 7, and then keep subtracting 7 from your answer until I tell you to stop…") Able (or not) to spell five-letter words such as "world" or "ocean" backward. (Usually, one of these tests will suffice)	Reticular activating system	Delirium primarily affects alertness and concentration
Memory	Direct questions	Ability to immediately recall three unrelated words that are not objects in the room (e.g., "umbrella," "car," "happiness") and to recall these words approximately 5 minutes later (if not spontaneously recalled, prompting or giving hints may suggest more impairment of memory retrieval than memory storage) Longer-term memory may be assessed by asking the last five presidents, etc.	Hippocampus (memory encoding), other parts of the cerebral cortex	Dementia results in memory impairment along with other cognitive findings. Cortical dementias are associated with memory storage difficulties, while subcortical dementias are associated with memory retrieval difficulties

Table 17.3 (continued)

Mental status examination component	How assessed	Sample descriptive terms	Part(s) of the brain being tested or neurobiologic mechanisms	Examples of practical clinical relevance
Abstraction	Direct questions	Ability (or not) to state similarities (e.g., apple and orange are both fruits, table and a chair are both furniture, newspaper and radio both tell the news, opera and a painting are both forms of art) or accurately interpret proverbs (though proverbs often test more than just abstraction)	Frontal lobe	Schizophrenia often is associated with frontal lobe maldevelopment
Judgment	Observation, possibly direct questions	Ability (or not) to exercise good judgment with regards self-care, behaving appropriately	Frontal lobe	As above
Insight	Observation, possibly direct questions	Insight into illness, need for treatment	Frontal lobe	As above
Suicidality, homicidality, violence	Direct questions	Presence or absence: ideations and/or intentions	Multiple areas	Important to explicitly cover, in the interests of safety

General medical conditions and substance-induced conditions, while often over-looked, are important to include in the differential diagnosis of many Axis I conditions.

The final step of the psychiatric assessment is to develop a treatment plan that adequately considers the formulation and differential diagnosis. Please refer to Chap. 1 for a diagrammatic illustration of how a successful plan addresses the various components of a bio-psycho-social-cultural-spiritual for-mulation. The following shown in Table 17.4 helps to develop a comprehensive plan.

We close, in Appendix, with a sample write-up of a fictitious patient (with grati-tude to George Lucas, creator of the Star Wars series, where many of the arbitrarily chosen fictitious names came from).

Table 17.4 Treatment planning template

	Biological	Psychological	Social/cultural
Additional information	Old records (e.g., to look at previous diagnoses and medication efficacy) Insure a recent physical exam Relevant labs, for example: Chemistry profile Complete blood count Thyroid function tests Tests to rule out infection (e.g., syphilis, HIV) Toxicology screen Neuroimaging	Additional interviews Speak with previous therapists, etc. Psychological testing: for example, intelligence testing, personality testing, projective testing (to evaluate for psychotic processes)	Talk to family, others if patient gives consent
Treatment	Continue effective medications, usually abstinence from substances	Individual psychotherapy to build rapport Groups—e.g., anger management, Alco-holics/Narcotics Anonymous	Family psychotherapy if appropriate Social services, stable living Structured setting—e.g., to remain safe, substance-free, etc. Other resources
Patient education (often covered above)	Education on benefits and side effects of medications	Psychoeducation on need for compliance, crisis resources, etc.	Family psychoeducation as appropriate

Review Questions

1. You are interviewing a patient, who suddenly becomes very quiet and possibly tearful when the topic of her childhood is discussed. The next most appropriate thing to do is to

    (a) Switch the topic to something less sensitive.
    (b) Immediately perform a cognitive examination.
    (c) Recognize the change in affect and empathically acknowledge the likely difficulty in discussing such a topic.
    (d) Immediately terminate the interview and postpone any further attempts at interview until the patient can regain composure.
    (e) Reassure the patient that you know exactly how she feels, and that it is perfectly okay to cry.

2. During the course of a diagnostic interview, your patient asks, for a second time, "Doctor, how old are you, anyway?" Which of the following is the best response?

    (a) "Once again, this interview is about you, not about me, so let's talk about something else."
    (b) "I'm old enough to be a physician and old enough to be interviewing you."
    (c) "I'm very uncomfortable talking about my personal life with patients."
    (d) "I notice that you're really interested in how old I am. I wonder what your thoughts are behind wanting to know."
    (e) "I'm somewhere between 20 and 60."

3. All of the following statements are correct EXCEPT

    (a) Affect describes one's observation of the patient's emotions during the interview.
    (b) Mood describes what the patient's emotional state has generally been.
    (c) Mood can be elicited through direct questioning of how the patient has been feeling.
    (d) Tangential thoughts never return to the original topic or question.
    (e) Circumstantiality is pathognomonic for a psychotic disorder.

4. Which of the following statements best describes the role of testing "serial 7's"?

    (a) Difficulties with this test may indicate delirium.
    (b) This test is intended to primarily test mathematical abilities.
    (c) Difficulties with this test always reflect dysfunction of the reticular activating system.
    (d) Psychotic individuals invariably have difficulty with this test.
    (e) This test must always be done in combination with asking the patient to spell "world" forward and backward and recall digit spans.

5. Which of the following statements about psychiatric assessment are correct?

    (a) A bio-psycho-social-cultural-spiritual formulation, because of its inherent inclusion of "psychiatric jargon" terms, is rarely useful for patients or other health professionals involved in patient care.

(b) Effective rapport is the foundation for all patient interviews, whether in psychiatry or in any other specialty of medicine.

(c) Psychiatrists should never perform physical examinations or order laboratory studies.

(d) Assessment of safety is merely an assessment of current suicidal or homicidal ideations.

(e) Learning disorders and pervasive developmental disorders are noted on Axis II.

Answers

1. c, 2. d, 3. e, 4. a, 5. b

Appendix Sample Write-Up

Name: Luke Skywalker, MS3
Attending Psychiatrist: Master Yoda, M.D.
Date: 05/01/2008
Identifying Data: Princess Leia is a 34-year-old cosmopolitan female, divorced, employed as a secretary.
Reason for Examination: Psychiatric consultation for patient on the general medical ward; medical student write-up #1.

> Summarize information relevant for eventual formulation and differential diagnosis

Referring Physician: Obi-Wan Kenobi, M.D. (internal medicine).
Source and Reliability: Patient, who appears fairly reliable. Chart also reviewed.
Chief Complaint: Acetaminophen overdose.

History of the Present Illness:

Ms. Leia is a 34-year-old female admitted last night for an acetaminophen, acetaminophen/oxycodone, and ibuprofen overdose. This overdose occurred late yesterday afternoon (Saturday) at her apartment. She ingested several extra strength acetaminophen tablets, a few acetaminophen/oxycodone tablets, and a few ibuprofen tablets following an argument with her boyfriend over his recent infidelity. This argument started on Friday night and caused her to essentially not sleep the whole night. Immediately following the ingestion, she called her boyfriend, who then brought her to the emergency room, from where she was subsequently admitted because of an acetaminophen level in the toxic range.

> Assess safety

Ms. Leia states that she thought that she would die as a result of the ingestion, but denies that she had been premeditating the act prior to yesterday's argument. She denies having left a suicide note and denies any history of giving away possessions in preparation for death. She says that what she did was "the dumbest thing I've ever done" and that she's "grateful to be alive." She cannot really say what has changed in their relationship, but says, "no matter what happens, it's not worth dying for."

Ms. Leia denies any past history of suicide attempts, command hallucinations telling her to commit suicide, or any intoxication at the time of the overdose. She notes that, for the past 4 months, she has had, more days than not, a depressed mood related to relationship difficulties, associated with: decreased enjoyment of usually pleasurable activities (e.g., going out with her friends, playing with her 6-year-old son at the beach), terminal insomnia (e.g., waking up at 3 am and not being able to go back to sleep), increased appetite with an unintentional 5-pound weight gain, decreased energy level, feelings of worthlessness, and difficulty concentrating in her job. She admits to some degree of sensitivity to perceived rejection—for example, crying when her friends go somewhere without her, or when her boyfriend is unable to make it for a planned date.

Past Psychiatric History:

> Pertinent positives and negatives

Ms. Leia reports that when she was around 28 years old, she experienced similar symptoms during the ending of her 5-year marriage to her ex-husband. In retrospect, she believes that her symptoms started within about 1 month following the birth of her son. She saw a psychiatrist (Dr. Qui-Gon Jinn) and took fluoxetine for around 9 months. She reports that the fluoxetine was helpful and stopped this medication because she felt she no longer needed it.

She denies any history of manic symptoms (e.g., sustained abnormally elevated mood, racing thoughts, decreased need for sleep, rapid speech, psychomotor agitation, grandiosity, impulsive spending).

She admits to sometimes feeling, especially in the past 4 months, a fast heartbeat and lightheadedness associated with feeling "stressed and overwhelmed with everything that's going on." These feelings would last less than a minute and would occur no more frequently than every few weeks. She denies any history of feeling any impending sense of doom during these instances, and she denies any worry about feeling these symptoms again in between these instances. She denies any history of repetitive, intrusive thoughts or behaviors. She also denies any history of anxiety in places where she may be under public scrutiny. In terms of any exposure to trauma, she reports having been involved in a car accident when she was 8 years old. Her mother's car was rear-ended on the freeway by a large truck, resulting in her mother needing to be hospitalized overnight. She says she coped reasonably well with this incident, and she denies any nightmares, flashbacks, or other re-experiencing phenomena related to this incident. She denies any past experience of physical or sexual abuse, and she denies any physical abuse in her current relationship.

She admits to drinking socially since age 18 or 19. The last time she had anything to drink was last week, with her friends. She reports only having one or two drinks each time. She denies any history of alcoholic blackouts, hallucinations related to drinking, or withdrawal seizures. She responded negatively to all components of the "CAGE" questionnaire. She denies any other history of substance use.

She denies any history of binging (e.g., eating large quantities of food in one sitting, feeling a lack of control over eating) or purging behavior.

Past Medical History:

Ms. Leia is otherwise healthy, without any chronic health problems. She denies any past history of seizures, major head trauma, or loss of consciousness. However, she notes that she had her wisdom teeth extracted 5 days ago and is still experiencing a significant amount of discomfort.

Ms. Leia has been pregnant only once, with her 6-year-old son. She reports a history of irritability and sadness before and during her menstrual periods. She has just started her menstrual period and denies any possibility of current pregnancy.

Current medications: acetaminophen/oxycodone.

Allergies: ALLERGIC TO PENICILLIN, WHICH CAUSES HIVES.

Family History:

Ms. Leia believes that her father (65 years old) may have developed depression following a heart attack. He was prescribed an antidepressant, which he took for about 1 year. Her brother also had a history of school difficulties and marijuana abuse as a teenager. She denies any other known family history of depression, completed suicides, other psychiatric disorders, or substance abuse. She has a maternal aunt with a history of hypothyroidism, for which she takes thyroid replacement on an ongoing basis.

(OPTIONAL graphic depiction)

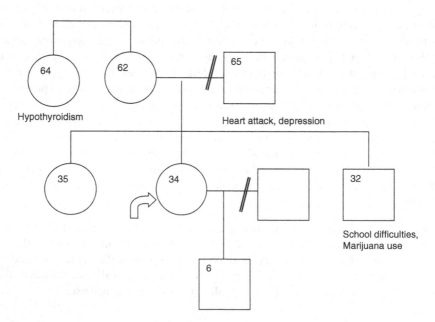

Developmental and Social History:

Ms. Leia grew up in Honolulu. Her parents divorced when she was 3 years of age. She denies that there was any domestic violence around the divorce, only arguing. She recalls being sad when her parents divorced, but admits that she does not really remember details. Her mother raised her. While growing up, she had infrequent contact with her father, who remarried. She reports that she did not get along well with her mother, because her mother was "too strict."

Ms. Leia reports having had difficulties in school, especially in math. She reports having been in special education for a few years. She denies any particular difficulty with concentrating/paying attention in school. She dropped out of 11th grade because she was "sick of school" and wanted to be with her boyfriend at the time. She completed her GED at age 18 years. She would like to return to school sometime and obtain a college degree, perhaps in education or psychology. She has held various jobs: as a cashier, food service provider, and office secretary. Most recently, she has worked as a secretary for a research company for the past 3 years.

Ms. Leia had been married to the father of her 6-year-old son for 5 years. Prior to that, she had only been in one long-term serious relationship (from high school). She reports that the marriage ended "mostly because he started getting more and more into drinking and I couldn't count on him to be around anymore." There had not been any domestic violence. She has been with her current boyfriend for the past 2 years. She reports that they had been arguing more especially in the past 5 or 6 months, generally over his ongoing friendship with ex-girlfriends.

Ms. Leia lives with her 6-year-old son. Her sister and brother help to provide childcare while she is at work. Her son stays with his father (who shares legal custody) during the weekends and was not with her during the time of the ingestion. She states that she misses her son when he is at his father's place. Her ex-husband pays child support, but still notes that it's "hard to make ends meet" especially now that her son has started private school at their local church. She currently sees her mother at least once per week and talks to her father around once every few months. She feels close to her older sister and sees her frequently during the week. Her sister has come to visit her in the hospital and has been supportive.

Ms. Leia is active in church and reports that her friends from church are also very supportive. When she stopped seeing Dr. Qui-Gon Jinn, she had hoped she could stay emotionally well if she prayed and talked regularly to her pastor.

Ms. Leia denies having any access to firearms or other weapons.

Review of Systems:

Constitutional: History of weight gain, decreased energy level.
Eyes: Negative.

ENT: History of recent extraction of wisdom teeth.

CV: For the past 4 months, occasional fast heartbeat and lightheadedness when she is anxious. No history of any chest pain, shortness of breath, or other cardiac symptoms.

Respiratory: Negative.

GI: Some nausea following overdose; otherwise negative.

GU: Regular urinary pattern, no discharge. Recently started menses.

Musculoskeletal: Negative.

Skin: Negative.

Neuro: Negative. No headaches, speech/gait abnormalities, weakness, numbness, paresthesias.

Psych: Depressed mood, suicidal ideation (see HPI).

Endocrine: No known history of thyroid disease. Endorses some history of feeling cold easily, even when others feel warm.

All others: Negative.

Physical examination:

Constitutional: Well developed, well nourished, no acute distress. Normal body habitus, no obvious deformities. Adequate groom; dressed in hospital gown. Vital signs: temperature 98.6 °F, pulse 72 per minute, BP 110/70, RR 18, SaO_2 100 % in RA.

Eyes: Pupils 3 mm, reactive.

Musculoskeletal: No abnormal movements, rigidity, or tremor. Appears to have normal use of all extremities.

Skin: Warm and dry, no diaphoresis.

Mental Status Examination:

Eye contact: Good. Cooperation with interview: Cooperated well.

Motor activity: No psychomotor agitation or retardation.

Speech: Normal rate, volume, clarity, and amount.

Mood: "Sad and depressed, not my usual self."

Affect: Congruent, depressed, and tearful at appropriate points of the interview (e.g., discussing recent relationship difficulties, discussing how she feels when her son is not there). Affect brightened somewhat upon discussing her son's achievements in school.

Thought process: Linear, goal-directed.

Thought content: No delusions or paranoid ideations. Conveys future orientation: return to work, see her son as soon as she is able.

Perceptions: Denies any auditory or visual hallucinations. Does not appear to be responding to hallucinations.

Orientation: Oriented to person, place, time, and situation.

Attention/concentration: Attended well to the interview and was able to spell "world" forward and backward without difficulty.

Memory: Able to register 3/3 unrelated words without difficulty and to remember 3/3 after 5 minutes. Able to name the past 5 US presidents in reverse chronological order.

Knowledge: Good fund.

Abstractions: Able to note similarities (apple/orange, table/chair, opera/painting) appropriately.

Judgment: Fair. She states that, if she were ever feeling suicidal again, she would call her sister or someone else who was able to assist her.

Insight: Fair. Able to recognize that her suicidal thoughts may be related to a recurrence of depression and that she may benefit from psychiatric care once again.

Suicidal ideations: Denies, even with repeated questioning. Verbally agrees not to do anything to harm herself in the hospital and agrees to inform staff if she were to feel distressed again.

Homicidal ideations: Denies.

Laboratory Studies (on Admission):

Urine toxicology: Positive for opiates, otherwise negative.

Electrocardiogram: Normal sinus rhythm, normal EKG.

Acetaminophen level: Borderline toxic range.

Acetylsalicylic acid level: negative.

CBC with differential: All values within normal range.

Comprehensive metabolic profile: All values within normal range, including LFTs.

PT/PTT: Within normal range.

Serum HCG: Negative.

Formulation:

In summary, Ms. Leia is a 34-year-old female admitted to the hospital for a potentially toxic intentional acetaminophen overdose and a history of depression.

Relevant biological factors include: a possible genetic predisposition to depression (family history), recent physical discomfort (status-post tooth extraction, sleep deprivation) just prior to the suicide attempt, and possible hormonal influences (history of postpartum onset of depression, history of mood changes before and during menses, which she is currently having). Other, less prominent (though possibly still relevant) factors include: current use of a pain medication that could affect mood (oxycodone) and infrequent use of alcohol (none in the past few days).

Relevant psychological factors include: the recent argument with her boyfriend, and possibly the fact that her son was not with her at the time of the suicide attempt (as the more recent, precipitating factors); a past history of losses and transitions, including her parents' divorce, a less-than-optimal relationship with the parent who raised her, and the breakup of a previous marriage; other factors (e.g., school difficulties) that could have led to a loss of self-esteem and predisposed her to depression; and what she describes as an increased sensitivity to perceived rejection. Also,

she is at a stage in life where she may be hoping for more stability in her relation-
ship/family life and financial situation than she currently has, and this may be an
additional factor contributing to depression.

Relevant social/cultural/spiritual factors include: ongoing financial stress and working in the single parent role. She describes receiving emotional and other support
from siblings and friends. She has maintained a stable job for the past few years.
Her beliefs about the nature and treatment of depression may be influenced by her
religious orientation. Her religious involvement is positive influence in her life.

Depicted graphically (with treatment interventions enclosed in ovals)—ALSO
OPTIONAL:

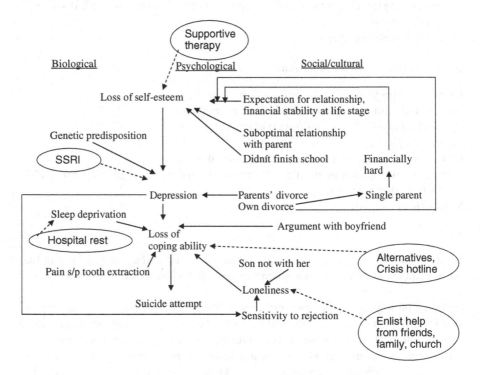

Differential Diagnoses:
On Axis I:

1. Major Depressive Disorder, Recurrent: patient meets DSM-IV criteria for this
   diagnosis. She also may meet the criteria for atypical features.
2. Bipolar II Disorder: a consideration given the history of recurrent major depressive episodes; however, no definite history of manic symptoms endorsed in this
   interview.
3. Adjustment Disorder with Depressed Mood: with the stressors being the relationship difficulties; however, because she meets the criteria for a Major Depressive
   Disorder, the latter diagnosis would supersede.

4. Panic Disorder: patient describes a history of fast heartbeat and lightheadedness; however, does not meet full criteria for panic attacks, and these symptoms occurred only in the context of what appears to be a major depressive episode.
5. Substance Abuse (Alcohol) and Substance-Induced Mood Disorder: based on the history provided, would not meet criteria for a substance use disorder; collateral information would be helpful in ruling out this possibility.
6. Premenstrual Dysphoric Disorder: patient describes some symptoms around menses that may be consistent with this condition; however, it is unclear that they were absent following menses and not merely an exacerbation of what is likely a Major Depressive Disorder.
7. Mood Disorder Due to a General Medical Condition (with depression): thyroid disorder (given family history) and primary heart condition (with anxiety symptoms) should be considered.
8. Mathematics or other Learning Disorder: given history of school difficulties and special education.

On Axis II:

1. Borderline Personality Traits: with sensitivity to abandonment; however, it is not clear that her history is necessarily characterized by "a pattern of unstable and intense relationships . . ." or "recurrent" suicidal behavior.
2. Dependent Personality Traits: discomfort with being alone; however, it is also not clear that criteria are met for this personality disorder.

On Axis III:

1. Status: post-overdose (acetaminophen, hydrocodone, ibuprofen)
2. Status: post-tooth extraction
3. PENICILLIN ALLERGY *(important to recall, though not necessarily directly relevant to current psychiatric status)*
4. Possible thyroid disorder: family history of thyroid disorder; history of cold intolerance.
5. Possible cardiac arrhythmia: given history of fast heartbeat, lightheadedness; however, the timing of these symptoms seemed to coincide with the episode of depression, and the EKG done on admission was negative.

Working diagnoses:

    Axis I Major Depressive Disorder, Recurrent
            Learning Disorder Not Otherwise Specified (Provisional)
    Axis II Deferred
    Axis III Status-post overdose
            Status-post tooth extraction with pain
    Axis IV Primary support, relationship difficulties, financial stressors
    Axis V Current GAF = 50; Highest GAF in past year = 75

Treatment Plan:

Treatment setting: Ms. Leia should remain in the hospital because she needs general medical treatment for the overdose. A standard hospital suicide risk assessment form has been completed, and orders have been written appropriate to her level of suicide risk, with removal of potentially injurious objects and frequent nursing checks.

Other specific interventions are as follows:

	Biological/medical	Psychological	Social
Additional information	1. Review past records from previous treating psychiatrist, with attention to medication issues 2. Consider checking a TSH	1. Meet again with patient to clarify diagnostic issues as noted above 2. Review past records from treating psychiatrist 3. Consider rating scales for depression and other mood disorders	1. With patient's permission, speak with family members for collateral information 2. Assess whether son (minor) is under appropriate care currently
Treatment	1. Medical treatment of overdose as per general medical team 2. Patient may be a candidate for re-starting of SSRI, such as fluoxetine, which had been helpful in the past. Consider monitoring response using standard rating scales for depression 3. Encourage adequate rest while in the hospital	1. Individual supportive psychotherapy to be provided during medical hospitalization, with focus on psychoeducation about depression and discussion of feelings about current and past stressors 2. In the longer term, may be a candidate for cognitive-behavioral psychotherapy (e.g., to address feelings of worthlessness, rejection) or interpersonal psychotherapy (e.g., to address role transitions, losses)	1. Enlist support from family members and friends where appropriate 2. Disposition (e.g., discharge to outpatient care versus psychiatric hospitalization) to be determined during follow-up visits

(Continued)

	Biological/medical	Psychological	Social
Patient education	1. Education about the alternatives to and potential benefits/risks of treatment with SSRI 2. Advise patient to avoid drinking alcohol at this time, as it may impair judgment and render her more vulnerable to self-destructive acts	1. Provide information on crisis phone numbers 2. Provide information on the importance of depression treatment, including ongoing medical follow-up	With patient's permission, enlist family's help in insuring safety in the environment (e.g., no large bottles of dangerous medications) and in encouraging patient to make use of available resources

Prognosis: Ms. Leia's prognosis at this point would seem to be fair to good. One important risk factor is current relationship instability. However, from the standpoint of completed suicide risk, she has a fairly favorable demographic profile (young, female, employed); no past history of suicide attempts; and no apparent substance abuse problem. From the standpoint of major depression, she has a history of good response to SSRI treatment in the past. Her social supports and church involvement may also be factors that weigh in her favor.

Bibliography

American Psychiatric Association. *Diagnostic and statistical manual of mental disorders, 4th ed.*, text revision. Washington, DC: American Psychiatric Press; 2000.

Guerrero APS, Hishinuma ES, Serrano AC, Ahmed I. Use of the "Mechanistic case diagramming" technique to teach the bio-psycho-social-cultural formulation to psychiatric clerks. Academic Psychiatry 2003; 27: 88–92.

Guerrero APS, Ling CYL, Ahmed I, Takeshita J, Bell CK. Development of a structured module to teach psychiatric interviewing competencies to medical students. Focus on Health Professional Education: A Multidisciplinary Journal (in press).

Chapter 18
Disorders of Childhood

Erika Ryst and Jeremy Matuszak

Childhood is a time of great vulnerability to psychiatric problems. This chapter will introduce three cases that will highlight some of the most common disorders and treatments.

At the end of this chapter, the reader will be able to

1. Describe the *fundamental* differences between a child and an adult psychiatric evaluation
2. Differentiate between the diagnostic criteria for adult and childhood psychiatric illnesses
3. Describe the epidemiology, phenomenology, etiology, and treatment for major childhood psychiatric diagnoses

Case Vignette 18.1.1 Presenting Situation: Sam

A mother brings in Sam, her 7-year-old boy, to you for a child psychiatric evaluation. She tells you that she is here at the insistence of the boy's classroom teacher, who notices an inability to sit still, decreased academic performance compared to his age-mates, and generally disruptive classroom behavior. These concerns have been going on for several months since the beginning of the school year. The mother seems a bit irritated that the school is requesting your evaluation. Sam is a cute, brown-haired boy with normal-appearing features. He gets up frequently from his seat but tends to hover in the immediate vicinity of his mother.

Please proceed with the problem-based approach!

E. Ryst
Assistant Professor of Psychiatry, University of Nevada School of Medicine

A. Guerrero, M. Piasecki (eds.), *Problem-Based Behavioral Science and Psychiatry*,
© Springer Science+Business Media, LLC 2008

Discussion

The psychiatric evaluation of a child differs from that of an adult in a number of fundamental ways. To start, children rarely present to your office with a chief complaint or treatment agenda. Rather, it is the parents/caregivers that will provide the reason for referral and evaluation. The process of evaluating a child/adolescent necessitates taking histories from not only the child, but the caregiver and school environments as well. When interviewing the child, it is important to communicate in a way that is appropriate to developmental level. The child may not be able to say in words what is wrong, but the observation of his behavior may give clues as to the diagnosis. A thorough chronological history including conception, childbirth, physical development/medical history, school functioning, and emotional development must be obtained to properly formulate the case. Special attention must be paid to any history of trauma (emotional, physical, or sexual) that may have precipitated the child's symptoms. Generating a differential diagnosis requires both time and caution, as symptoms of different disorders may present in the same way (for example, irritability could reflect a biological mood disorder or an environmental stressor such as child abuse). Therefore, the DSM-IV-TR, while a useful diagnostic guideline, may not be as applicable to children as it is to adults.

Differential diagnosis at this time is broad, but includes: attention deficit hyperactivity disorder (ADHD), pervasive developmental disorder (PDD), mental retardation (MR) or learning disorder, mood or anxiety disorder, environmental causes (e.g., being bullied at school), and oppositional defiant disorder (ODD).

Case Vignette 18.1.2 Continuation

Sam's school sends evaluation results. He has a high IQ with academic performance in the expected range for age. However, on the Weschler Intelligence Scale for Children (WISC), the working memory and attention scales show current impairment. A WISC performed 1 year ago showed a slightly higher IQ with attention and memory in the average range. During your classroom observation, you observe that Sam is highly distractible, particularly in high-stimulation situations. He jumps at loud noises and then has trouble returning to his schoolwork. At times, he gazes out of the window and seems to be lost in his own world. You are able to speak with Sam's first-grade teacher (he is now in the second grade) and she indicates that none of the current behavioral and cognitive problems existed 1 year ago.

 Please proceed with the problem-based approach!

This new information should now narrow the differential diagnosis. ADHD has now moved lower in the differential as these symptoms were not present before age 7. Additionally, it is now evident that the changes in attention and cognition are of a more acute onset (i.e., <1 year), thus placing a pervasive developmental disorder lower on our differential *as* well. Normal IQ effectively rules out mental retardation. At this time, a mood disorder, anxiety disorder, or an environmental cause to these behaviors must still be considered.

Although ADHD is lower on our differential, it is worth discussing here. DSM-IV-TR requires a pattern of either inattentive symptoms or hyperactivity–impulsivity lasting at least 6 months. These symptoms must be both maladaptive and inappropriate for developmental age. To make a formal diagnosis, some of these symptoms must have been present before age 7. Additionally, there must be evidence of impairment in social, academic, or occupational function in two or more settings. Again, taking a comprehensive school/home/individual history is needed to make an informed diagnosis.

The prevalence of ADHD has been suggested to fall between 3 and 7 % in school-age children. Twin studies have shown the heritability of this disorder to be as high as 80 %. Likewise, if a parent meets criteria for ADHD, there is a 50 % chance that the child will as well. In searching for the genetic basis for ADHD, it is evident that there are disruptions in both the norepinephrine and dopamine neurotransmitter systems. Among these systems, irregularities in the cingulate gyrus, caudate, and cerebellum (each with a corresponding dopamine pathway) have been implicated.

Psychostimulants, which effect both norepinephrine and dopamine systems, are the mainstay for treatment of ADHD. Medications that work on norepinephrine alone (e.g., atomoxetine), while more effective than placebo, do not appear to be quite as effective. These treatments have been so effective that approximately 75 % of subjects receiving *a first trial* of stimulants show academic *and* behavioral improvement compared to 0–25 % receiving placebo. Up to 90 % of children with ADHD respond if a second trial of medication is tried or medication dosage is altered. It is important to mention here that the risk of dependence on low-dose oral stimulants is remarkably low.

One of the most rigorous studies in child psychiatry, the Multimodal Treatment Study of ADHD (MTA), established a strong evidence base for the medication treatment of ADHD in children. This large-scale, NIMH-sponsored study was originally designed to test whether medications alone, psychosocial treatments alone, or a combination of the two best treated the symptoms of ADHD. The study found that while medication was the best treatment for the core symptoms of ADHD, combined treatment was superior to the other groups in addressing some of the associated problems of ADHD such as poor social skills and disrupted family relations. Helpful adjunctive psychosocial treatments include psychoeducation, parent training in behavior management skills, school advocacy and social skills training (Arnold et al., 1997).

While it used to be felt that the majority of children would "grow out of" their ADHD symptoms, recent studies indicate that ADHD continues at least into early adolescence in the majority of cases. Due to a paucity of data regarding adult outcomes, as well as methodological differences between the few existing studies, it is not at this time clear how frequently ADHD persists into adulthood. However, there is some evidence that many adults continue to suffer from some, if not all, of the symptoms of ADHD. Persistent ADHD is also associated with significant comorbidity including lower educational achievement, conduct disorder and antisocial personality disorder, major depression, car accidents, and cigarette smoking.

Case Vignette 18.1.3 Conclusion

You speak with the pediatrician, who has known Sam since birth and who is very happy that Sam is now under psychiatric care. His parents separated when he was three months of age, and Sam's mother has always given the impression of being a sensitive and caring caregiver. However, the pediatrician has noticed a change in the mother's overall demeanor over the last year, which has coincided with the entry of a new boyfriend into the home. Since then, the pediatrician has felt that Sam's mother has seemed more distant and closed. On one occasion, the boyfriend accompanied the family to an appointment, and the pediatrician thought he may have smelled alcohol on his breath. Just last week, the pediatrician had been able to speak separately with the mother, who admitted, after initially denying any problems, that her boyfriend, when intoxicated, would become physically abusive toward her and verbally belittling toward Sam. He had consulted with child protective services and planned to see Sam in follow-up.

 Please proceed with the problem-based approach!

When child abuse is suspected, the first and foremost concern is the child's ongoing safety. As a physician, you are legally mandated to report child abuse (even if only suspected and not confirmed) to Child Protective Services (CPS). If needed, the police can be called or the child can be admitted to the hospital to protect him/her while awaiting a CPS evaluation. Failure to report could result in further injury or even the child's death. Child abuse is common across all ages, socioeconomic classes, and ethnic groups; 2.9 million cases of child abuse were reported in 1999 alone, with 826,000 of these reports found to be true. Child abuse leads to approximately 1,100 deaths a year in the United States alone. Please refer to Chap. 7 for a further discussion of child abuse. Given its prevalence, child abuse needs to be considered in the differential diagnosis for any behavioral disorder in a child.

A victim of child abuse may display a number of changes including anxiety, depression, aggression, or post-traumatic stress disorder (PTSD). One study demonstrated that as high as 64 % of children who experience sexual abuse and 42 % of children who have been physically abused go on to develop PTSD. The criteria for PTSD (see Chap. 22, Anxiety Disorders) were designed for an adult population and, although there is an overlap in the symptoms of PTSD in children and adults, children understandably respond to trauma differently than adults and therefore diagnostic criteria of PTSD in children is somewhat different. Children may re-experience their trauma through post-traumatic play, play reenactment of the event, nightmares, flashbacks/dissociations, and distress at reminders of the event. Avoidance in children may be evidenced by constricted play, social withdrawal, restricted range of affect, *and* loss of previously acquired developmental skills. For the diagnosis of PTSD in children, Criterion D may be met by the child having night terrors, sleep difficulties, night walking, poor concentration, hypervigilance, *or* an exaggerated startle response.

Once safety issues are addressed, there are a number of psychotherapeutic and biologic treatments available. Psychotherapeutic treatments should facilitate the child feeling safe and being able to recall the traumatic events without feeling powerless. Medication options include treatment with SSRIs or alpha-2-agonists (clonidine or guanfacine), which can attenuate impulsive behaviors arising from the event and limit arousal symptoms. As noted in Chap. 21, SSRIs use in adolescents and children is controversial.

Case Vignette 18.2.1 Presenting Situation: Teddy

Teddy is a 9-year-old Caucasian boy who presents to his pediatrician with a 4-month history of bowel incontinence. These episodes only occur while awake and never during sleep. Teddy had been previously bowel trained at the age of 4 years, though his mother recalls that toilet training had been a struggle. Since he was a young child, Teddy has suffered from intermittent constipation, which has required medical intervention including hospitalization for bowel clean-out. However, except during episodes of severe constipation (when he has had some leaking), he has been able, for the most part, to stay clean. His mother is now concerned because over the last few months she has noticed significant fecal staining of Teddy's underwear, which includes formed stools as well as leaking.

 Please proceed with the problem-based approach!

The DSM-IV-TR defines encopresis as: repeated (at least once per month for at least 3 months) passage of feces into inappropriate places (e.g., clothing or floor) in a child who is 4 years or older. This should not be exclusively the result of a substance/medication or general medical condition except if constipation is the intermediary mechanism. There are two subtypes for encopresis: with (retentive) and without (non-retentive) constipation and overflow incontinence. If continence has never been achieved, this is called primary encopresis. On the other hand, as in Teddy's case, there has been a period of continence with subsequent bowel incontinence, so his condition is called secondary encopresis. Several studies cite the prevalence of encopresis between 1 and 2 % in children between 7 and 10 years old. It is more common in males.

The differential diagnosis of encopresis at this time includes spinal cord injury (leading to dysregulation of the anal sphincter), Hirschsprung disease, anal stenosis, imperforate anus with fistula, or psychological in nature.

The etiology of encopresis can be physiologic, psychological, or a combination of both. In physiologic encopresis, chronic constipation leads to a vicious cycle of ongoing bowel problems and incontinence. For example, the child avoids making bowel movements because they are hard and painful; more and more fluid gets re-absorbed from the bowel, and the retained feces becomes harder and harder. Over time the child becomes obstructed, and liquid waste leaks around the retained feces causing soiling. In psychologically mediated encopresis, unresolved psychological issues get played out in the realm of bowel movements. For example, a child with a strong need for control (who perhaps is in conflict with a controlling parent), exasperates the parent by willfully defecating at inopportune times and inappropriate places. Finally, physiological and psychological processes often go hand-in-hand, as encopresis may start out as a willful behavior on the part of the child, but develops into a problem of chronic constipation as a result of the child's habit of holding in feces.

Case Vignette 18.2.2 Continuation

Physical examination, including rectal examination, is unremarkable. A plain film of the abdomen fails to reveal any obstruction and/or impaction. There is neither recent nor remote history of trauma. Teddy's mother relates to you that she and Teddy's father were divorced shortly before these problems began. Since their separation, Teddy has had little contact with his father.

Although the initial history is consistent with retentive encopresis, Teddy's current presentation is somewhat different. There is no mention of recent bouts of constipation consistent with retentive constipation. Furthermore, physical examination is unremarkable. Given this, a biologic cause is lower on the differential and one must look closely for psychological contributors to this problem.

The treatment of encopresis in children is multi-pronged. The use of laxatives (either short or long term) may relieve the constipation that frequently causes pain in this disorder. A behavioral approach is also commonly employed, including a structured bowel training program (using the restroom at set intervals) and a program of biofeedback which teaches the child to relax the external anal sphincter successfully. Psychological treatment, such as play therapy to allow the child to work out unresolved conflicts, may also be appropriate if there are significant psychological factors involved.

It is important to effectively rule out any potential medical cause for encopresis before concluding that it is psychologically based. When it is psychologically based, however, the underlying motivator is frequently control. Children are dependent on caregivers in nearly every aspect of their lives—food, clothing, shelter, when to wake up, when to go to bed. One thing a child *does* have control over is his or her bowels. By holding in feces or soiling themselves, children may employ the little autonomy they do have in a very tangible way. For this reason, encopresis often reflects a child's attempt to regain control over feelings of helplessness (such as when a child is being hurt or abused). Alternatively, it may embody the dynamics of a control struggle between child and parent. Psychological treatment allows further exploration of these issues and identification of the unique meaning of the encopretic symptom for the child and his or her family. If unconscious conflicts driving this symptom are uncovered, the symptom itself resolves. Please see Chap. 27 on Eating Disorders for related topics.

Case Vignette 18.3.1 Presenting Situation: Michael

You are a pediatrician and have been treating Michael, a 3-year-old boy, since his birth. Michael's mom is a first-time parent, and you have perceived her as relatively anxious and insecure about her parenting experience. She is bringing Michael to you for his 3-year-old check-up. At this visit, when reviewing normal developmental milestones, it becomes clear that Michael's language is significantly delayed. He has a few words, such as "baba" for milk, which his mother is able to understand but is unintelligible to others. He has trouble getting his needs met because he does not point or gesture for what he wants.

 Please proceed with the problem-based approach!

At this point, a differential diagnosis could include language delay, mental retardation, pervasive developmental disorder (including autistic disorder), and various general medical causes of the lattermost two diagnoses. The investigation should therefore include a comprehensive review of

- Birth history (e.g., problems with pregnancy, prenatal exposures, anoxia at birth)
- Previous development (e.g., regression in milestones versus earlier hints of developmental delay, development in other areas).
- Temperament as an infant (e.g., colicky, responsive/non-responsive/cuddly)

- Social development and interaction between mother and infant (e.g., was there give-and-take or social reciprocity? Was there a social smile at 2 months, peek-a-boo play at around 7 months, back-and-forth connection with parent at 9–11 months, and pointing to indicate a desire to share interests at 12–18 months?)
- Language milestones (e.g., vocalizations as an infant, one-word utterances at 1 year, two-word phrases at 2 years?)
- Medical assessment: seizure history; sensory deficits (hearing/vision); signs/symptoms of specific genetic disorders such as Fragile X, audiometry, and visual exam; routine lead screening
- Physical examination with attention to growth, developmental status, and facial features/dysmorphology
- Laboratory tests in the presence of global developmental delay:

  - Chromosomal analysis
  - Fragile X testing
  - Neuroimaging

- Other laboratory tests, selected based on physical findings

  - Wood's Lamp of the Skin (tuberous sclerosis)
  - Urinary amino acids
  - Blood organic acids
  - Biochemical tests for any suspected inborn errors of metabolism
  - EEG

- Psychoeducational testing

  - Occupational therapy/physical therapy assessment
  - Speech and language testing (vocabulary, syntax/grammar, articulation/oral-motor skills, pragmatic skills)
  - Intelligence testing
  - Adaptive testing (e.g., Vineland Adaptive Scales)

Case Vignette 18.3.2 Continuation

Michael's work-up yields the following results. All laboratory tests are within normal limits. There is no evidence of dysmorphology on physical examination and chromosomal testing reveals a normal karyotype. Speech and language testing shows significant language delay—currently at the 12-month level (2 years language delayed). Adaptive skill testing shows both fine motor and gross motor delays, though not as severe as the language and social developmental delays.

Michael's mother reports normal pregnancy and delivery, but has always felt that "something is wrong with my child." As a newborn, he wasn't as "cuddly" as other babies. He slept a lot and appeared to get overstimulated very easily. His mother doesn't recall playing "peek-a-boo" or other types of give-and-take games. Michael does not use non-verbal gestures (such as pointing) to communicate or indicate interest. Upon direct observation, he is minimally interactive, even with his mother. He maintains minimal eye contact and does not appear to be curious about toys in the office. Michael plays repetitively with cars and lines them up in sequence over and over. His mother reports that he does this at home, too, for hours at a time. Additionally, there is no use of fantasy play and he is very inflexible. For example, he gets upset if the examiner tries to engage him in playing with the car. The examiner also notices that the child seems to self-stimulate himself by twisting and turning his body.

Please proceed with the problem-based approach!

At this point, because of the significant social developmental and communication delays, the most likely diagnosis is a pervasive developmental disorder (PDD), specifically autistic disorder. Also, because of what appear to be global developmental delays, the child likely also meets the criteria for mental retardation (MR).

The DSM-IV-TR defines mental retardation as an IQ of approximately 70 or below with deficits in adaptive functioning in at least two of the areas of self-care or interpersonal functioning. The deficits must be present by age 18. Most people with mental retardation have mild mental retardation and may not be diagnosed until after entering school. More severe levels of mental retardation, as indicated in Table 18.1, have more obvious functional deficits.

The cardinal features of autistic disorder, as defined by the DSM-IV-TR, include: impairment in social interactions (e.g., in the use of non-verbal behaviors, peer relationships, shared interest/attention with others, social/emotional reciprocity), impairment in communication (e.g., language delay, impairment in ability to converse, stereotyped or repetitive or idiosyncratic language use, lack of spontaneous developmentally appropriate make-believe play or social imitative play), and restricted repetitive and stereotyped behaviors (including rituals, motor mannerisms, and preoccupation with object parts). Of note, language delay is not enough in itself to make a diagnosis of autism; most important is the demonstration of specific deficits in social interaction.

Table 18.1 Categories of mental retardation

IQ score range	Diagnosis	Functioning
55–70	Mild mental retardation	Deficits may be mild, may live independently with supports
40–55	Moderate mental retardation	Obvious deficits, may live in a group home
25–40	Severe mental retardation	Limited communication skills
<25	Profound mental retardation	Constant care requirements

For autistic disorder, the criteria cannot be met for either Rett's disorder or childhood disintegrative disorder, both of which have deterioration in functioning. Rett's disorder occurs usually in females and is associated with hand-wringing behaviors. The other conditions in the pervasive developmental disorder group are: Asperger's disorder (in which there is relative preservation of language ability) and pervasive developmental disorder not otherwise specified.

The prevalence of pervasive developmental disorders approaches 1 %, with nearly 1/4 of this population meeting criteria for true "autism." The etiology of autistic disorder is, at this time, unknown. Current hypotheses suggest both a genetic and environmental contribution to this disorder.

Evidence supporting a genetic etiology includes robust data on concordance between identical twins, which is 60–90 %, compared to only 3–10 % concordance of autism in fraternal twins. There is also growing evidence with regards to underlying brain differences between autistic and normal children. Specifically, neuroimaging studies show reduced size and number of cells in the cerebellum, and PET scan studies show abnormalities in brain serotonin.

From an environmental perspective, intrauterine infections have been suggested to predispose a child to autism, as have environmental exposures to substances such as mercury. A lingering controversy has been whether or not childhood vaccinations lead to an increased risk of autism, but research has failed to suggest such a link.

There is no specific treatment for autism, but intervention is focused on improvement of function, which includes a multimodal treatment plan such as: social skills

Table 18.2 Other diagnoses specific to children and adolescents

	Diagnostic features	Special features
Disruptive behavioral disorders of childhood		
Oppositional defiant disorder	A pattern of hostile, irritable, and defiant behavior	Must be more oppositional than developmental peers
Conduct disorder	Aggressive, destructive, delinquent (criminal) behaviors	Can be precursor to antisocial personality disorder in adults
Learning, motor disorders and language disorders		
Reading disorder	Low reading achievement on standardized tests	Reading ability below expected for IQ
Mathematics disorder	Low math achievement on standardized tests	Math ability below expected for IQ
Disorder of written expression	Low level of writing skills	Writing ability below expected for IQ
Developmental coordination disorder	Low levels of coordination/motor performance	Possible delays in developmental milestones
Language disorders	Limited vocabulary; errors in grammar Difficulty understanding words	Expressive language and mixed receptive–expressive language subtypes
Phonological disorder	Difficulties in speech sound production	
Tourette's disorder	Motor and vocal tics	Onset before age 18

training, speech/language services, occupational therapy, functional behavioral analysis and behavior management training, educational interventions/advocacy, and, sometimes, medication to treat associated symptoms such as anxiety or aggression. Recently several exciting studies suggest that some medication treatments (such as risperidone) help not only with reducing aggression and agitation associated with autism, but may in fact also promote small developmental gains (Williams, 2006).

While children who are identified and helped early have the best prognosis, intervention at any age can promote developmental gains and improve functioning. The key in any intervention plan is to employ as many modalities as possible to promote the child's growth. Each child with autistic disorder requires a comprehensive assessment to identify areas of deficit, which should then inform a targeted and multi-faceted treatment plan.

The diagnostic breadth of childhood psychiatric illness is as broad as (if not broader than) their adult counterparts. In addition to a number of disorders unique to those persons under the age of 18 as outlined in Table 18.2, there are diagnoses common to both age groups but that may have different presentations in childhood, as outlined in Table 18.3. It is important to understand the fundamental differences in presentation and diagnostic criteria of these disorders.

Table 18.3 Adult disorders that may present in childhood

Disorder	Diagnostic features	Special features in children
Major depression	Same as adults	Mood may be irritable instead of sad; failure to make expected weight gains
Dysthymic disorder	One year duration	Mood may be irritable
Bipolar disorder	Same as adults	Controversial
Phobia	Minimum duration 6 months; anxiety may be expressed by crying, tantrums, or freezing	May not recognize fear as unreasonable; animal and natural environment phobias usually are childhood onset
Generalized anxiety disorder	One symptom of anxiety in children for at least 6 months	Formerly called overanxious disorder of childhood
Social phobia	Minimum duration 6 months; anxiety may be expressed by crying, tantrums, or freezing	May not recognize fear as unreasonable; anxiety in peer and adult settings
Obsessive–compulsive disorder	Same as adults	May not recognize obsessions or compulsions as unreasonable; association with strep infections
Personality disorders	Same as adults	Usually not diagnosed in children due to developmental variations
Schizophrenia	Same as adults	Rare
Gender identity disorder	Four or more opposite sex preferences; rejection of gender-related activities	Onset in childhood

Review Questions

1. The psychiatric evaluation and diagnosis of a child:

   (a) Is primarily obtained from the observation of the child
   (b) Must always conform to DSM-IV-TR criteria
   (c) Must include at least three settings of problematic behavior to diagnose ADHD
   (d) Should include a thorough history including school functioning, developmental milestones, and conception
   (e) Two of the above

2. Which of the following statements is true about treatment of ADHD?

   (a) Atomoxetine (Strattera) exerts its main effects on the serotonin neurotransmitter system.
   (b) It is especially controversial because of a lack of large-scale, non-pharmaceutical industry-sponsored studies.
   (c) Methylphenidate should be avoided because of its addictive properties.
   (d) Should focus exclusively on the dopamine neurotransmitter system.
   (e) None of the above.

3. Which of the following statements is true regarding child abuse?

   (a) Abuse can result in symptoms of play reenactment of the event, restricted affect, night walking, and avoidance.
   (b) CPS should be notified only if suspicion for abuse is high, because they have a responsibility to always separate the child from suspected perpetrators.
   (c) If the family admits to one isolated case of abuse, you can delay notifying CPS in order to maintain the therapeutic alliance which must be maintained for successful intervention and treatment.
   (d) More than half of all CPS-reported cases are confirmed as real.
   (e) Studies show that child abuse is considerably more common in low socioeconomic class, minority communities.

4. All of the following diagnoses must have symptoms, if not full features prior to age 18 EXCEPT:

   (a) Antisocial personality disorder
   (b) Autistic disorder
   (c) Disorganized schizophrenia
   (d) Gender identity disorder
   (e) Tourette's disorder

5. A 4-year-old female patient is brought in by her mother because of recent observations that her daughter is less sociable, withdrawing from friends, wringing her hands, and toe-walking. The child is reported to have developed normally for the first 2 years of life, though she may have shown some decreased eye contact at around 18 months. The patient is reported to have much less irritability in the

last year; crying, speaking, and asserting herself less. On exam, you discover her head circumference has fallen from its previously normal position on the growth curve. Regarding this patient

(a) Autistic disorder is the most likely diagnosis because the patient shows clear deficits in social interaction, including language delay.
(b) Autistic disorder is most likely diagnosis because symptoms were first noticed in the second year of life.
(c) Autistic disorder is not likely because full DSM-IV-TR diagnostic criteria have not been elicited in the history.
(d) The diagnosis of autistic disorder is not likely because of other findings in this case.
(e) None of the above.

Answers

1. d, 2. e, 3. a, 4. c, 5. d

Appendix: Partially Populated Tables

Case table 18.1.1

Facts	Hypotheses	What information do I want at this time?	Learning issues
Referral was initiated by the school Poor school performance, hyperactivity, and behavior problems at school Mother seems irritated that an evaluation has been requested	Attention deficit hyperactivity disorder (ADHD) Pervasive developmental disorder (PDD) Mental retardation (MR) Learning disorder mood or anxiety disorder Environmental causes (e.g., being bullied at school) oppositional defiant disorder (ODD)	Collateral information including history from teacher, direct observation of the child in the classroom, input from the child's pediatrician A more detailed history including: (1) in what environment(s) do these behaviors occur, (2) are there other symptoms that might narrow the differential including sleep disturbances, change in appetite, loss of interests in activities, moodiness, tearfulness, anxiety, etc. (3) Are these new or old behaviors? (4) What is the child's level of function in different areas (e.g., home, school, with friends), (5) social/environmental details, (6) family history. IEP (Individualized Education Program) evaluation to assess IQ and academic functioning	

Case table 18.1.2

Facts	Hypotheses	What information do I want at this time?	Learning issues
High IQ, no impairment in academic performance Deficits in working memory and attention scales as demonstrated by the WISC Child is highly distractible Hypervigilant to loud noises Symptoms have started within the last year; previous school functioning was normal	ADHD, PDD, and MR are less likely Mood disorder Anxiety disorder Environmental cause	More thorough social history	

Case table 18.1.3

Facts	Hypotheses	What information do I want at this time?	Learning issues
Pediatrician's impression of the mother is overall favorable The patient's mother has become more withdrawn since a new boyfriend has moved into her home Pediatrician believes he smelled alcohol on the boyfriend's breath during an in-office visit	Child abuse Witness to domestic violence	Is there physical evidence of child abuse? e.g., multiple bruises in different stages of healing, fractures not consistent with normal injury Direct questioning of child and parent regarding possible child abuse	

Case table 18.2.1

Facts	Hypotheses	What information do I want at this time?	Learning issues
Previously bowel trained History of intermittent constipation requiring medical intervention Encopresis does not occur at night	Spinal cord injury Hirschsprung disease Anal stenosis Imperforate anus with fistula Psychogenic origin	Physical examination Plain film of the abdomen Anorectal manometry sometimes useful History of trauma suggesting spinal cord injury Detailed social history	

Case table 18.2.2

Facts	Hypotheses	What information do I want at this time?	Learning issues
→ Physical examination is unremarkable → Onset of problems coincided with the divorce of Teddy's parents	Retentive encopresis less likely Psychological etiology more likely	Further exploration of psychological causes such as central issues	

Bibliography

Arnold LE, Abikoff HB, Cantwell DP, Conners CK, Elliott G, Greenhill LL, Hechtman L, Hinshaw SP, Hoza B, Jensen PS, Kraemer HC, March JS, Newcorn JH, Pelham WE, Richters JE, Schiller E, Severe JB, Swanson JM, Vereen D, Wells KC. National Institute of Mental Health Collaborative Multimodal Treatment Study of Children with ADHD (the MTA). Design challenges and choices. *Arch Gen Psychiatry* 1997; 54(9): 865–70.

Cheng K, Myers KM. Child and Adolescent Psychiatry: The Essentials. Lippincott Williams & Wilkins, 2005.

Filipek PA, Accardo PJ, Ashwal S, Baranek GT, Cook EH Jr, et al. Practice parameter: Screening and diagnosis of autism. Report of the Quality Standards Subcommittee of the American Academy of Neurology and the Child Neurology Society. *Neurology* 2000; 55(4): 468–79.

Mikkelsen EJ. Modern Approaches to enuresis and encopresis. In Melvin Child and Adolescent Psychiatry: A Comprehensive Textbook. Lippincott Williams & Wilkins, 2002; Lewis (ed.), 700–711.

Pliszka S. Practice Parameter for the Assessment and Treatment of Children and Adolescents With Attention-Deficit/Hyperactivity Disorder. AACAP Work Group on Quality Issues - *J Am Acad Child Adolesc Psychiatry* 2007; 46(7): 894–921.

Tanguay PE. Pervasive developmental disorders: A 10-year review. *J Am Acad Child Adolesc Psychiatry*, 2000; 39(9): 1079–95.

Williams SK. Risperidone and adaptive behavior in children with autism. *J. Am. Acad. Child Adolesc. Psychiatry* 2006; 45(4): 431–9.

Chapter 19
Substance Use Disorders

William F. Haning III and Anthony P.S. Guerrero

Multiple illnesses comprise the substance use disorder spectrum. The management of any illness within the spectrum relies heavily on the availability of diagnostic and treatment resources and upon the level of participation by the patient. The two cases in this chapter demonstrate different problems and approaches to these challenging disorders.

At the end of this chapter, the reader will be able to

1. Discuss the epidemiology, mechanisms, clinical presentation, clinical evaluation, differential diagnosis, treatment, and prevention of substance-related disorders, with particular attention to alcohol, tobacco, cannabis, opioids, and stimulants
2. Describe medical co-morbidities and counter-transference issues that need to be considered when caring for patients with substance use disorders

Case Vignette 19.1.1 Grant Lifeson

Grant Lifeson is a 50-year-old male admitted to the orthopedic service yesterday after jumping off of a four-story building. He sustained a significant leg fracture and multiple bruises and contusions. A psychiatric consultation was ordered for evaluation of suicidal behavior. In the emergency room, Mr. Lifeson was noted to smell of alcohol and to have "track marks" on his arms. His blood alcohol level was 0.31 and his urine toxicology screen was positive for alcohol, cocaine, and opiates. Before you enter the room, the attending orthopedic surgeon, who appears quite worried, informs you that the patient is threatening to leave the hospital and has even tried to climb out of his bed.

Mr. Lifeson is superficially cooperative and gives only minimal answers. He appears diaphoretic and seems to have difficulty focusing on your questions. He says blandly that he wants to leave the hospital because he is tired and wants to rest. He gives the same answer when the same question is repeated and cannot state

W.F. Haning III
Associate Professor of Psychiatry, Program Director, Addiction Psychiatry/Addiction Medicine
Director, Graduate Affairs, University of Hawai'i John A. Burns School of Medicine

A. Guerrero, M. Piasecki (eds.), *Problem-Based Behavioral Science and Psychiatry*,
© Springer Science+Business Media, LLC 2008

what may happen to him if he were to refuse the recommended care. He states that he jumped off the ledge of his apartment building because he was "just fed up with it all . . . but I guess I learned my lesson now."

 Please proceed with the problem-based approach!

Epidemiology

Substance use and addiction is common in the USA. Consider these facts:

- According to the Centers for Disease Control and Prevention (CDC, 2007), approximately 8 % of persons in the USA aged 12 years or older have used any illicit drug in the past month.
- Approximately 6 % of persons in the USA aged 12 years or older have used marijuana in the past month.
- With regard to substances that are currently legal, smoking prevalence varies from approximately 10 to 33 % across the USA and territories.
- In the USA, over 50 % of the adult US population drank alcohol in the past 30 days; approximately 5 % of the total population drank heavily; and 15 % of the population binge drank (defined as more than four drinks).

The morbidity and mortality related to legal and illegal drug use in the USA is also significant. For example,

- Annually in the USA, cigarette smoking results in serious illnesses in approximately 8.6 million people and death in 440,000 people. It is the most preventable cause of premature death in the USA.
- In 2001, there were approximately 75,000 deaths in the USA attributable to excessive alcohol use, which is the third leading lifestyle-related cause of death in the USA.
- According to the Office of National Drug Control Policy (2004a), the economic cost of drug abuse is around $180.9 billion, which represents the cost of health and crime consequences and the loss of productivity from death and inability to work (see summary below).
- In 2004, poisoning was second only to motor-vehicle crashes as a cause of death from unintentional injury in the USA. Nearly all of these deaths were from drugs, and most of the drugs involved were prescription and illegal drugs.
- Costs of substance abuse vs. other morbidities:

    - Social/health cost to the US society: $ $\frac{1}{2}$ trillion/year
    - Illicit drugs: $181 billion/year

- Tobacco: $168 billion/year
- Alcohol: $185 billion/year
- ($534 billion/year for substance abuse)
- Diabetes: $132 billion/year
- Cancer: $210 billion/year

Mechanisms, Clinical Manifestations, and Acute Treatment

Substance abuse and its medical sequelae are common in general medical settings, as illustrated in the case of Mr. Lifeson. While his urine toxicology was positive for alcohol, opiates, and cocaine, it is important to identify which of these substances— in intoxication or withdrawal—may be producing his symptoms. It is also critical to identify the intoxication or withdrawal syndrome that is the most life threatening and requires the most urgent treatment. Table 19.1 provides a summary of mechanisms and key clinical findings associated with intoxication and withdrawal of the major substances of abuse.

Mr. Lifeson presents with apparent confusion, which could be explained by several of the intoxication or withdrawal symptoms listed above, and certainly by alcohol withdrawal delirium, which may be life threatening. The consulting physician needs to ask Mr. Lifeson about his pattern of substance use and past medical history, with attention to co-morbid general medical conditions that could increase his risk of complications from intoxication and/or withdrawal. Mr. Lifeson's physicians also need to monitor his vital signs and to note any other symptoms of intoxication and withdrawal on his physical examination. They will also obtain laboratory studies to screen for co-morbidities.

Case Vignette 19.1.2 Continuation

Mr. Lifeson says that he had been drinking "a lot" for the past "week or so," and that he has been a "good drinker" since he was "a boy." He denies any past history of withdrawal seizures. He admits to almost daily heroin use, but says he only uses cocaine "once in a while." He says that he was on methadone "about five years ago" but can't remember his dose, only that it was "high." He denies current use of other drugs, including barbiturates and prescription medications.

His past medical history is significant for cellulitis of his arm from injecting drugs. He takes no medications regularly. He smokes two packs per day of cigarettes. In the hospital, he is on Demerol (mepridine) p.r.n. for pain.

Physical exam:

Vital signs: Temperature 99.8°F, R 22 per minute, HR 112 per minute, BP 146/92. He rates his pain a 5 out of 10.

Table 19.1 Mechanisms and clinical manifestations of the major substances of abuse

Substance	Mechanism	Clinical manifestations in intoxication (potentially life-threatening ones are bolded)	Clinical manifestations in withdrawal (potentially life-threatening ones are bolded)
Alcohol and sedative/hypnotics, including benzodiazepines and barbiturates	Facilitation of GABA binding to its receptor	**Respiratory depression**, slurring of speech, lateral nystagmus, sedation, disinhibition, nausea/vomiting	**Alcohol withdrawal delirium ("delirium tremens"), seizures,** hypertension, tachycardia, diaphoresis, tremors (*withdrawal risk higher with chronic heavy use and sudden cessation, as well as with concurrent illness or trauma*)
Cocaine, methamphetamine, and "stimulants"	Increased release of catecholamines and/or blockage of catecholamine reuptake	**Cardiac arrhythmias,** hypertension, vasospasm, agitation, mydriasis	Depression, sedation, lethargy
Ecstasy or methylene-dioxymethamphetamine (MDMA)	Release of catecholamines and serotonin	As above (with stimulants) and dehydration	Withdrawal uncommon; some characteristics associated with stimulants, when present
Gamma-hydroxy-butyrate (GHB)	GABA and dopamine and receptor agonism	**Seizures (synergistically with alcohol), coma (synergistically with stimulants)**	Uncommon, but resembles benzodiazepine withdrawal when present
Inhalants	Cell membrane disruption	**Cardiac arrhythmias,** encephalopathy	Lethargy, anhedonia, irritability
Hallucinogens, including lysergic acid diethylamide (LSD)	Serotonin receptor agonism	Agitation, delirium	No syndrome described
Marijuana	Cannabinoid receptors	Delirium uncommonly, not associated with coma or death; sedation, confusion	Irritability, insomnia, distractability and inattention, anxiety
Opioids (including heroin)	Opioid receptor agonism	**Respiratory depression/apnea,** miosis, hypotension, constipation, **sedation/coma**	Autonomic hyperactivity, mydriasis, pain, diarrhea (*withdrawal risk higher with chronic heavy use and sudden cessation*)
Phencyclidine	N-methyl-D-aspartic acid (NMDA)	Agitation, fever, muscle rigidity	No syndrome described

General appearance/mental status: Mr. Lifeson is disheveled, with poor eye contact. His speech is soft and minimally slurred and his mood is mildly irritable. His affect is anxious. Mr. Lifeson denies any auditory or visual hallucinations or current suicidal or homicidal ideations. He appears to have a hard time following your questions. He is able to state his name, but he gives the wrong name of the hospital and is unable to give the date. He is unable to repeat more than three digits forward and two digits backward.

HEENT: Pupils 5 mm.

Neck: Supple.

Abdomen: Liver edge appreciated 2 fingerbreadths below the ribcage.

Neurologic: Tremors of outstretched hands. He has difficulty with finger-to-nose testing. Gait cannot be assessed due to the leg fracture.

Skin: "Track marks" are present. He is diaphoretic. There is no jaundice.

Review of labs and other studies:

CBC: Mild anemia with a mildly elevated mean corpuscular volume.

Chemistry panel: Elevated gamma glutamyl transferase and other liver function tests.

Head CT scan: Normal.

EKG: Normal except for sinus tachycardia.

The psychiatric consultant contacts the admitting physician to discuss immediate recommendations, which include:

1. *Patient should not be allowed to leave the hospital, as he appears to be delirious and to lack decisional capacity.*
2. *A sitter at bedside.*
3. *Initiation of a benzodiazepine protocol to manage alcohol withdrawal.*
4. *Thiamine, vitamins, and folic acid.*
5. *Initiation of a patient-controlled analgesia unit, with close monitoring of pain control and pupil size.*
6. *Close monitoring of vital signs and placement of a pulse oximeter.*
7. *Consideration of other laboratory tests, including HIV and hepatitis.*
8. *Close attention to hydration, nutrition, and overall health.*

Over the next few days, with intensive treatment, Mr. Lifeson's mental status improves, and his vital signs normalize. Although he still seems to have some difficulty with finger-to-nose testing, he is much less tremulous. He is able to remain alert and oriented, with an improved capacity to perform digit spans.

Please proceed with the problem-based approach!

The tachycardia, elevated blood pressure, tremulousness, and confusion all are consistent with *alcohol withdrawal delirium*, in combination with *opioid withdrawal* and *cocaine intoxication*. At this point, it is important to review the treatment of intoxication and withdrawal of the major substances, summarized in Table 19.2 (see APA, Practice Guidelines for treatment, 2006).

While a discussion of the organ systems affected by alcohol is beyond the scope of this textbook it is worth noting that Mr. Lifeson likely had medical complications of alcohol use, including elevated liver function tests, macrocytic anemia, and cerebellar dysfunction. Because of the multi-organ effects of substances of abuse

Table 19.2 Treatment of intoxication with and withdrawal from the major substances of abuse

Substance	Treatment of intoxication	Treatment of withdrawal
Alcohol and sedative/hypnotics, including benzodiazepines (BZs) and barbiturates	Supportive care, including attention to airway, breathing, circulation; benzodiazepine antagonist (flumazenil) for BZs only	Thiamine, magnesium sulfate, anticonvulsants arguably, benzodiazepine-based protocols (for alcohol); BZs for BZ and other sedative-hypnotic dependence
Cocaine, methamphetamine, and "stimulants"	Benzodiazepines for agitation, appropriate cardiac antiarrhythmic medication	Under investigation, present recommendations off-label. In interim, support sleep (trazadone, antihistamines, sedatives circumspectly); feed/hydrate
Ecstasy/MDMA	As for stimulants	None generally required; as for stimulants if syndrome present
Gamma-hydroxy-butyrate (GHB)	Respiratory support	None
Heroin and opioids	Naloxone (Narcan) acutely	Opioid agonists (buprenorphine, methadone); α_2-Agonists (clonidine), antiemetics (promethazine)
Inhalants	Respiratory support	None
Hallucinogens, including lysergic acid diethylamide (LSD)	Antipsychotic medication (risperidone, haloperidol), benzodiazepines	None
Marijuana	Conservative	None
Phencyclidine	Antipsychotic medication (risperidone, haloperidol), benzodiazepines	None

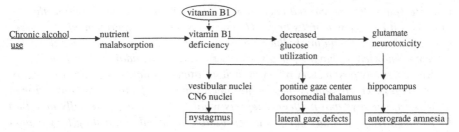

Fig. 19.1 Mechanisms and signs and symptoms associated with Wernicke's encephalopathy and alcohol-induced persisting amnestic disorder

and the poor access to care that patients who abuse substances often experience, it is important to thoroughly evaluate such patients for medical complications of substance abuse. For Mr. Lifeson, an electrocardiogram was obtained to rule out cardiovascular sequelae of cocaine abuse, and neuroimaging was obtained in order to rule out intracranial pathology (perhaps from unrecognized trauma) as a cause of the delirium. Finally, tests for hepatitis and HIV were obtained because of the history of intravenous drug abuse.

In addition, without treatment with thiamine (to be given *before* any dextrose-containing solution) and effective management of the alcohol withdrawal, Mr. Lifeson may be at risk for Korsakoff's syndrome (alcohol-induced persisting amnestic disorder), typically associated with Wernicke's encephalopathy. The mechanisms and signs and symptoms associated with this condition are indicated in Fig. 19.1.

Beyond acute management, Mr. Lifeson's physicians will gather further history about Mr. Lifeson to formulate a comprehensive management plan to include posthospital care (ASAM Patient Placement Criteria 2nd Ed.).

Case Vignette 19.1.3 Continuation

Mr. Lifeson reports that he has been feeling very depressed for the past week, after losing a job that he had held for almost 1 year. He had been drinking more heavily than usual. He reports a history of regular drinking, mostly after work, usually six beers each evening, for the past 25 or so years. He went through an alcoholism rehabilitation program about 8 years ago, and attended Alcoholics Anonymous (AA) for a few months afterward. His longest period of sobriety from alcohol was 10 months, during and after the rehab, but he continued to use other drugs "a little" during that period. He acknowledges one driving under the influence (DUI) conviction and gives positive responses to all four "CAGE" items (need to cut down, annoyance with criticism, guilt about drinking, use of alcohol as an "eye opener"). Mr. Lifeson gives further details about his heroin use: he had relapsed after having been on methadone for about 1 year and occasionally was involved in selling drugs to support his habit. He denies any other history of illegal activity or trouble with the law. He states that he snorted cocaine on the day prior to admission and that he only uses it every few months or so. He admits to having experimented with other drugs in the past, including hallucinogens during the 1970s: "You name it, I tried it." He acknowledges having friends who "are worse drug addicts than I am."

He denies any past history of psychiatric treatment, suicide attempts, or diagnosis of depression. He admits that he had been thinking of suicide the day prior to admission, but says that he deeply regrets what he had done, especially now that he is sober. He denies any persistent depression or anhedonia lasting longer than 2 weeks prior to having lost his job. He denies any past history of manic symptoms unrelated to cocaine intoxication. He denies having experienced any hallucinations or delusions.

Mr. Lifeson lives by himself in a small apartment in town. He had been homeless in the past. He has one half-brother in Hawai'i, with whom he has limited contact, but otherwise his family is on the mainland. His 7-year marriage ended 15 years ago, and he has limited contact with his previous wife and teenage son. He believes that several of his uncles had problems with alcoholism. He says: "I sure hope my son doesn't turn out like I did."

The order for a bedside sitter is discontinued.

As Mr. Lifeson's medical status improves, he is switched from PCA morphine to a modest daily dose of methadone (given in liquid form in orange juice) and offered disulfiram, which he politely refuses now but says he will consider later. You also recommend the use of the medication acamprosate and offer community resources for substance abuse treatment and general medical follow-up.

Mr. Lifeson is visibly relieved to learn that his tests for HIV and hepatitis were negative. You discuss safe sex and HIV prevention guidelines, which he says he will follow ("I need to get my life together"). He asks you if and when he should have his HIV test repeated.

You also advise him on the importance of smoking cessation. Although he is not yet ready to set a quit date, he is open to hearing your advice regarding the "5 R's": Relevance of quitting smoking, Risks of smoking, Rewards of quitting smoking, perceived Roadblocks to quitting smoking, and importance of Repetition. He promises to discuss this issue at his medical follow-up visit. He also asks whether or not the nicotine patch or bupropion might be appropriate for him.

Differential Diagnoses

The *Diagnostic and Statistical Manual for Mental Disorders*, fourth edition, text revision (2000) offers a categorical description of substance use disorders, summarized below in Table 19.3.

At the time of his admission, in addition to the acute intoxication and withdrawal syndromes discussed above, it is likely that Mr. Lifeson meets criteria for alcohol and opioid dependence and cocaine abuse.

The mechanisms to explain Mr. Lifeson's current presentation are shown in Fig. 19.2.

Table 19.3 Relevant categories of substance use disorders specified in the *Diagnostic and Statistical Manual of Mental Disorders*, fourth edition, text revision (2000)

Disorder	Highlights
Substance dependence	• Maladaptive, with clinically significant impairment or distress • Three or more of the following within a 12-month period: tolerance, withdrawal, increasing amount and duration, failure to cut down/control use, significant time spent in obtaining/using/recovering from substance, interference with usual activities, continuation despite physical or psychosocial problems • Specifiers: with/without physiological dependence • Other specifiers if in remission: early/sustained full/partial remission in controlled environment and/or on agonist therapy
Substance abuse	• Also maladaptive, with clinically significant impairment or distress • Only need one of the following: failure to fulfill role obligations, continuation despite physical hazard, legal problem, persistent/recurrent interpersonal problems • No criteria met for substance dependence (which takes precedence as a diagnosis)
Substance withdrawal or intoxication delirium	• Other criteria for delirium, namely: disturbance of consciousness and attention; change in cognition (e.g., memory, orientation) or perceptual disturbances not better accounted for by dementia; acute onset with fluctuation in symptoms • Temporally related to substance withdrawal or intoxication
Substance-induced persisting amnestic disorder	• Significant memory impairment that represents a decline from previous functioning • Not fully explained by delirium, dementia, or substance withdrawal • Etiologically related to the persisting effects of substance use

Comprehensive Management and Prevention

As indicated in Fig. 19.2, long-term management will need to include a bio-psycho-social approach, which is essential for the treatment of all substance use disorders. Table 19.4 summarizes the medication interventions that may be appropriate for each specific substance of abuse.

For Mr. Lifeson, methadone might address both opioid withdrawal and his need for pain management, given the recent injuries. The conscientious clinician in this case also made sure to address the tobacco use, which (in spite of its legality) is a serious health risk in the long term. The clinician can refer to treatment resources in US Public Health Service (2003).

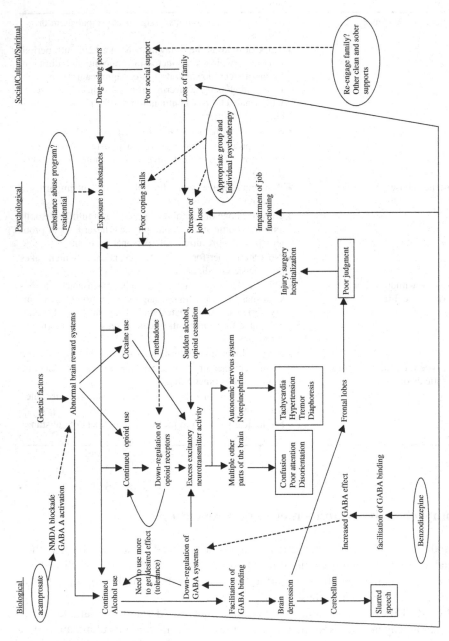

Fig. 19.2 Mechanisms to explain Mr. Lifeson's current presentation

Table 19.4 Pharmacotherapy of addictions (limited list)

Class	Medication	Indication	Efficacy	Considerations
Agonist	Methadone	Opioid withdrawal/maintenance (controlled substance CII)	High	Dispensing restrictions beyond CII; overdose risk; lengthy withdrawal
	Buprenorphine	Opioid withdrawal/maintenance (controlled substance CIII)	High	Milder restrictions than with methadone; little risk of overdose, lower risk or of diversion
	Nicotine replacement therapy (NRT)—gum, patch, nasal insufflation	Nicotine dependence	Low–moderate	Best in conjunction with adjunctive therapy (bupropion)
	Benzodiazepines—diazepam, alprazolam, etc.	Alcohol or sedative-hypnotic withdrawal (GABA agonist)	High	Risk of overdose in outpatient setting
Antagonist	Naloxone	Opioid overdose	High	Abrupt withdrawal, profoundly dysphoric; I.V. only
	Naltrexone	Opioid dependence; some efficacy in alcohol dependence	Moderate	Blocks effects of self-administered opioids, useful in monitored abstinence. Oral and long-acting injection
	Flumazenil (Mazicon)	Benzodiazepine overdose	High	Abrupt withdrawal, dysphoric; short-acting so principally diagnostic; expensive
Aversive agents	Disulfiram (Antabuse)	Alcohol dependence	Moderate	Interrupts alcohol metabolism to create acetaldehyde accumulation; profoundly distressing: N/V, HA, hypotension, dysphoria when challenged with ethanol intake

Table 19.4 (continued)

Class	Medication	Indication	Efficacy	Considerations
Other (anticraving agents, satiety agents, others of unknown mechanism)	Naltrexone—diminution of craving, early alcohol satiety (harm reduction strategy as well as abstinence enhancement)	Alcohol dependence	Low–moderate	Available as oral (daily) or injectable (Vivitrol—monthly), though expensive
	Acamprosate—NMDA blocker, GABA-A activation	Alcohol dependence	Moderate	Low risk, some SEs (HA/N), best initiated in abstinence
	Bupropion—antidepressant with catecholaminergic and dopaminergic agonism, nicotinergic antagonism	Nicotine dependence, ?stimulant dependence (criteria not yet refined)	Low–moderate	Reduces seizure threshold. With nicotine dependence, best employed with concomitant nicotine replacement therapy (NRT)
	Varenicline (Chantix)—nicotine receptor partial agonist	Nicotine dependence	Moderate	May be best employed with bupropion; use with NRTs increases side effect profile
	Clonidine—alpha-2 adrenergic agonist	Opioid withdrawal—symptom management without controlled substances	Moderate	Best employed with antinauseant (promethazine), anticonvulsants
	Anticonvulsants—divalproate/Depakote, others	Alcohol and sedative-hypnotic withdrawal (where benzodiazepenes not indicated)	Moderate	Incomplete efficacy in controlling seizures; not indicated for delirium. Consider adjunctive use of clonidine, other sedating agents (trazadone, promethazine) for sleep

Prevention

Finally, Mr. Lifeson raised the important issue of how to best prevent his son from having the same substance use problems that he had. As reviewed by the National Institute on Drug Abuse (2003), effective prevention principles include enhancement of protective factors (e.g., parental support), reduction of risk factors (e.g., psychosocial adversity and negative peer influences), and enhancement of academic and social competence through prevention-based curricula in the schools. From the clinician's standpoint, it is important to detect substance abuse risk factors as well as substance abuse itself as early as possible in order to optimize outcome. The next case illustrates the importance of this principle.

In contrast to the previous case, the following is a description of an outpatient setting, where the "patient" is not the one recognizing the problem or seeking help.

Case Vignette 19.2.1 Carlisle Van Heusen

You are the primary care physician for Dr. Carlisle Van Heusen, a 55-year-old male physician with progressive impairment in multiple spheres in his life. He is famous in the medical community for once having successfully sued the major community hospital for restraint of trade issues centering on his medical staff privileges.

On a busy Friday, Jenny Van Heusen drags in her reluctant husband to your office during an overbooked slot. She wants to talk to you about "his behavior," which may have something to do with drinking. She says, "I thought of bringing him in to see the local addiction specialist, but Carlisle would be paranoid seeing a psychiatrist. He would be worried about what people might think: patients, other doctors."

On further questioning (limited by Dr. Van Heusen's presence in the room) Jenny reports the following:

Home life: His behavior has been reclusive. He has taken to driving home and going directly to his study. On weekends, he no longer hikes. There are two teenage children who avoid him because he is unfriendly, judgmental, and sometimes punitive.

- *Not reported: He has struck Jeremy, one son, in an argument over how he was speaking to Jenny.*
- *Not reported: His daughter, Carmen, has a friend who is Carlisle's patient. Carlisle fondled the friend during a recent physical examination. A Licensing Board complaint has been filed.*

Professional life: Carlisle is constantly paged at home, yet never seems to need to go to the hospital; he manages most of his practice by calling in medications.

- *Not reported: He splits meds with his patients; he offers to "discard legally" unused pills and then diverts them to his own use ("diversion").*

- *Not reported: Self-prescribed zolpidem until 3 years ago, when it became a controlled substance.*
- *Health: He has gained weight. She thinks he has hypertension but he never sees a doctor; he tells her, "It's under control."*
- *Not reported: He obtains tramadol at three pharmacies; he prescribes it widely but keeps all samples.*

Behavior: He is angry when she asks about his drinking.

- *Not reported: She is terrified of asking him.*

"What is your concern or fear?," you ask. She answers that she is worried because Carlisle's father was alcoholic.

You begin by having Carlisle sign releases for communication with several key people: his wife, a colleague, the children. Regardless of how you met Carlisle, your management of his problems follows a Change Model of intervention (please refer to Chap. 10: Adherence in Medicine).

You proceed with a comprehensive history and examination.

 Please proceed with the problem-based approach!

From a primary care standpoint, useful resources for assessment of alcohol and other substance abuse are listed below:

- See Treatment Improvement Protocols, Center of Substance Abuse Treatment of Substance Abuse and Mental Health Services Administration: TIPs 24 and 34 http://www.kap.samhsa.gov/products/manuals/tips/index.htm.
- CAGE Questionnaire (Appendix 1).
- Michigan Alcohol Screening Test (MAST) (Appendix 2).
- Structured Clinical Interview for DSM-IV TR (SCID).

Case Vignette 19.2.2 Continuation

Dr. Van Heusen's first-person history is significant for the following:

- *Raised to a Taiwanese mother and a German-Dutch father, Carlisle had four siblings. Two survive. His father was a military officer whose social life centered on alcohol use; when he retired, it became the centrally organizing theme in his life.*
- *Carlisle's mother lived with the father until his death; she remarried, to a Native American casino owner.*
- *Carlisle resolved at an early age to never drink or smoke.*

- *He moved to Hawai'i for residency in family practice, married another doctor—she is a pathologist—and developed a demanding community and hospital practice in a large-group partnership.*
- *In 1998, he decided to go solo.*
- *He has suffered headaches most of his adult life. They are commonly disabling.*
- *For medical care, he used to see whomever of his partners was available; he has provided his own care to himself, since.*
- *In 1998, in a suit to get out of his previous practice agreement, he alleged misconduct against two of his colleagues. One, a recovering alcoholic, he accused of "always being drunk." His contention was that he left because of increased joint liability. The suit was withdrawn when the partnership agreed to settle.*

Salient findings:

- *Carlisle acknowledges that his headaches have worsened, and that they frequently do not respond to opioids.*

  - *Not reported: He has been ordering and using injectable Stadol/butorphanol through the mail.*

- *He agrees that he has given up most of his social and athletic interests. He indicates that this is because his practice is too busy.*

  - *Not reported: He spends as much time as always at work. His productivity has fallen 20 % since 2005.*

- *He believes that his wife will leave him if he doesn't recover; he states that he wants the marriage to continue.*

  - *Not reported: He has always felt that Jenny was a superior physician and the more successful partner in the marriage. He sees this illness as yet another acknowledgment of his inferiority to her. He is actually ambivalent about the marriage.*

- *He thinks that he has an ulcer. He has been taking cimetidine (Tagamet).*

  - *Not reported: Hematemesis 2 weeks ago after a binge.*

- *He is short of breath on exertion, but ascribes this to cigarettes, 20 pack-years.*

  - *Not reported: He has edema.*

You perform a physical examination and appropriate laboratory studies and draw diagnostic conclusions. Your impression is: alcohol dependence, severe, with opioid abuse and benzodiazepine abuse.

Carlisle is willing to see an addiction specialist, who develops a treatment plan predicated on his level of readiness for change:

1. *Inductive care (residential, day treatment, or outpatient as appropriate and available). Psychotherapies in the treatment of addictions include: cognitive-behavioral therapy, 12-step facilitation, and contingency management. These*

occur in the context of group psychosocial rehabilitation. A patient's required level of care can be identified using a level of care algorithm developed by the American Society of Addiction Medicine. (Patient Placement Criteria 2nd Ed.)

2. *Medication therapy.*
3. *Community reinforcement (also known as Network Therapy, is a contractual management for behavioral monitoring, treatment adherence, and relapse prevention; Marc Gallanter).*
4. *Peer identification, such as physician support groups.*
5. *Recovering community identification such as Alcoholics Anonymous and Narcotics Anonymous.*
6. *Family treatment (reflecting family unit disruption and "contagion," associated with substance use disorder).*
7. *Medical care (somatic consequences of substance use disorder) and psychiatric care (neuropsychological co-morbid consequences of substance use disorder).*

Situations like Dr. Van Heusen's are clinically, ethically, and legally complex. Physicians in need of addiction treatment should be referred to an addiction specialist. The number of physicians involved in the care of a physician should be generous, and their communications with one another should be frequent. At least one objective of this is to prevent the colleague from resuming the role of self-physician.

Review Questions

1. Which of the following statements is FALSE about the epidemiology of substance use disorders?

   (a) Smoking prevalence varies from approximately 10 to 33 % across the 50 states, the District of Columbia, Guam, Puerto Rico, and the US Virgin Islands.
   (b) Excessive alcohol use is the third leading lifestyle-related cause of death in the USA.
   (c) Annually in the USA, cigarette smoking results in serious illnesses in approximately 8.6 million people and death in 440,000 people.
   (d) The percentage of persons in the USA aged 12 years or older who have used any illicit drug in the past month is approximately 3 %.
   (e) None of the above.

2. A patient on the medical/surgical unit requests "something to take the edge off of my alcohol withdrawal." Following many years of heavy, regular drinking, he had his last drink 4 days prior to his admission for pneumonia. He has tachycardia, elevated blood pressure, and difficulty sustaining attention. The most appropriate treatment(s) at this time is (are)

   (a) Thiamine, multivitamins, and benzodiazepines
   (b) Alpha-2-adrenergic agents such as clonidine or guanfacine
   (c) Therapeutic prescription for beer to be given with each meal

(d) Either naltrexone or acamprosate to reduce cravings

(e) All of the above

3. A 15-year-old patient uses marijuana nearly every day in order to "mellow myself out so that I can function." She describes significant anxiety symptoms, almost to the point of panic, if she is unable to have access to marijuana. She obtains the marijuana mostly through trafficking it in her high school. She states that, for the past several months, she has used significantly more of the drug "because I can afford it now." Her academic record reflects an ability to "get straight A's when I put my mind to it." She is often in trouble with her parents for staying out late with her drug-using peers. She denies any past psychiatric symptoms other than "hating her parents" prior to the age of 13, when she first began using marijuana. The most likely diagnosis is

(a) Cannabis abuse

(b) Cannabis dependence

(c) Panic disorder with self-medication

(d) Antisocial personality disorder

(e) None of the above

4. Which of the following is NOT a component of the CAGE questionnaire?

(a) Cut down (use)

(b) Anger (with discussion)

(c) Anxiety (with cessation of drinking)

(d) Guilt (over use)

(e) Eye opener

5. A 23-year-old male is brought to the emergency room with combativeness, paranoia, and pressured speech. His heart rate and blood pressure are elevated. Which of the following is (are) likely substance(s) to explain these findings?

(a) Cocaine

(b) MDMA

(c) Inhalants

(d) All of the above

(e) (a) and (b) only

Answers

1. d, 2. a, 3. b, 4. c, 5. e

Appendix 19.1: CAGE Questionnaire (Ewing, 1984):

(High sensitivity and specificity in most medical populations. Manner of questioning influences outcome, questioner should avoid leading the answer with affect. Recommended that more neutral risk screening be conducted first, e.g., diet/exercise/seat belts/smoking.)

Has the patient any of these responses, to the suggested questions?

Cut down (or discontinued) use

- Because symptoms worsened
- Because a doctor or therapist or advisor suggested

Angry when using or annoyed when drug or alcohol use discussed

- Anger or altercation during use
- Hostile defensiveness surrounding use

Guilt surrounding use

- Guilt, or shame regarding behaviors while using
  Any suicidal gesture

Eye-opener

- Effort to medicate withdrawal, e.g., alcohol or sedatives to suppress hangover symptoms or to permit function at work

A score of two or more positive responses suggests alcohol dependence (Buchs-baum et al., 1991) and warrants re-screening with MAST (Michigan Alcohol Screening Test) or S-MAST (Short MAST) or full diagnostic review with the SCID (Structured Clinical Interview for DSM-4TR).

Appendix 19.2: Short MAST (Seltzer et al., 1975):

1. Do you feel you are a normal drinker?   Yes **No**
2. Do your spouse or parents worry or complain about your drinking?   **Yes** No
3. Do you ever feel bad about your drinking?   **Yes** No
4. Do friends or relatives think you are a normal drinker?   Yes **No**
5. Are you always able to stop drinking when you want to?   Yes **No**
6. Have you ever attended a meeting of Alcoholics Anonymous?   **Yes** No
7. Has drinking ever created problems between you and your spouse?   **Yes** No
8. Have you ever gotten into trouble at work because of drinking?   **Yes** No
9. Have you ever neglected your obligations, your family, or your work for 2 or more   **Yes** No
    days in a row because you were drinking?
10. Have you ever gone to anyone for help about your drinking?   **Yes** No
11. Have you ever been in the hospital because of drinking?   **Yes** No
12. Have you ever been arrested even for a few hours because of drinking?   **Yes** No
13. Have you ever been arrested for drunk driving or driving after drinking?   **Yes** No

Scoring: 1 point for each of answers in bold
2 points = possible problem in use of alcohol
3 points = probable alcohol problem in use of alcohol

References

American Psychiatric Association. Diagnostic and Statistical Manual for Mental Disorders IV-TR. American Psychiatric Press, New York, 2000.

American Psychiatric Association, Work Group on Substance Use Disorders. Practice Guideline for the Treatment of Patients with Substance Use Disorders, Second Edition, 2006. http://www.psych.org/psych_pract/treatg/pg/SUD2ePG_04-28-06.pdf. Accessed 10/9/07.

Buchsbaum DG, Buchanan RG, Centor RM, Schnoll SH, Lawton MJ. Screening for alcohol abuse using CAGE scores and likelihood ratios. *Annals of Internal Medicine* 1991;115(10):774–7.

Centers for Disease Control and Prevention, Annual Smoking-Attributable Mortality CDC. MMWR 2005;54(25):625–8. http://www.cdc.gov. Accessed 9/2/07.

Ewing JA. Detecting alcoholism: the CAGE questionnaire. *JAMA: Journal of the American Medical Association* 1984;252:1905–7.

Harwood H., Updating estimates of the economic costs of alcohol abuse in the United States, H. Lewin Group for the NIAAA, 2000.

Mee-Lee D. ASAM Patient Placement Criteria, Second Edition (PPC-2), 2005. http://coce.samhsa.gov/cod_resources/PDF/ASAMPatientPlacementCriteriaOverview5-05.pdf. Accessed 11/1/07.

National Institute on Drug Abuse. Preventing Drug Use Among Children and Adolescents, Second Edition, 2003. http://www.drugabuse.gov/pdf/prevention/RedBook.pdf. Accessed 10/9/07.

Office of National Drug Control Policy. The Economic Costs of Drug Abuse in the United States, 1992–2002. Executive Office of the President, Washington, DC, 2004a (Publication No. 207303). http://www.whitehousedrugpolicy.gov/publications/economic_costs/economic_costs.pdf. Accessed 9/2/07.

Seltzer MA, Vinokur A, Van Rooijen LJ. A self-administered Short Michigan Alcohol Screening Test (SMAST). *Journal of Studies on Alcohol* 1975;36:117–26.

US Public Health Service, Treating Tobacco Use and Dependence, 2003. http://www.surgeongeneral.gov/tobacco/. Accessed 10/9/07.

Chapter 20
Psychotic Disorders

Steven J. Zuchowski and Ryan Ley

At the end of this chapter, the reader will be able to

1. Recognize symptoms and signs of the most common psychotic disorders and discuss a differential diagnosis
2. Discuss the appropriate assessment of new onset psychotic disorders, including a description of the general medical work-up of a patient presenting for the first time with psychotic symptoms
3. Outline a comprehensive treatment plan for a patient with a chronic psychotic disorder, utilizing the biopsychosocial model

Case Vignette 20.1.1 Helen Harter Presenting Situation

Ms. Helen Harter is a 19-year-old woman who presents to the emergency department where you are on call, accompanied by her mother. Her chief complaint is "twisted ankle." The mother explains that her daughter stepped on her ankle wrong as she was descending the stairs at home and developed pain, swelling, and erythema. You send the patient to x-ray and, while she is there, her mother approaches you with a different concern.

Ms. Harter's mother explains that for the past several months, her daughter hasn't been the same. She has been keeping to herself more. She lost her job at Starbucks about 3 months ago and began avoiding her friends. Lately, she has begun isolating herself from her family as well, staying in her bedroom with the door closed for many hours at a time. Last weekend, when her favorite aunt was visiting from Ohio, Ms. Harter hardly came out for nearly 48 hours. As far as her mother knows, she no longer talks on the telephone, reads or watches TV. While in her room, she lies in bed and listens to heavy metal music. She hasn't been showering or brushing her hair or putting on makeup. Ms. Harter has had no interest in seeking another job, which has led to arguments between her and her father, who feels she is being lazy. Throughout high school, Ms. Harter was quite outgoing, had many friends, talked

S.J. Zuchowski
Assistant Professor, University of Nevada School of Medicine

A. Guerrero, M. Piasecki (eds.), *Problem-Based Behavioral Science and Psychiatry*,
© Springer Science+Business Media, LLC 2008

on the telephone almost non-stop during waking hours, and was very interested in the latest styles and fashions.

Please proceed with the problem-based approach!

Case Vignette 20.1.2 Conclusion

During the interview, Ms. Harter admits to you that she hears a single male voice that is often derogatory toward her and sometimes "bosses her around." She describes her mood as "okay" and does not appear significantly depressed. Her thinking seems to flow logically. However, she hints that her mother is putting tiny amounts of poison in her food in an attempt to kill her. Most nights, she sleeps through the night without awakening. She has not thought of suicide or violence. She states that if her mother keeps trying to poison her, she will simply move out into her own apartment.

Ms. Harter's physical and neurological exam is normal. However, she appears unkempt and has a noticeable body odor. Routine labs are within normal limits and her urine toxicology screen is negative. She denies all drug and alcohol use.

Learning Issues

An apparent personality change like described in Ms. Harter's case is a very worrisome finding at any age. While some variability in how outgoing a person feels is normal, new findings of social isolation and poor personal hygiene point toward a significant psychiatric or general medical problem. However, these symptoms are non-specific. They could represent the early stages (prodrome) of a severe psychotic disorder such as schizophrenia or a mood disorder such as major depressive disorder. Substance dependence could also present this way. General medical causes, such as hypothyroidism, must also be considered and ruled out.

The loss of her job could have triggered her illness or may have been the result of her symptoms. For example, she may have started coming in late to work, frequently missing work, or coming in looking unkempt. Sometimes patients and families will seem to grasp at straws to find an understandable explanation for the onset of psychiatric symptoms and may seek to place all of the blame on a specific event. Clinicians should withhold judgment on causes and attempt to get as complete a database as possible before drawing conclusions.

Psychotic Symptoms

The most obvious and well-known manifestations of the psychotic disorders are delusions and hallucinations. Delusions are fixed, false beliefs, often of a paranoid nature. These false beliefs are, by definition, inflexible even in the face of evidence to the contrary that most people would find overwhelmingly convincing. For example, a psychotic individual might believe that he/she is being followed and watched by someone that wants to harm him/her. No amount of discussion or pointing out of inconsistencies to the patient is likely to make a dent in their belief system. Bizarre delusions are false beliefs that are also impossible (e.g., that aliens are beaming radio signals to electrodes planted in people's teeth), while non-bizarre delusions are possible though still false (e.g., that the government is spying on one's activities).

Hallucinations are false sensory perceptions, most commonly auditory hallucinations such as hearing voices. As a rule, true psychotic hallucinations are somewhat persistent and not just fleeting misperceptions. The fleeting misperceptions that all normal people experience from time to time are called illusions. An example of an illusion is thinking that you hear your name being called when you are in the shower. People with hallucinations might hear a running commentary on their behavior, or they may experience a critical, insulting, or threatening voice that may wax and wane.

Risks Associated with Psychosis

Statistically speaking, people with mental illness are no more likely than people without mental illness to commit acts of violence. However, sometimes people with mental illness do commit acts of violence and it is imperative that a physician always consider violence risk and do what is possible to mitigate it (for instance, by hospitalizing the patient when necessary). While most people even with paranoid delusions are not violent, the presence of paranoid delusions, like in Ms. Harter's case, is one factor that increases violence risk. Command hallucinations of a violent nature present another risk factor. Although patients rarely if ever act like automatons in response to every command hallucination, they may feel compelled to comply with a voice that persistently barks orders or threatens harm if the commands are not followed.

Finally, a patient's mother is statistically the most likely victim of patient violence, likely because the mother is most often the most intimate caregiver. Thus, in Ms. Harter's case, her risk of violence to others—particularly toward her mother—must be carefully considered. In most cases, psychiatric hospitalization—against the patient's wishes if necessary and if legally possible—is the chosen intervention if the risk of harm to self or others is significantly elevated.

Other risks in patients with psychosis are the risks of self-harm and the risks associated with being so ill that basic needs cannot be met. For example, if a patient with schizophrenia has disorganized thoughts and behaviors, he/she may not be able to access shelter, food, and medical care in the community. Every state has specific criteria for involuntary hospitalization for mentally ill people who are a risk to themselves or others.

Case Vignette 20.2.1 Jack Langdon Presenting Situation

Mr. Langdon is a 23-year-old man who presents to your primary care office as a new patient. His chief complaint is, "I cut my arm." When questioned about this, he relates going to the supermarket the other night to buy some ice cream and bacon. He apparently doesn't like to go during the day because "There are too many people there." Mr. Langdon starts a detailed, somewhat rambling narrative about being followed by secret service agents because of his ability to read minds. At first you think you are not following his story and feel confused. Then you realize that the source of confusion is Mr. Landon's loosened thought processes and not you.

During the first few minutes of the interview, you see he has an incision on his left forearm, approximately 8 cm long. When questioned about this, he responds, "They were following me." You ask again how he came to have the cut on his arm. He makes reference to sonic blasts, which pushed him into a window. Clearly several days have passed since the incident, given the presentation of the cut. Mr. Langdon then asks you for a prescription for methylphenidate, to treat his symptoms of ADHD, which was diagnosed 9 months ago. The primary symptoms he reports is "trouble focusing."

 Please proceed with the problem-based approach!

Case Vignette 20.2.2 Continuation

Mr. Langdon seems slightly distractible and occasionally glances about the room. His medical history is unremarkable, and he has never had any seizures, head trauma, or loss of consciousness. He has no allergies and no prior surgeries, accidents, or hospitalizations.

Mr. Langdon's psychiatric review of systems is notable for recent anxiety that developed when he was working in the construction industry. He smokes $\frac{1}{2}$ pack of cigarettes per day, drinks a couple of beers on the weekend, and smokes methamphetamine "every now and then." He lives in an apartment and lost his job recently. He came into the office with his mom and you ask him for permission to talk to her alone. He reluctantly agrees.

Case Vignette 20.2.3 Continuation

Mr. Langdon's mother tells you her son has recently been keeping more to himself. He lost his job in construction because he had some anger management issues and had quite a bit of impatience when others didn't perform their jobs well. She notes he was a bit socially aloof growing up. Although he did have a few friends, they were not particularly close. He neither excelled nor failed in school. She was aware of his diagnosis of ADHD and acknowledged he seems to have trouble concentrating, but wondered if this was a "real diagnosis."

Mr. Langdon's mother also tells you her son did more than smoke methamphetamine occasionally: he used it heavily for approximately 2 years and was involved in selling it. He spent some time in jail but has been sober for 6 months. His parents have urged him to attend Crystal Meth Anonymous meetings, but he resists. Over the course of the past 2 months his parents have been paying his rent and giving him money for groceries because he has had trouble finding work. His paranoid symptoms seemed to start about 4 weeks ago.

You perform a physical exam and note some early cellulitis from the incision on his arm, with some minimal redness, swelling, and weepy drainage. His physical exam is also notable for tachycardia, temperature of 100.3, and some lateral gaze nystagmus. He has "sleeve" tattoos. His medical review of systems reveals an ongoing headache for the past day or so, but is otherwise negative. He hasn't traveled anywhere recently, has no sick contacts, and is feeling pretty well. You order a CBC with differential, chemistry panel, urine drug screen, and T4/TSH. You consider RPR and HIV, but he has minimal risk factors.

Mr. Langdon is dressed in jeans, a white T-shirt, and suede sneakers. He is neat and well groomed, though he has tousled hair. He is alert and oriented to the place and date. He is polite, pleasant, and cooperative. His speech is of a regular rate and rhythm with normal volume and latency. His eye contact is brief; he engages and looks away. He describes his mood as "good, all right." His affect is mood-congruent with a slightly decreased range of expression. He has had no thoughts of self-harm or harm to others. He denies experiencing voices or visual hallucinations, though he does mention a government conspiracy against him. There were no observed responses to internal stimuli. The remainder of the mental status exam shows a possible deficit in abstraction, with concrete interpretations of proverbs. His short-term memory is intact and insight is compromised. His judgment appears fair in that he is seeking medical attention for the cut on his arm.

Learning Issues

Although delusions are commonly of a paranoid (threatening) nature, they may fall in a variety of other categories. For example, psychotic patients may demonstrate grandiose delusions, such as the belief that they are extremely wealthy and powerful. There are delusions of jealousy (e.g., that a spouse is cheating him), erotomanic delusions (e.g., that a high-status person is in love with him), or somatic delusions (e.g., that the patient's heart has stopped). Delusions of reference are beliefs that events in the environment have special meaning referable to the patient (e.g., the light turning green was a message to call the president). Psychotic patients often have combinations of delusions that do not fit classification.

In addition to delusions and hallucinations, there are also less obvious manifestations of psychotic illnesses. Patients may not only demonstrate clear abnormalities in the content of their thought, as described above, but also exhibit disorders in the process of their thinking. For example, a patient's thinking may be disorganized and loose, not linear and logical as we expect. Psychotic patients may also demonstrate negative symptoms; they may be distractible and inattentive or may seem emotionless in their facial expressions (referred to as having a "flat affect"). Their speech may seem relatively devoid of meaningful content and interviewing these individuals may feel like trying to "pull teeth." Patients with psychotic disorders may have all or none of these secondary manifestations.

The differential diagnosis for Mr. Langdon's clinical presentation and constellation of symptoms includes substance-induced psychosis, schizophreniform disorder, schizophrenia, and schizotypal personality disorder. The distinguishing characteristics of the psychotic disorders and other common differential possibilities are summarized in Table 20.1.

Clearly Mr. Langdon's pattern of substance use would make methamphetamine dependence a possibility. Please refer to Chap. 19 for a further discussion of substance use disorders. The urine drug screen will be useful to ascertain if he has been using recently. Mr. Langdon's treatment plan will have to address multiple issues and should be individualized to his particular stressors and needs.

Neurobiology of Psychosis

Psychotic symptoms are thought to have a common neurobiological basis: an excess of dopaminergic activity in certain parts of the brain. Evidence for the dopamine theory of psychotic disorders includes the following:

1. Drugs that block central nervous system (CNS) dopamine receptors reduce psychotic symptoms.
2. Drugs that block CNS dopamine receptors have side effects similar to Parkinson's disease. Parkinson's disease is caused by a lack of dopamine in the basal ganglia.
3. The medications used to treat psychotic disorders are dopamine receptors antagonists (blockers).
4. High doses of amphetamines can cause schizophrenia-like symptoms in otherwise normal individuals.

A diagram of the possible pathophysiology of psychotic symptoms is shown in Fig. 20.1.

Table 20.1 Psychotic Disorders and Related Diagnoses

Diagnosis	Key features	Would presence of delusions support this diagnosis?	Would hallucinations support this diagnosis?	Would disorganized thoughts, behavior, and/or significant impairment support this diagnosis?	Would prominent mood symptoms support this diagnosis?	Time course
Schizophrenia	Active symptoms must include at least two of the following (only one needed if delusions are bizarre or hallucinations are commentating or conversing voices): delusions, hallucinations, disorganized speech, grossly disorganized or catatonic behavior, negative symptoms (including flat affect)	Yes	Yes	Yes	No	At least 6 months, with at least 1 month of active symptoms
Schizophreniform disorder	Active symptoms of schizophrenia	Yes	Yes	Yes	No	At least 1 month, but less than 6 months
Brief psychotic disorder	At least one of the following: delusions, hallucinations, disorganized speech, grossly disorganized or catatonic behavior	Yes	Yes	Yes	Usually not	At least 1 day but less than 1 month

Table 20.1 (continued)

Diagnosis	Key features	Would presence of delusions support this diagnosis?	Would hallucinations support this diagnosis?	Would disorganized thoughts, behavior, and/or significant impairment support this diagnosis?	Would prominent mood symptoms support this diagnosis?	Time course
Schizoaffective disorder	Active symptoms of schizophrenia plus either a major depressive, manic, or mixed episode (see Chap. 21: Mood Disorders and Suicide)	Yes	Yes	Yes	Yes, however, there needs to be psychotic symptoms present for at least 2 weeks without any prominent mood symptoms	
Delusional disorder	Non-bizarre delusions for at least 1 month	Yes—but must be non-bizarre delusions	No—except for tactile or olfactory hallucinations related to delusional theme	No	No	At least 1 month
Paranoid personality disorder	See Chap. 24	No—there is distrust and suspiciousness, without outright delusion	No	Usually not (though this disorder can be premorbid to schizophrenia)	No	Pervasive
Schizotypal personality disorder	See Chap. 24	No—there are only social/interpersonal deficits, perceptual distortions, and eccentricities	Illusions (though not frank hallucinations) are possible	Circumstantiality and odd behavior are possible; can also be premorbid to schizophrenia	No	Pervasive

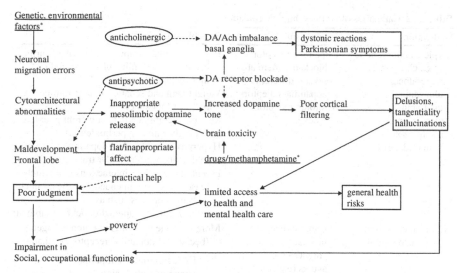

Fig. 20.1 Diagram showing the possible pathophysiology of psychotic symptoms

The medications that have been developed for psychotic disorders are summarized in Table 20.2. In most situations, atypical antipsychotics (other than clozapine) are the medications chosen for initial treatment of psychotic disorders.

The mechanisms and treatments of the extrapyramidal side effects are described in Table 20.3.

Profiles of selected antipsychotic agents are summarized in Table 20.4.

Recommended monitoring for side effects of antipsychotic agents is summarized in Table 20.5.

Psychosis Due to Substances and General Medical Conditions

The presence of psychotic symptoms alone is not pathognomonic for any specific disorder or diagnosis. Patients with a wide variety of general medical and psychiatric disorders may manifest psychotic symptoms, and reversible general medical causes must always be considered first when someone presents with a new onset of psychosis. For example, psychotic symptoms may be traced back to a brain tumor, a seizure disorder, a high calcium level, or hyperthyroidism.

The "psycho-mimetic" effect of amphetamine is well known; however, recreational drugs of all types can trigger hallucinations and delusions. Even prescribed medications, taken precisely as directed by a physician, can sometimes result in psychotic symptoms.

Table 20.2 Categories of Antipsychotic Medications

Medication	Mechanisms	Possible side effects
Atypical antipsychotics (e.g., clozapine, risperidone, olanzapine, quetiapine, ziprasidone, aripiprazole, paliperidone)	Dopamine receptor blockade (there are several different dopamine receptors) Serotonin receptor blockade	Extrapyramidal symptoms (described further below) via dopamine blockade in the nigrostriatal stract Weight gain and sedation (via histamine receptor blockade) Metabolic complications of weight gain (e.g., hyperglycemia, hyperlipidemia) Hyperprolactinemia (via dopamine blockade in the tuberoinfundibular tract) Potential drug–drug interactions (for which reason it is recommended that the clinician consult databases such as http://medicine.iupui.edu/flockhart/table.htm
Typical antipsychotics (e.g., haloperidol)	Dopamine receptor blockade: higher in "higher potency" agents (e.g., haloperidol, fluphenazine) and lower in "lower potency" agents (e.g., thorazine)	More prominent in "higher potency" agents (because of dopamine receptor blockade): Extrapyramidal symptoms Hyperprolactinemia More prominent in "lower potency " agents (because of other receptor blockade): Anticholinergic side effects Sedation Hypotension (due to alpha-adrenergic antagonism) Cardiac rhythm disturbances (particularly QT prolongation)

Schizophrenia and Subtypes

If general medical and substance-related causes have been ruled out as a cause of psychotic symptoms, the patient may be suffering from a primary psychotic disorder. Schizophrenia affects 1 % of the population and usually has its onset in the late teens or early adulthood. There are five subtypes of schizophrenia: paranoid, disorganized, catatonic, undifferentiated, and residual type.

Paranoid type is something of a misnomer, as the patient does not need to have paranoid ideation. The criteria for this subtype include preoccupation with delusions or voices in the absence of disorganized speech or behavior, catatonia, or affect withdrawal. The delusions may be persecutory, and patients with this subtype may mistrust others. Examples of some delusions might include the CIA stalking them, someone poisoning their food, someone taking pictures of them or spying on them, or their thoughts being broadcast on television.

The experience of voices is sometimes present in paranoid schizophrenia, and often these voices will be engaged in making derogatory comments about the person, commenting on their activities, or murmuring. Sometimes they can be command type, telling the person to do things that may involve self-harm or harm to

Table 20.3 Major Categories of Antipsychotic Side Effects

Syndrome	Manifestations	Mechanism	Treatment
Neuroleptic malignant syndrome	Hyperthermia, muscle rigidity, autonomic instability, rhabdomyolysis and renal failure	Functional denervation (from dopamine blockade) of the sympathetic nervous system from central control	Supportive care, dantrolene, bromocriptine
Acute dystonia	Acute muscle spasm; may involve the eye muscles (oculogyric crisis) and or neck muscles	Relative excess of acetylcholine relative to dopamine effect in the basal ganglia	Anticholinergics
Akathisia	Significant motoric restlessness and discomfort		Beta-adrenergic blockers, benzodiazepines
Parkinsonism		Relative excess of acetylcholine relative to dopamine effect in the basal ganglia	Anticholinergics
Tardive dyskinesia	Slow, writhing movements; may involve lip-smacking or other orofacial movements	Possibly oxidative damage in the basal ganglia secondary to chronic dopamine blockade and unregulated excitatory neurotransmission	In theory, antioxidants

others. Although there can be agitation or behavioral disturbances that can even progress to violence, most patients with schizophrenia are not violent. And with appropriate treatment and a supportive environment, patients with this subtype can function quite well.

Disorganized subtype of schizophrenia contrasts with the paranoid subtype. The criteria for the disorganized subtype is: prominent disorganized speech and behavior, with a flattened or inappropriate affect.

Catatonic subtype of schizophrenia describes dramatically altered behavior. Typically, patients with this subtype experience immobility and lack of responsiveness to the environment. They may also have flailing and rocking behaviors. "Waxy flexibility" refers to the postures that patients will maintain for hours if placed by others.

Benzodiazepines can improve symptoms of catatonia, and this subtype may also respond to ECT.

The undifferentiated subtype of schizophrenia is used whenever the constellation of symptoms does not fit paranoid, catatonic, or disorganized types.

Residual type refers to an attenuated form of schizophrenia. There may be an absence of delusions, visual hallucinations, voices, or disorganized speech in a patient who still has negative symptoms such as decreased range of affect and monotone speech.

Table 20.4 Common Antipsychotic Medications

Medication	Available forms	Long-acting preparation?	Special side effects	Other comments
Risperidone	Oral, rapidly disintegrating, liquid	Yes	Higher rate of extrapyramidal symptoms and hyperprolactinemia	Currently the only atypical antipsychotic with Food and Drug Administration approval for use in children and adolescents
Olanzapine	Oral, rapidly disintegrating, intramuscular	No	Higher rates of sedation and weight gain	
Quetiapine	Oral	No	Theoretical risk of corneal clouding	
Ziprasidone	Oral, intramuscular	No	Slightly higher risk (compared with the other atypical antipsychotics) of QT prolongation	Lowest risk of weight gain and metabolic sequelae among the atypical antipsychotics
Aripiprazole	Oral	No		Lower risk of weight gain and metabolic sequelae among the atypical antipsychotics
Clozapine	Oral	No	Higher rates of sedation and weight gain Agranulocytosis is a potentially life-threatening complication	Used in cases refractory to other atypical antipsychotics
Haloperidol	Oral, intramuscular, intravenous	Yes	Risks of typical antipsychotics as described above	Of the antipsychotics, haloperidol is the one with the most data for use in delirium (see Chap. 25: Cognitive Disorders) Also, haloperidol is the antipsychotic with the most data for use in pregnancy

Table 20.5 Guidelines for Monitoring Patients on Antipsychotics

Measure	Minimum frequency
Fasting lipids	Every 6 months
Fasting blood sugar	Every 6 months
Formal assessment for extrapyramidal movements	Every 6 months (for typical antipsychotics) and every 12 months (for atypical antipsychotics), using the Abnormal Involuntary Movement Scale (AIMS)
Eye examination	Every year for quetiapine
Electrocardiogram	At baseline and as indicated for medications that may prolong the QT interval
Body mass index	At each visit for the first 6 months, then quarterly thereafter

Case Vignette 20.3.1 Presenting Situation: Vera Franklin

Mrs. Vera Franklin is a 59-year-old woman who presents to the ER with a chief complaint of "These parasites are eating me up, it's really driving me crazy. Just look at my legs, it's awful." She points to her lower legs, which show some generalized xerosis, mild erythema, and changes associated with venous stasis. She leans down to scratch her right shin while looking at you.

A review of systems reveals some occasional lower extremity edema, intermittent pain, and pruritis. Mrs. Franklin is appropriately attentive to your questions, but is quite concerned about what she thinks may be an "infestation."

Her eye contact is good, with a clear, open gaze. She wonders if she has had more headaches recently and complains that she has had a lot of trouble sleeping. She has had both early and middle insomnia. Mrs. Franklin describes experiencing some minimal sadness over the course of the past several weeks.

Her vitals are relatively unremarkable, except her blood pressure which is elevated to 162/86. She is afebrile, with a pulse of 78.

Please proceed with the problem-based approach!

Case Vignette 20.3.2 Continuation

Mrs. Franklin used to travel extensively as a flight attendant in her twenties and thirties, including travel to Africa and the Far East, but has had no recent travel. She lives by herself in a relatively new condo and has had the carpets steam-cleaned this year. Her condo is free of pests. She hasn't started using any new detergent, shampoo, soaps, or moisturizers. She has no pets.

Repeat blood pressure measurements are 145/88 and 142/84. Mrs. Franklin has been undergoing quite a bit of stress recently. She and her husband were divorced a few years ago, and she was kicked out of her bridge group for being intoxicated and disruptive. Her 401K lost 45 % of its value in the last quarter, and she is worried about her future finances.

Mrs. Franklin enjoys watching the Discovery Channel and first started experiencing itchy legs after watching several shows devoted to malaria and other diseases affecting the African sub-continent. At first she didn't think anything of this, attributing her symptoms to "just being nervous and over-reacting." Gradually though, her symptoms began to worsen. The past several weeks she has had significant itching. Her legs also seemed to become quite dry, despite using moisturizers. She came to the ER because she was worried about some sort of skin infection. She seems to have little doubt this is what is causing her symptoms. She notes, "Sometimes it feels like they're crawling on me."

Physical exam reveals the changes on her legs that were previously noted. She is well nourished. Her heart sounds are a bit distant, but otherwise unremarkable. The remainder of her exam is within normal limits.

She was alert and oriented to date and place on the Mental Status Exam. She was dressed in jeans, a western-style snap blouse, and wore light eye shadow. Her eye contact was appropriate. Her speech was of a regular rate and rhythm with normal volume and latency. She seemed engaged and provided developed answers to questions. Her attitude was cooperative and slightly bemused. She described her mood as "good, but a little worried about my legs." She often scratches her legs during the exam.

Her affect was mood-congruent, lively, and pleasant. She denied any anxiety. She had no thoughts of self-harm. She denied any voices, visual hallucinations, special powers, or beliefs. She laughed at this question and showed a well-developed sense of humor. She denied any paranoia or suspiciousness. Cognitive testing was without deficits. Her judgment was positive.

Mrs. Franklin is a smoker and has a 25 pack-year history. She noted she "drinks a glass of wine or two with dinner," but uses no illicit substances.

Blood tests were all normal, and you take a skin scraping to assess for a fungal infection.

Please proceed with the problem-based approach!

Case Vignette 20.3.3 Case Conclusion

The result of the skin scraping is negative. Close inspection of her legs reveals no apparent source of infection. There are no burrows, noticeable fomites, or open sores. Her legs are somewhat erythematous, but that could be secondary to scratching. There is no induration or warmth, and minimal pain.

Mrs. Franklin has never been diagnosed with a psychiatric disorder, although she has been experiencing some increased stress and anxiety of late. She has no positive psychiatric family history.

Learning Issues

The differential diagnosis would have to point strongly toward either lichen simplex chronicus or delusional disorder. Psychic factors are significant in both. The possibility of parasitic infection should not be entirely ruled out, but is considerably less likely. A delusional disorder is characterized by non-bizarre delusions. Although her thoughts about infection may be odd, they could represent a true life experience. Bizarre delusions are those that are clearly outside the realm of normal human experience such as alien abduction or brain implants that transmit thoughts.

A person with a delusional disorder may present quite normally, and indeed one of the criteria for delusional disorder is the absence of prominent mood or psychotic symptoms. Functioning is not markedly impaired, and behavior is not bizarre. Criterion A symptoms of schizophrenia cannot have been met (i.e., disorganized speech or behavior, flattening of affect, or hallucinations). Subtypes of delusional disorder include erotomanic, persecutory, somatic, mixed, grandiose, jealous, and unspecified.

Mrs. Franklin may be cautiously open to considering antipsychotic medication, after a careful explanation of rationale. A low-dose atypical antipsychotic may help decrease somatic symptoms that have been distressing and is likely to help with sleep and mood. Antidepressants have also been used in patients with somatic delusions and might be considered as well. A topical steroid cream could also help calm the inflammation and provide some relief from her ongoing itching.

Treatment resistance can be difficult to overcome, especially if a patient denies he/she has a problem. Most patients with somatic delusions treated with pharmacotherapy report some improvement in symptomotology, and many of these patients may experience complete resolution. Psychotherapy may also be useful in developing coping strategies, a stronger sense of self, and emotional resilience.

This case illustrates some of the subtleties of psychiatric diagnosis and the interplay between physical and psychic symptoms. Mrs. Franklin may have mild systolic hypertension and chronic tension headaches in addition to feeling as though her legs are infected with bugs. Her condition will be difficult to treat in the emergency setting, and referral to a psychiatrist will be helpful. The information that she is unlikely to be suffering from an infestation must be conveyed gently. An direct approach that is delivered with sensitivity and sincerity is most likely to be successful.

Review Questions

1. A previously healthy 19-year-old man presents with 7 months of hearing derogatory voices, social isolation, and the belief that the government is monitoring him wherever he goes. He denies all drug and alcohol use. The most likely diagnosis is

    (a) Schizophrenia
    (b) Bipolar II disorder
    (c) Schizoaffective disorder
    (d) Major depressive disorder

2. To rule out other possible causes of this patient's symptoms, which of the following tests should be considered?

    (a) Brain imaging
    (b) Routine blood work (CBC, electrolytes, liver and kidney functions)
    (c) Urine toxicology screen for illicit drugs
    (d) All of the above

3. A 62-year-old woman presents with the isolated complaint of feeling parasites crawling under her skin. Examination and tests reveal no evidence of parasites but she is not reassured. Other than a preoccupation with the parasite infestation, she functions normally. The most likely diagnosis is

    (a) Schizophrenia
    (b) Bipolar I disorder
    (c) Delusional disorder
    (d) Major depressive disorder

4. What kind of treatment would you offer this patient?

    (a) Antipsychotic medication
    (b) Psychotherapy
    (c) Physical exams of her skin every 3 months to rule out actual infestation
    (d) All of the above

5. A 45-year-old man, new to the city, presents with a long history of partially controlled schizophrenia. He has been in and out of treatment over the years and has been hospitalized over a dozen times in other states, mainly due to medication non-adherence. The treatment plan for this man should include all of the following elements as priorities EXCEPT

    (a) Continued psychotropic medication and attention to adherence
    (b) Attempts to ensure stable housing
    (c) Assistance in obtaining general medical follow-up
    (d) Insight-oriented psychotherapy

Answers

1. a, 2. d, 3. c, 4. d, 5. d

Populated Tables

Case table 20.1 Helen Harter

What are the facts?	What are your hypothesis?	What do you want to know next?	What specific information would you like to learn about?
19-year-old woman with ankle injury and 1 year of progressive social isolation and decreased attention to personal hygiene and grooming	Major depressive disorder Schizophrenia Substance dependence General medical condition	Does she hear voices or see visions? Is she paranoid? Does she feel someone is trying to harm her or monitor her? How is her mood? Suicidal or homicidal thoughts? How is her sleep? Appetite? Energy level? Concentration? Any sense that others can read her mind? She can read minds? Personal messages from TV, music, etc.? Physical exam Mental status exam Screening blood work (CBC, CMP, TSH/T4) Urine toxicology screen	
19-year-old who admits to auditory hallucinations in the form of a derogatory voice Apparent paranoid delusion of being poisoned by her mother No disorder of thought process	Schizophreniform disorder (duration between 1 month and 6 months) Major depressive disorder with psychotic features Substance dependence (less likely but should always be kept in mind) Occult general medical condition (becoming more unlikely)	Any other hallucinations or delusions? Does the voice ever command her to do violent things or to commit suicide? Does she have any delusions of being controlled by an outside force? Brain CT or MRI scan?	

Case table 20.2 Jack Langdon

What are the facts?	What are your hypothesis?	What do you want to know next?	What specific information would you like to learn about?
23-year-old man with 8 cm laceration on forearm, obtained under unusual circumstances	Schizophrenia or schizophreniform disorder	When was last use of methamphetamine or other drugs? Any periods of heavy use?	
Believes he can read minds and that he was being followed by Secret Service because of this ability	Methamphetamine-induced psychotic disorder	Duration of symptoms? Prior episodes?	
Uses methamphetamine "every now and then."	Mood disorder with psychotic features	Mood symptoms? Detail about his ability to read minds? Hears voices? What are they like?	
Lost job recently	Psychotic disorder due to general medical condition	Suicidal or homicidal thoughts?	
Unremarkable medical history		Why did he lose job? Urine toxicology screen Screening blood work (CBC, CMP, TSH/T4, might add RPR) Brain imaging—consider especially with focal signs, history of head trauma, inexplicable	
Per mother, no meth use × 6 months but was heavy user × 2 years	Substance-induced psychotic disorder	Results of urine toxicology screen, screening blood work, brain imaging	
Psychiatric symptoms began 4 weeks ago	Schizophreniform disorder	How is he doing with living independently?	
Signs of early infection of forearm wound	Schizotypal personality disorder	Condition of his apartment? Financial situation? Access to medical care?	
Lateral gaze nystagmus	Timeframe is too short for schizophrenia (minimum 6 months)		
Headache	Mood disorder is unlikely		
No suicidal or homicidal thoughts	Mild soft tissue infection unlikely to lead to psychotic symptoms		
Denies hallucinations			

Case table 20.3 Vera Franklin

What are the facts?	What are your hypothesis?	What do you want to know next?	What specific information would you like to learn about?
59-year-old woman who feels she has a skin infection Bilateral lower extremity edema pruritis, erythema, and xerosis Headaches and elevated bp Multiple allergies	Lichen simplex chronicus (scratch dermati-tis/neurodermatitis) Atopic dermatitis Contact dermatitis Somatoform disorder NOS Delusional disorder Parasitic infection	How long has she experienced her symptoms? How did they evolve? CBC, chem panel, TSH/T4 Repeat blood pressure measurements Does she have any associated symptoms with her headaches? Has she had any strange thoughts, or atypical sensory experiences? Is anyone out to get her? Does she feel paranoid or suspicious of others? Social history Mental status exam	
Symptoms began shortly after watching television shows, and progressively worsened She has had significant stress recently No recent travel or pest exposure No new cosmetic, skin, or laundry products No atypical thoughts or experiences	Lichen simplex chronicus (scratch dermati-tis/neurodermatitis) Delusional disorder Parasitic infection	Does she have any psychiatric history? Is there any family psychiatric history? Results of skin scraping Is she open to considering psychiatric medication?	

Bibliography

American Psychiatric Association. Diagnostic & Statistical Manual of Mental Disorders, Fourth
    Edition, Text Revision, American Psychiatric Association, New York, 2000.
American Psychiatric Association. Treating Schizophrenia: A Quick Reference Guide, 2004.
    http://www.psych.org/psych_pract/treatg/quick_ref_guide/SchizophreniaQRG_04-15-05.pdf.
    Accessed 10/17/07.
Applebaum PS, Robbins PC & Monahan J. Violence and Delusions: Data from the MacArthur
    Violence Risk Assessment Study. American Journal of Psychiatry 2000; 157:566–572.
Sadock BJ & Sadock VA. Synopsis of Psychiatry, Ninth Edition, Lippincott, Williams & Wilkins,
    Philadelphia, 2003.

Chapter 21
Mood Disorders and Suicide

Mireille Anawati

This chapter covers a very important group of disorders in psychiatry as well as suicide, which is one of the leading causes of death in the United States. At the end of this chapter, the reader will be able to

1. Discuss the epidemiology, mechanisms, clinical presentation, clinical evaluation, differential diagnosis, and treatment of mood disorders
2. Appreciate the mechanisms and adverse effects of antidepressants
3. Discuss epidemiology and appropriate intervention for suicide attempts

Case Vignette 21.1.1 Caroline Atwater

Caroline Atwater, a 27-year-old woman comes to you, her primary care physician (PCP), for an annual checkup. You review the Beck Depression Inventory, a checklist screening form she filled out in the waiting room and see that Ms. Atwater has been feeling depressed, having difficulty sleeping for several weeks and has lost 10 pounds in the past 2 months. She also doesn't seem to have much of an appetite, and quit playing tennis a few months ago because she "doesn't have enough energy for that anymore."

 Please proceed with the problem-based approach!

At this point, a differential diagnosis should include

- Major depressive disorder
- Dysthymic disorder
- Substance-induced mood disorder

M. Anawati
Fourth-year Medical Student University of Hawai'i John A. Burns School of Medicine

A. Guerrero, M. Piasecki (eds.), *Problem-Based Behavioral Science and Psychiatry*,
© Springer Science+Business Media, LLC 2008

- Mood disorder due to a general medical condition
- Malignancy
- Hypothyroidism

It is important to distinguish major depressive disorder from dysthymic disorder, substance-induced mood disorder, and mood disorder due to a general medical condition. While the latter two are somewhat self-explanatory, let us discuss and clarify between the former. Major depressive disorder describes one or more major depressive episodes. The diagnostic criteria for a major depressive episode include a period of two or more weeks with depressed mood or loss of interest or pleasure. The period of mood disturbance also includes four or more of the following symptoms: changes in appetite or changes in weight, difficulty sleeping (i.e., insomnia or hypersomnia), low energy or fatigue, feelings of guilt or worthlessness, poor concentration, agitation, and recurrent thoughts of suicide. In contrast, dysthymia is a chronic mood disorder characterized by depression for most of the day, more days than not, accompanied by fewer symptoms than in a major depressive episode. Dysthymia's minimum time criterion is at least 1 year in children and at least 2 years in adults (American Psychiatric Association, 2000; Moore & Jefferson, 2004)

Case Vignette 21.1.2 Continuation

You complete a physical exam and find nothing significant. Ms. Atwater has no lymphadenopathy, tibial edema, or thyromegaly. Digital rectal exam was hemoccult negative. You order diagnostic labs such as urine toxicology, free T4, thyroid-stimulating hormone, hemoglobin, and hematocrit. All labs were within the normal limits.

 Please proceed with the problem-based approach!

This scenario is meant to generate critical analysis. Was the approach of this physician appropriate? Was there a leap to a physical exam and labs before completing a thorough history? A masterful interview allows for both improved diagnostic accuracy and improved patient–doctor relationships.

Important aspects of the history in considering differential diagnoses include PMH of thyroid disease, cancer, and other chronic medical conditions (see Table 21.1); past psychiatric history of eating disorders, depression, manic episodes, or substance abuse; family history of cancer, depression, substance abuse, suicide attempts; and social history for childhood physical or sexual abuse, recent loss of a loved one, homelessness, financial instability, stress levels at work/school, relationships, and social support. In the review of systems, the physician may ask about appetite as well as weight changes, heat/cold intolerance, energy level,

Table 21.1 Medications and general medical conditions associated with depression

Medications	Analgesics (e.g., ibuprofen, indomethacin, opioids, phenacetin)
	Antibiotics (e.g., ampicillin, sulfamethoxazole, clotrimazole, tetracycline, griseofulvin, metronidazole, nitrofurantoin, streptomycin)
	Antihypertensive agents (e.g., hydralazine, methyldopa, prazosin, propanolol, reserpine, clonidine)
	Antineoplastic agents (e.g., bleomycin, vincristine, vinblastine)
	Steroids and hormones (e.g., corticosteroids, oral contraceptives, prednisone, triamcinolone)
	Stimulants and appetite suppressants (amphetamine, fenfluramine)
Medical conditions	Neurologic: chronic subdural hematoma, dementia, epilepsy, Huntington's disease, migraine headaches, normal pressure hydrocephalus, narcolepsy, Parkinson's disease, stroke, temporal lobe epilepsy, Wilson's disease
	Infectious: encephalitis, HIV, infectious hepatitis, influenza, mononucleosis, subacute bacterial endocarditis, syphilis, trauma, tuberculosis
	Neoplasms: bronchogenic carcinoma, CNS tumors, pancreatic cancer, lymphoma
	Metabolic/endocrine: Addison's disease, anemia, Cushing's disease, diabetes, hepatic disease, electrolyte abnormalities (e.g., hypokalemia or hyponatremia), hypoparathyroidism, hypopituitarianism, hypothyroidism, menses related, pellagra, porphyria, thiamine/B12/folate deficiencies, uremia
	Collagen-vascular disease: Rheumatoid arthritis, sjögren's arteritis, systemic lupus crythematosus
	Cardiovascular: Chronic heart failure
	Respiratory: Obstructive sleep apnea

sleep cycle, mood changes, irritability, neurological function, gait, coordination, and academic or occupational performance. When there is a suspicion of a mood disorder, the interview should also query for manic symptoms such as grandiose thinking, decreased need for sleep, elevated mood, spending sprees, and pressured speech to screen for bipolar disorder appearing as unipolar depression.

An Annual visit for patients with no significant medical problems potentially leaves time for health risk screening. Does she see a gynecologist annually for cervical cancer screening? What is her living environment like? Does she go to school or have a job? Does she have a significant other? Has she been exposed to domestic violence or sexual abuse? According to data collected by the CDC in 2000, the three most common causes of death in men and women of all races, ages 25–34, are unintentional injury (e.g., motor vehicle accidents), suicide, and homicide (www.cdc.gov).

Mood disorders include a rather wide spectrum of diagnoses. Typically, they are divided into depressive disorders, bipolar disorders, and mood disorders secondary to another cause (i.e., due to general medical condition or substance induce) (American Psychiatric Association, 2000). The various mood disorders are summarized in Table 21.2. In this case, symptoms and duration are consistent with a major depressive disorder.

Table 21.2 Mood disorders

Depressive disorders
- Major depressive disorder
- Dysthymic disorder
- Depressive disorder not otherwise specified

Bipolar disorders
- Bipolar I disorder
- Bipolar II disorder
- Cyclothymic disorder
- Bipolar disorder not otherwise specified

Mood disorder due to a general medical condition
Substance-induced mood disorder
Mood disorder not otherwise specified

Depression is extremely common and commonly undiagnosed. Nearly 50 % of all cases of depression, similar to those with adult-onset diabetes, remain undetected for years or inadequately controlled (Sadock, 2005). Silent conditions such as hypertension are detected with routine screening and tend to be treated much earlier, with significant reductions in complications such as myocardial infarction and stroke.

Depressive disorders afflict approximately 20 % of women and 10 % of men at some time during their lives (Sadock, 2005). The median age of onset is 40 years, but depression may occur at any age. There is no evidence to suggest that prevalence is related to ethnicity, education, income, or marital status. However, adult and adolescent females are two to three times as likely to have major depressive disorder as are adult and adolescent males (www.cdc.gov).

There are several models that explain the pathophysiology of depression. Figure 21.1 incorporates various aspects of these models to explain the current beliefs behind the multifactorial components which lead to the development of depression in any given individual. The biogenic amine model is based on retrospective understanding from the pharmacological action of antidepressant and thymoleptic agents. These pharmacologic agents have revolutionized the treatment of depression. However, the fundamental biochemistry of mood disorders is still far from being understood (Sadock, 2005).

Case Vignette 21.1.3 Conclusion

After discussing her symptoms in greater detail, you learn that her insomnia and difficulty concentrating resulted in the loss of her job, and she is planning to move back in with her parents to save money. Ms. Atwater feels isolated and calls herself a "failure" several times throughout the interview, but denies suicidal ideations. She also mentions a recent discussion between she and her boyfriend about getting pregnant.

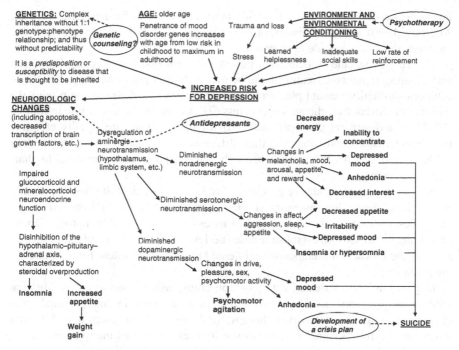

Fig. 21.1 Mechanistic diagram showing the pathophysiology of depression. Treatment options are indicated by *dashed lines*

Since she meets criteria for a major depressive episode, you prescribe a selective serotonin reuptake inhibitor, after discussing possible adverse effects and the expected delay in efficacy. You schedule an appointment in one week.

The DSM-IV criteria require that the symptoms during a depressive episode be significant enough to impair function to meet the threshold for major depressive episode for appropriate diagnosis (American Psychiatric Association, 2000). In this case, her symptoms are clearly affecting her function and her social life. The functional impairment increases the importance of early symptom recognition and treatment to avoid further complications, especially a suicide attempt. There is typically a period of approximately 3 years between the onset of mood disorder and first suicide attempt (Brent, 2004). During that window of opportunity, it is critical to identify and treat depressive disorders and thus prevent the onset of suicidal behavior.

Sixty percent of depressed patients have suicidal ideations, and 15 % commit suicide (Sadock, 2005). Although depressive disorders are more commonly seen in women and women attempt suicide more often, more men actually die of suicide.

The risk of suicide increases with a diagnosis of major depression, active alcoholism, separation divorce, and cocaine use. Educational achievement appears to be inversely associated with risk of suicide attempt (Petronis, Samuels, Moscicki & Anthony, 1990). A family history of mood disorders and/or suicide attempts also increases the risk of suicide attempts.

The risk of suicide in depressed patients is managed with regular follow up and adequate treatment. Treatment can be medication or psychotherapy. The major categories of antidepressant pharmacologic agents are selective serotonin reuptake inhibitors (SSRIs), tricyclic antidepressants (TCAs), monoamine oxidase inhibitors (MAOIs), and atypical antidepressants. All of these classes are equally effective in treating major depression, but they differ in safety and adverse effects (see Table 21.3). Up to 70–75 % of patients with major depression will respond to pharmacologic therapy.

Several depression scales (e.g., Center for Epidemiological Studies Depression Scale, Beck Depression Inventory, or Hamilton Rating Scale for Depression) are available to screen for depression and to assess the severity of symptoms. These scales are useful tools to establish a baseline level of depression and subsequently monitor the efficacy of therapeutic regimens, but cannot substitute for a diagnostic interview.

Depression is often treated with psychotherapy, either alone or in combination with antidepressants. Evidence-based interventions include interpersonal psychotherapy, cognitive-behavioral therapy, and some of the marital and family interventions. Interpersonal psychotherapy focuses on current interpersonal problems and seeks to recognize depressive precipitants such as interpersonal losses, role disputes and transitions, social isolation, or deficits in social skills. Cognitive-behavioral therapy is based on the premise that helping patients to recognize and correct erroneous beliefs can relieve their negative thoughts and behaviors. Marital and family problems are common in the course of mood disorders; thus, marital and family therapies can help educate families about mood disorders and facilitate support and communication. Factors contributing to the success of these various modalities include mild to moderate illness; a stable environment; and the patient's motivation, capacity for insight, psychological mindedness, and capacity to form a relationship. Therapeutic alliance is also pivotal for the effectiveness of treatment (Ebert, Loosen, and Nurcombe, 2000).

Another alternative treatment modality is electroconvulsive therapy (ECT). ECT is an effective treatment (with about 70–85 % efficacy) for treating severe depression, particularly depression in the elderly and with delusions and agitation. ECT causes a generalized central nervous system seizure; however, the exact mechanism for its antidepressant effects is unknown. The patient undergoing ECT is anesthetized and given a muscle relaxant. Then, electrodes are placed on the temples and a current is generated. The patient is awake within 5–10 min. Treatments are usually given every other day for 6–14 sessions. The most common side effects are memory disturbance and headache (Ropper & Brown, 2005). Improvements from ECT are temporary, and patients must receive maintenance treatment to avoid relapse.

Major depressive disorder may occur as a single episode or may be recurrent. The average, untreated depressive episode lasts for about 10 months. At least 75 % of the affected patients have a second episode of depression, usually within the first

Table 21.3 Pharmacology of antidepressant medications

Pharmacologic class, examples, and indications	MOA	Adverse Effects
All antidepressants		Patients should be counseled about the potential for rare, serious side effects, including allergic or other life-threatening reactions; increase in suicidal ideations; and unmasking of mania
SSRIs (e.g., fluoxetine, citalopram, escitalopram, fluoxamine, paroxetine, sertraline) First-line agents for depression; also used in various anxiety disorders such as panic disorder and OCD	Inhibit reuptake of 5HT from the synaptic cleft by blocking reuptake transporters; more 5HT selectivity at lower doses Different SSRIs have different profiles of inhibiting cytochrome P450 enzymes. The reader is encouraged to consult available resources including: http://medicine.iupu i.edu/flockhart/table .htm	Significantly fewer adverse effects than other antidepressants; side effects include nausea, diarrhea, insomnia, sedation, headache, sexual dysfunction; serotonin syndrome[a]
TCAs (e.g., amitriptyline, nortriptyline, imipramine, desipramine) Used in depression, anxiety disorders, and as adjuncts in bulimia and chronic pain disorders	Inhibit reuptake of 5HT and NE from synaptic cleft by blocking reuptake transporters	Lack of specificity leads to greater range of adverse effects *Anticholinergic effects*: dry mouth, blurred vision, constipation, urinary retention, heat intolerance, tachycardia, nausea/vomiting *Antiadrenergic effects*: orthostatic hypotension, dizziness, reflex tachycardia *Antihistaminergic effects*: sedation, weight gain Potential for cardiotoxicity and neurotoxicity
MAOIs (e.g., phenelzine, tranyl-cypromine) Effective for refractory depression and refractory panic disorder, also good for depression with atypical features (e.g., psychosis), and other anxiety disorders including social phobia, OCD	Block deamination of monoamines by inhibiting monoamine oxidase, thus increasing cytoplasmic levels of 5HT and NE in the presynaptic neuron	MAOIs: tyramine toxicity: indirect sympathomimetic effects stimulate release of stored catecholamine when foods with tyramine are consumed (e.g., cheese, red wine, fava beans, cured meats) MAOIs + SSRIs: Serotonin syndrome[a] MAOIs = TCAs: Hypertensive crisis[b]

Table 21.3 (continued)

Pharmacologic class, examples, and indications	MOA	Adverse Effects
Atypicals		
NDRI: bupropion Indications: depression, smoking cessation aid, seasonal affective disorder, ADHD	Like amphetamines, inhibits NE reuptake and DA reuptake	Insomnia, headache, constipation, dry mouth, nausea, and tremor are most common; of note: no sexual side effects (advantage over SSRIs) Slightly greater tendency (versus the other antidepressants) of lowering the seizure threshold, particularly in patients with eating disorders
SNRIs: venlafaxine, duloxetine Indications: depressive disorders, anxiety disorders, ADHD, chronic pain management	Selective inhibitor of serotonin and NE reuptake	Similar to SSRIs, see above May raise blood pressure
SARI: nefazodone Indications: refractory major depression, insomnia, PTSD, chronic pain	Inhibits presynaptic 5HT reuptake and blocks postsynaptic serotonin receptors ($5HT_2$ so as to minimize anxiety as a side effect)	Nausea, dry mouth, dizziness, sedation, agitation, constipation, weight loss, and headache are common Rare hepatotoxicity
NASA: mirtazapine Indications: depressive disorders, especially patients who need to gain weight	Blocks $5HT_2$ and $5HT_3$ receptors (so as to minimize anxiety and gastrointestinal upset as side effects) and acts as a selective alpha 2 adrenergic *ant*agonist, thus increasing NE and beneficial 5HT transmission	Sedation, weight gain, dry mouth, constipation, fatigue, and dizziness are common Rare bone marrow suppression

SSRI: selective serotonin reuptake inhibitor, OCD: obsessive-compulsive disorder, 5HT: serotonin, TCA: tricyclic antidepressant, MAOI: monoamine oxidase inhibitor, NE: norepinephrine, DA: dopamine, NDRI: NE/DA reuptake inhibitor, SNRI: 5HT/NE reuptake inhibitor, SARI: 5HT antagonist and reuptake inhibitor, NASA: NE/5HT reuptake inhibitor, ADHD: attention deficit hyperactivity disorder, AE: adverse effects

[a]Serotonin syndrome is typically seen with combined use of MAOIs and SSRIs, initially consisting of lethargy, restlessness, confusion, flushing, diaphoresis, tremor and myoclonic jerks, and eventually can result in hyperthermia, hypertonicity, rhabdomyolysis, renal failure, convulsions, coma, and death

[b]Hypertensive crisis can result in headache, tachycardia, nausea, cardiac arrythmias, and even stroke

6 months after the initial episode (Sadock, 2005). As mentioned above, 15 % of depressed patients eventually commit suicide. For those who survive, the prognosis of major depression is variable, with 50 % of patients recovering, 30 % partially recovering, and 20 % with a chronic course (Sadock, 2005).

In the case above, Ms. Atwater mentioned pregnancy toward the end of her visit. Pregnancy can complicate the course of a depressive disorder because of the potential adverse effects of medications on the fetus and the risk of postpartum depression. Given that the prevalence of depression peaks between the ages of 20–40 years, depression during pregnancy likewise is common. Women with a previous history of depression are at an increased risk. As with depression in general, depression during pregnancy remains under-recognized and under-treated. It is particularly difficult to diagnose depression during pregnancy because of overlap in somatic complaints common to both conditions, such as sleep disturbances, eating disturbances, weight gain, irritability, fatigue, and lack of energy (Sadock, 2005).

Postpartum depression occurs in up to 15 % of postpartum women and has the same diagnostic symptoms as major depressive disorder. Risk factors include past history or family history of depression, past history of premenstrual dysphoric disorder, or previous postpartum depression. These findings suggest that certain women are sensitive to changes in reproductive hormone levels, such as those occurring premenstrually and during the postpartum or perimenopausal periods (Sadock, 2005). Unlike "postpartum blues," which is usually transient, mild, and common, postpartum depression results in clinically significant impairment and may impact the well-being of both the mother and the baby (see Chap. 3).

Case Vignette 21.2.1 Josh Traner

Josh Traner is an 18 year old senior in high school coming to see your primary care colleague Dr. Stanton because of "mood swings." His mother accompanies him and describes his moods as alternating weeks of irritability and "goofy behavior," followed by weeks of stomachaches, isolation and refusal to attend school. No major recent events or family stressors have occurred to trigger this behavior. He lives at home with his two sisters, mother, and father. He was doing extremely well in school until about 1 year ago, when his grades began to drop.

Dr. Stanton completes a very thorough physical exam, and orders for basic laboratory studies, including a thyroid stimulating hormone test. After feeling sure that this young man did not have a general medical cause that could explain the symptoms, Dr. Stanton refers Josh to you for psychiatric consultation and evaluation.

Please proceed with the problem-based approach!

At this point, a differential diagnosis should include

- Attention deficit hyperactivity disorder
- Bipolar II disorder
- Substance-induced mood disorder
- Mood disorder due to a general medical condition
- Learning disorder
- Somatization disorder
- Physical or sexual child abuse
- Oppositional defiant disorder

Case Vignette 21.2.2 Continuation

You meet with Josh and his mom. As soon as you walk into the room, you notice that Josh has taped bandages covering both wrists. He is ripping pages out of a magazine, throwing them everywhere and making a mess.

When you ask him to tell you a little bit about how he has been feeling, he starts to describe "really bad stomach pains." He speaks very fast and repeats himself often. You also notice that he loses his focus, and his train of thought changes to a question about the office building then a comment about your tie.

His mother explains that she is concerned about his sleep habits. She read in a recent newspaper article that adolescents and teens require a lot of sleep, but her son hasn't been sleeping much lately, and she always hears him getting up and making noise as if he is organizing things in the middle of the night. He hasn't been to school in 2 weeks.

He has no other medical conditions and no other psychiatric history.

His grandfather has bipolar disorder, diagnosed when he was in his 20s.

There is no history of substance abuse.

 Please proceed with the problem-based approach!

An important risk factor for bipolar disorder is family history of bipolar disorder (as seen in this case) (Ebert, Loosen, and Nurcombe, 2000). Nearly 50 % of patients with bipolar illness have a family history of the disorder (Belmaker, 2004). Peak age of onset for the first episode is in the teens and early twenties (Moore & Jefferson, 2004). The lifetime prevalence of bipolar disorder is approximately 1 %, affecting over three million people in the United States. Ten to fifteen percent of adolescents with recurrent major depression may eventually be diagnosed with bipolar disorder (Ebert, Loosen, and Nurcombe, 2000). The gender distribution for bipolar disorder is almost equal among males and females, but females tend to have more serious, rapid-cycling, bipolar disorder.

Only one manic episode is needed for the diagnosis of bipolar illness, as long as the manic symptoms are not due to a general medical condition such as pheochromocytoma or amphetamine abuse (see Table 21.4; Belmaker, 2004). According to the DSM-IV classification, bipolar disorder (aka "manic depression") can be classified into bipolar I disorder, consisting of episodes of mania with or without depressive episodes; bipolar II disorder, consisting of episodes of hypomania cycling with depressive episodes; and cyclothymic disorder, consisting of hypomania and less severe episodes of depression (American Psychiatric Association, 2000). Hypomania is defined as mild manic episodes without psychotic symptoms or dangerousness to oneself or to others (Belmaker, 2004).

Schizophrenia and bipolar disorder were among the first multigenic traits to be analyzed by genetic linkage analysis, and it is now believed that bipolar disorder results from the effects of a small number of mutant genes (Kandel, 2000). In addition to genetic predisposition, environmental and neurobiological components also contribute to bipolar disorder, as they do for unipolar depression. Patients with bipolar disorder may experience depressive episodes due to low levels of neurotransmitters as outlined in Fig. 21.2. The major difference is that bipolar disorder involves episodes of mania as well, which are associated with increased levels of dopamine and other neurotransmitters. A possible model for the pathophysiology of bipolar disorder is shown in Fig. 21.2.

As described in the DSM-IV, a manic episode is described as a distinct period of elevated, expansive, or irritable mood that lasts for a week or longer, associated with three or more of the following symptoms: inflated self-esteem, more talkative than usual, decreased need for sleep, distractibility, flight of ideas, increase in goal-oriented activity, and excessive involvement in pleasurable activities that have a high potential for painful consequences, such as careless shopping sprees. A mixed episode, on the other hand, meets criteria for both a manic episode and a major

Table 21.4 Medications and general medical conditions associated with mania

Medications	Amphetamines	Cocaine	Levodopa
	Anticonvulsants	Corticosteroids	Methylphenidate
	Baclofen	Decongestants	Opioids
	Barbituates	Disulfiram	Phencyclidine
	Benzodiazepines	Hallucinogens	Tricyclic
	Bromocriptine	Hydralazine	antidepressants
	Cimetidine	Isoniazide	Yohimbine
Medical conditions	Neurologic: epilepsy, Huntington's disease, migraine headaches, multiple sclerosis, poststroke, trauma, Wilson's disease		
	Infectious: AIDS, Influenza, neurosyphillis, Q fever, herpes simplex encephalitis		
	Neoplasms: diencephalic glioma, parasagittal meningioma, pheochromocytoma, right intraventricular meningioma, tumor of floor of the fourth ventricle		
	Metabolic/endocrine: hemodialysis, menses related, postoperative and postpartum states, thyroid disorders		
	Collagen-vascular disease: systemic lupus erythematosus		

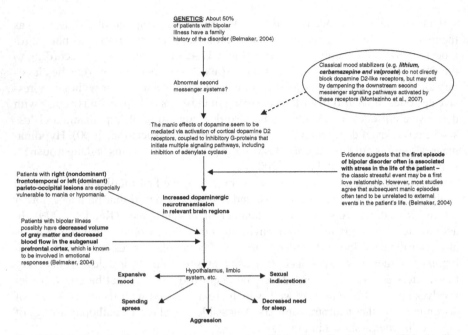

Fig. 21.2 Mechanistic diagram showing a proposed model for the pathophysiology of bipolar disorder. Treatment options are noted by *dashed lines*

depressive episode nearly every day during the week or longer (American Psychiatric Association, 2000).

Case Vignette 21.2.3 Conclusion

You take time to explain the diagnosis of bipolar disorder and the treatment options available, as well as expectations for the future, to both the patient and his mom. You then address any further questions they have and give them a handout about bipolar disorder to read at a later time, in order to reinforce some of the points you have made. Most importantly, you make a follow-up appointment for them in one week, to address any questions that may arise and also to assess the efficacy and tolerance of the medication you prescribe.

As described above, bipolar disorder consists of depressive episodes as well as distinct manic episodes that may last for weeks or months. The primary goal of treatment is the prevention of these episodes with the use of mood stabilizers (i.e., lithium, valproate, and carbamazepine) and some of the new atypical antipsychotic drugs (olanzapine or quetiapine). It is important to treat bipolar disorder effectively, considering the substantial public health problem associated with aggressive episodes of mania which many patients experience (Belmaker, 2004). Medication treatments are summarized in Table 21.5.

Table 21.5 Examples of medications used in bipolar disorder

Pharmacologic agent	MOA and pharmacokinetics	Adverse effects	Labs to monitor
Lithium (mood stabilizer) First-line in bipolar disorder; more effective in manic states than depressive states; used in both acute and maintenance Also used for schizoaffective disorder and severe cyclothymia	Main MOA involves G-proteins by blocking inositol-1-phosphatase in neurons, with subsequent interruption of the phosphatidylinositol second messenger system Excreted unchanged by the kidney; half life: 20 h Monitor drug levels to keep in 0.8–1.2 mEq/l range	Most common cause of noncompliance is impaired cognition, and impaired social/occupational function Common side effects: GI distress, weight gain, fine tremor, and cognitive impairment. Tremor can be treated with propanolol Other: Nephrotic syndrome, diabetes insipidus, sick sinus syndrome, insulin-like effects, psoriasis, hypothyroidism	Basic metabolic profile, including renal function Complete blood count Thyroid stimulating hormone Lithium level Urinalysis Electrocardiogram
Valproic acid (anticonvulsant-mood stabilizer) Used with lithium or alone in bipolar disorder and schizoaffective disorder; more effective in rapid cycling and mixed episodes Can also be used in schizophrenia Also used as a single agent for migraine headache	Suppresses high frequency, repetitive neuronal firing by blocking voltage-dependent sodium channels and also affects neuronal signal transduction through actions on protein kinase C Also increases brain GABA levels by inhibition of GABA catabolism by transaminases Metabolized by liver, but not affected much by P450; half life is 6–16 h; highly protein bound, ideal serum level is 50–125 μm/ml	Common side effects: alopecia, weight gain, sedation, dizziness gastrointestinal upset (e.g., nausea and vomiting), and elevated transaminases Rare: hepatitis, pancreatitis, thrombocytopenia, ataxia, tremor, hyperammonemic encephalopathy	Liver function tests Complete blood count Valproic acid level
Carbamazepine (anticonvulsant-mood stabilizer) For acute and maintenance in bipolar disorder; more effective than	Alters neurotransmission by inhibiting pre-synaptic Na+ channels; also inhibits glutaminergic neurotransmission Metabolized by the liver	Most common side effects are GI complaints (nausea, vomiting, constipation, diarrhea, loss of appetite) and CNS complaints (sedations, dizziness, confusion, ataxia) Can cause	Complete blood count

Table 21.5 (continued)

Pharmacologic agent	MOA and pharmacokinetics	Adverse effects	Labs to monitor
lithium in rapid cycling and mixed episodes Also used for cyclothymia, schizoaffective, and some impulse-control disorders	(CYP3A4); excreted renally; P450 inducer; initially half life is 25–65 h, then can decrease to 12–17 h Titrate to serum level of 8–12 μm/ml	life-threatening thrombocytopenia, agranulocytosis, aplastic anemia Other: rash, urticaria, hepatitis, cholestatic jaundice, SIADH	
Lamotrigine (anticonvulsant-mood stabilizer) More effective for depressive phases of bipolar; not effective against mania or rapid cycling	Affects Na+ channels to modulate the release of glutamate and aspartate; also has a weak inhibitory effect on 5HT receptors Hepatically metabolized with subsequent renal excretion; half life: 25 h	Common: dizziness, sedation, headache, diplopia, blurred vision, ataxia, and decreased coordination Side effect most likely to result in discontinued use is rash (10 % incidence). Severe Stevens–Johnson syndrome can occur Other: weight gain, nausea/vomiting, agitation	
Olanzapine[a] (atypical antipsychotic) Approved for treatment of schizophrenia, acute bipolar mania, and maintenance treatment of bipolar disorder	Antagonist of serotonin-2A, DA-1,2,3,4, alpha-1, histamine–1, and muscarinic–1 receptors Hepatic metabolism via CYP1A2; Half life is 21–50 h; levels are decreased by tobacco use and carbamazepine	Common: drowsiness, sedation, dry mouth, akathisia, insomnia, weight gain, constipation, and elevated lipids and plasma glucose Less frequent: orthostatic hypotension, lightheadedness, nausea, tremor	Fasting blood sugar and lipids
Quetiapine (atypical antipsychotic) Used for schizophrenia and acute bipolar mania; also effective in delirum, dementia, agitation, anxiety disorders, and OCD	Antagonist of serotonin-2A, DA-2, alpha-1 and 2, and histamine-1 receptors Hepatic metabolism via CYP3A4; half life is 6 h	Orthostatic hypotension, somnolence/sedation, weight gain, dyspepsia, abdominal pain, and dry mouth Very low incidence of extrapyramidal symptoms. Lens opacification a potential concern	Fasting blood sugar and lipids Eye examinations

MOA: mechanism of action, DA: dopamine, 5HT: serotonin, CYP: cytochrome P450; OCD: obsessive-compulsive disorder

[a]Can be used alone or in combination with a mood stabilizer; also commonly used together with fluoxetine

A manic episode, although ultimately self-limited, could last months or years if not treated effectively (Belmaker, 2004). Untreated manic episodes generally last about 3 months. The course is usually chronic with relapses. As the disease progresses, episodes occur more frequently. Appropriate therapy or prophylaxis between episodes helps to decrease the risk of relapse. However, not all patients experience significant improvement in symptoms with treatment. Patients respond differently to optimal therapy. For example, those who have four or more episodes of mania, depression, or mixed episodes per year are considered to be "rapid cyclers," and rapid cycling is difficult to treat.

When discussing expectations with patients and/or their parents, different populations may require specific recommendations. For example, women with bipolar disorder should be advised that the postpartum period is a time of considerable risk (Belmaker, 2004). Alternatively, all patients should be advised that acute mania is a medical emergency, and if a manic patient is not treated rapidly, he or she is liable to engage in activities that may endanger the patient's marriage, job, and possibly their own life (Belmaker, 2004).

In a study conducted by Oquendo et al., no significant difference was seen between suicide attempters and nonattempters in the following categories: total years of education, race, marital status, life events, employment status, and number of children. However, patients with a history of suicidal behavior were more than twice as likely to be male (Oquendo, 2000).

Review Questions

1. Name five medical conditions or medications associated with depression.
2. How do you distinguish dysthymia from a major depressive episode?
3. What are the three risk factors for a suicide attempt?
4. Describe three classes of antidepressant medications and the adverse effects associated with each.
5. Name three medical conditions or medications associated with mania.
6. A lack of which neurotransmitter(s) is associated with depression?
7. An excess of which neurotransmitter(s) is associated with mania?
8. Name two medications used for bipolar disorder and describe their mechanisms of action.

References

American Psychiatric Association. (2000). *Diagnostic and statistical manual of mental disorders* (4th ed., text revision). Washington, DC: Author.

Belmaker, R. H. (2004). Medical progress: Bipolar disorder. *New England Journal of Medicine 351*, 476–486.

Brent, D.A., Oquendo, M., Birmaher, B., Greenhill, L., Kolko, D. et al. (2004). Familial transmission of mood disorders: Convergence and divergence with transmission of suicidal behavior. *Journal of the American Academy of Child and Adolescent Psychiatry 43*(10), 1259–66.

Ebert, M. H., Loosen, P. T., & Nurcombe, B. (2000). Mood disorders. In: *Current diagnosis and treatment in psychiatry*. New York: McGraw-Hill

Kandel, E.R., Schwartz, J.H., & Jessell, T.M. (2000). *Principles of neural science*. 4th ed. New York: McGraw-Hill.

Montezinho, L.P., Mørk, A., Duarte, C.B., Penschuck, S., Geraldes, C.F., Castro, M.M. (2007). Effects of mood stabilizers on the inhibition of adenylate cyclase via dopamine D(2)-like receptors. *Bipolar Disorder 9*(3), 290–297.

Moore, D.P., & Jefferson, J.W. (2004). Major depressive disorder. In: *Handbook of medical psychiatry*. 2nd ed. Pennsylvania: Mosby, Inc.

Oquendo, M. A., Waternaux, C., Brodsky, B., Parsons, B., Haas, G.L. et al. (2000). Suicidal behavior in bipolar mood disorder: Clinical characteristics of attempters and nonattempters. *Journal of Affective Disorders 59*(2), 107–117.

Petronis, K. R., Samuels, J. F., Moscicki, E. K., & Anthony, J. C. (1990). An epidemiologic investigation of potential risk factors for suicide attempts. *Social Psychiatry and Psychiatric Epidemiology 25*(4), 193–199.

Ropper, A. H., & Brown, R. H. (2005). Reactive depression, endogenous depression, and manic-depressive disease. In: *Adams and Victor's principles of neurology*. (8th ed.). New York: McGraw-Hill.

Sadock, B. J. & Sadock, V.A. (2005). *Kaplan and Sadock's comprehensive textbook of psychiatry*. 8th ed. New York: Lippincott Williams & Wilkins. Volumes I & II.

Chapter 22
Anxiety Disorders

Mireille Anawati

This chapter addresses the most common group of disorders in psychiatry and general medical practice. The impact of an anxiety disorder can range from a nuisance (such as with a phobia) to severe disability (such as with post-traumatic stress disorder). A listing of the various anxiety disorders is provided in Table 22.1.

At the end of this chapter, the reader will be able to

1. Discuss the epidemiology, mechanisms, clinical presentation, clinical evaluation, differential diagnosis, and treatment of common anxiety disorders
2. Describe the mechanisms of action and potential adverse effects of anxiolytics

Case Vignette 22.1.1 Alicia Giri

Alicia Giri, a 19-year-old freshman, presents to you at her college health center. Her main complaint is of nightmares and difficulty concentrating for the past 4 months. She typically gets in bed at 10 p.m. and cannot fall asleep for hours. Once she finally does, she wakes up shortly thereafter from a bad dream, sweating, with palpitations. This happens five to six times each week. During the day, Alicia feels tired and has a hard time concentrating in class. She cannot focus on her homework or study for exams, and her grades have diminished from straight As in her first semester to Cs this semester. She dropped one class after failing the midterm. Prior to these last 4 months, she slept well through the night and always felt well rested during the day. Alicia has tried over-the-counter sleeping pills, a glass of wine before bed, and listening to soothing music, none of which have worked.

 Please proceed with the problem-based approach!

M. Anawati
Fourth-year Medical Student, University of Hawai'i John A. Burns School of Medicine

A. Guerrero, M. Piasecki (eds.), *Problem-Based Behavioral Science and Psychiatry*,
© Springer Science+Business Media, LLC 2008

Table 22.1 Anxiety disorders

Panic disorder
Specific phobia
Social phobia
Obsessive-compulsive disorder
Post-traumatic stress disorder
Acute stress disorder
Generalized anxiety disorder
Anxiety disorder due to a general medical condition
Substance-induced anxiety disorder
Anxiety disorder not otherwise specified

At this point, a differential diagnosis should include:

- Primary insomnia
- Caffeine or substance-induced disorder
- Adjustment disorder (i.e., college)
- Post-traumatic stress disorder
- Acute stress disorder
- Anxiety due to a general medical condition (i.e., hyperthyroidism)
- Other anxiety disorders
- Depression

Case Vignette 22.1.2 Continuation

You obtain further history: Alicia has no known medical conditions and her only medication is oral contraceptive pills. She has never had a surgery or been hospitalized. There is no family history of suicide, depression, or anxiety. She lives in a dorm room with a good friend from high school where she graduated with honors. She has many friends at school and also plays for an intramural volleyball team. She drinks alcohol on social occasions but does not smoke cigarettes or use any other drugs. She does not currently have a sexual partner. When asked about her romantic relationships she gets very quiet and tears begin to form. After a few moments of silence, Alicia tells you about her senior prom night. After leaving the ballroom, she and her boyfriend of 2 years were hit by another student, who was drunk and ran a red light. Both she and her boyfriend were injured. She suffered a broken arm and several lacerations. Her boyfriend died en route to the hospital.

Please proceed with the problem-based approach!

Post-traumatic stress disorder (PTSD) may occur in anyone who has been exposed to a traumatic event. Traumatic experiences may include a life-threatening accident, torture, a natural disaster, or some other extraordinary event. Patients with PTSD may re-experience the event over and over again as if unable to lay it to rest. Since trauma may occur at any age, so too can PTSD. The most common precipitating traumas, such as combat or accidents, occur in early adult years; thus, most cases have an onset in the twenties. Symptoms may appear either acutely or immediately, within days or weeks after the trauma, or in a delayed fashion up to years after the initial incident (Moore and Jefferson, 2004).

Most studies of PTSD have found higher rates in women than in men (Olff et al., 2007). There are no conclusive data suggestive of inherited susceptibility or specific gene involvement. The pathophysiology is somewhat obscure as well, and is summarized in Fig. 22.1. Biochemical and endocrinologic studies of patients have shown that noradrenergic activity is clearly abnormal. In fact, Vietnam War veterans with PTSD excrete high levels of norepinephrine in their urine, suggesting higher circulating levels (Kandel et al., 2000). Patients with PTSD have a generalized increased sympathetic nervous system and cortisol response. Yohimbine, a noradrenergic agonist, can provoke "flashbacks" or panic attack in PTSD patients (Moore and Jefferson, 2004; Kandel et al., 2000). Brain areas implicated in the stress response include the amygdala, hippocampus, and prefrontal cortex. Traumatic stress can be associated with lasting functional and possible structural changes in these brain areas (Bremner, 2006).

Common presenting symptoms of PTSD may include recurrent thoughts, images, or distressing dreams, avoidance of situations or activities that stimulate recollections of the trauma, a restricted range of affect, a sense of foreshortened future,

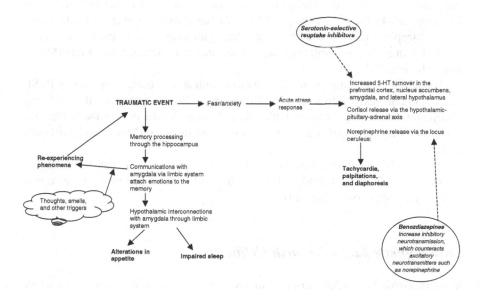

Fig. 22.1 Mechanistic diagram showing the pathophysiology of PTSD

and/or difficulty concentrating and insomnia. According to the DSM-IV, there are six diagnostic criteria for PTSD. The first is an extreme traumatic stress accompanied by intense fear, horror, or disorganized behavior. The next three are: (1) persistent re-experiencing of the traumatic event such as repetitive play or recurring intrusive thoughts; (2) avoidance of cues associated with the trauma; and (3) persistent physiological hyper-reactivity or arousal. The last two diagnostic criteria quantify how long and how disabling the symptoms are. Signs and symptoms must be present for more than 1 month following the traumatic event and cause clinically significant disturbance in functioning. When evaluating a patient's symptoms, it is helpful to differentiate between PTSD and acute stress disorder. The latter describes similar symptoms as those seen in PTSD, which only last for a minimum of 2 days and a maximum of 4 weeks and occur within 4 weeks of the traumatic event (Pelkonen et al., 2006).

Case Vignette 22.1.3 Conclusion

After allowing Alicia to express her emotions and collect her thoughts, you find that her nightmares relate to her accident on prom night. You explain that her symptoms are consistent with PTSD and that there are medications available to help control the insomnia and poor study habits, and you also recommend that she see someone in student counseling services for psychotherapy. She then asks about her prognosis and how long she will suffer these symptoms.

Medications most commonly used in the treatment of PTSD are antidepressants. Typically, selective serotonin-reuptake inhibitors (SSRIs) are used, such as fluoxetine, paroxetine, and sertraline, all of which have been found effective (Moore and Jefferson, 2004). Please see Chap. 21 for a further discussion of these medications. Benzodiazepines may be used to treat acute symptoms. Pharmacologic treatment for nightmares may include cyproheptadine, prazosin, or anticonvulsants (Moore and Jefferson, 2004).

About half of the time, more often in those with acute onset, symptoms of PTSD remit spontaneously within months. However, a chronic course of illness is not uncommon, especially in those with delayed onset. When the course is chronic, symptoms may wax and wane for years or even decades (Moore and Jefferson, 2004).

If Alicia did not have a history significant for a traumatic event, the diagnosis of adjustment disorder would be high on the differential, primarily because it is relatively common (see Chap. 29).

Case Vignette 22.2.1 Kenneth Uchitelle

Kenneth Uchitelle, a 20-year-old male presents to the emergency room where you are working with chest pain, tachycardia, palpitations, shortness of breath,

tachypnea, tremors, and visual disturbances described as the "room going black."
His chief complaint is that he "thinks he is going to die."

 Please proceed with the problem-based approach!

At this point, a differential diagnosis should include

- Cardiac event or arrhythmia
- Substance intoxication or overdose
- Panic attack/disorder
- Generalized anxiety disorder
- Hyperthyroidism
- Hypoglycemia
- Phobia
- Anxiety due to a general medical condition

Case Vignette 22.2.2 Continuation

Kenneth has no past medical history and takes no medications. He was hospitalized once for surgical correction of a left ankle fracture.

He has no family history of depression, anxiety, substance abuse, or other mental illness, and no family history of thyroid disorders.

He lives at home with his mom, dad, and younger sister. Kenneth denies any alcohol, cigarette, and illicit drug use. He attends the community college and works fulltime.

Your physical exam reveals: Vital signs: Temp 98.7, HR: 115, BP: 136/90, RR: 35, O2 sat: 99% on room air. Gen appearance: a 20-year-old well-groomed tremulous male, in moderate distress. Skin: diaphoretic. No bruising or rashes. HEENT: Head is atraumatic. Eyes are without conjunctival injection. Pupils are 3 mm bilaterally and equally reactive to light. Mouth has moist mucous membranes. CV: Tachycardia, with regular rhythm. No murmurs. Resp: No accessory muscle use. Tachypnea. Lung sounds are clear to auscultation bilaterally, without wheezing or rhonchi. Abdomen: non-distended. No masses. Extremities: Good tone. Strong radial and dorsalis pedis pulses bilaterally.

An accucheck reveals glucose of 103 mg/dL.
Urine toxicology is negative.
ECG shows sinus tachycardia.
TSH and T4 are within normal limits.

Please proceed with the problem-based approach!

Kenneth Uchitelle is suffering from a panic attack, described by the DSM-IV as a discrete period of intense fear or discomfort, in which symptoms develop abruptly and reach a peak within 10 minutes. Panic attacks typically last 20–30 minutes and occur at an average of two times per week in most patients. However, some patients experience several attacks per day whereas others may only have attacks once or twice a year. Symptoms typically seen during these attacks include: palpitations, tachycardia, diaphoresis, trembling, shortness of breath, chest pain, dizziness, nausea, and fear of dying. Kenneth would be diagnosed with panic disorder if he has (1) recurrent panic attacks without any obvious precipitating factor and (2) is persistently worried about effects of the attacks, fears another attack, or experiences a significant change in behavior related to the attacks, for 1 month or longer after this episode (American Psychiatric Association, 2000).

In contrast, generalized anxiety disorder (GAD) describes persistent, excessive anxiety or worry for at least 6 months, associated with symptoms such as irritability, sleep disturbances, muscle tension, restlessness, or difficulty concentrating (American Psychiatric Association, 2000). The onset is typically before age 20, and is twice as common in women. Up to 90 % of patients with GAD have a coexisting mental disorder such as major depression, social or specific phobia, or panic disorder; thus, it is important to screen for various symptoms and treat them accordingly. The most effective treatment for GAD is a combination of behavioral psychotherapy and pharmacotherapy (e.g., anxiolytics).

The lifetime prevalence of panic disorder is 2 % and that of generalized anxiety disorder is about 5 %, both having a female to male ratio of about 2:1 (Moore and Jefferson, 2004). Onset of both anxiety disorders is usually in adolescence or childhood years; however, it may also appear in early adult years.

Panic disorder appears to run in families. Family and twin studies support a genetic role in generalized anxiety disorder. These anxiety disorders are associated with abnormalities in GABAergic and noradrenergic activity, namely increased noradrenergic activity and decreased serotonin and GABA activity (Moore and Jefferson, 2004). The pathophysiology of panic disorder is summarized in Fig. 22.2.

Certain substances such as caffeine and nicotine can induce panic attacks or exacerbate anxiety in patients with panic disorder. It is important to counsel patients about potential aggravators.

Case Vignette 22.2.3 Continuation

The nurse working your shift gives Kenneth one oral dose of lorazepam and his symptoms gradually resolve. When he feels better, he is intensely curious about what

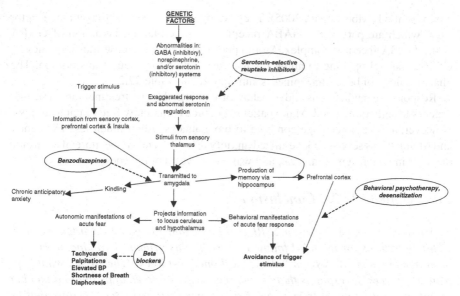

Fig. 22.2 Mechanistic diagram showing the pathophysiology of panic disorder

he experienced and why this happened. You do your best to explain that he has suffered a panic attack and explain the likelihood that he would suffer another one. You discharge Kenneth home without medications and with instructions to follow up with his PMD the following day. He asks if he should see a psychiatrist.

Please proceed with the problem-based approach!

The goal of treatment in panic disorder is twofold: to prevent future attacks and to relieve anticipatory anxiety that patients may have. Both cognitive–behavioral treatment and medication can be effective. Pharmacologic therapy is primarily used in prevention of future attacks.

Pharmacologic long-term treatment for panic disorder and generalized anxiety disorder is very similar. Benzodiazepines have a rapid onset of action and few side effects. Because they are potentially addictive, benzodiazepine use is usually restricted to short term or acute management. SSRIs are currently considered first-line therapy for panic disorder. Starting SSRIs at low doses and increasing the dose slowly will minimize activating side effects or anxiety-like symptoms (Moore and Jefferson, 2004). Please refer to Chap. 21 on further discussion of the antidepressant medications.

Benzodiazepines, which belong to the category of anxiolytic medications, are typically used to treat symptoms associated with anxiety disorders, such as panic disorder, social phobia, generalized anxiety disorder, and adjustment disorder with anxious mood (Albers et al., 2005). They act by binding to benzodiazepine receptor sites, which are part of the GABA receptor, and facilitating the action of GABA at the GABA receptor complex. More specifically, they increase the frequency of GABA channel opening to allow for increased inhibitory neurotransmission. The pharmacology of benzodiazepines is summarized in Table 22.2.

Response to medications and to behavioral psychotherapy treatment in panic disorder is usually quite good. Many patients become completely free of panic attacks. However, a large percentage continue to have attacks, albeit much less frequently and of much less severity. Generalized anxiety disorder tends to be more of a chronic disorder in which symptoms wax and wane over years or decades.

Case Vignette 22.2.4 Conclusion

Two months after he starts an SSRI antidepressant for panic disorder, Kenneth Uchitelle returns for his third follow up visit to this primary care doctor. He has been free of panic attacks, but "almost had one" last week. When asked what happened last week, he explains that he has recently considered applying to a number of colleges but he has a tremendous fear of flying. He is so scared to fly that he will only attend a college to which he can drive from his hometown. When his mom suggested trying to fly and they started looking into airplane tickets to go look at a few campuses, he began getting "insanely anxious."

Fear is an appropriate response to a known threat. A phobia is an irrational fear that leads to avoidance of the feared object or situation. A *specific phobia* refers to fear of a specific object or situation, whereas a *social phobia* (aka social anxiety disorder) is a fear of social situations (e.g., speaking in public, using public bathrooms). Phobias are the most common mental disorders in the United States; up to 25 % of the population has one or more specific phobia (Sadock et al., 2005). Specific phobias are more common than social phobias. The average age of onset is in the mid-teens. Females are more commonly affected than males in specific phobias, but social phobias are equally common in men and women (Sadock et al., 2005).

Table 22.2 Pharmacology of benzodiazepines

Benzodiazepine	Pharmacokinetics	Adverse effects
Alprazolam (Xanax®) *short-acting*	Hepatic metabolism via CYP3A4; half-life is up to 12 hours but clinical duration of action is short; fast onset with quick relief	Common: sedation, dizziness, ataxia, impaired fine motor coordination
Lorazepam (Ativan®) *short/mid-acting*	Metabolism is not P450 dependent, and only affected when hepatic dysfunction is severe; half-life 14–15 hours	
Diazepam (Valium®) *long-acting*	Hepatic metabolism via CYP450; half-life up to 100 hours; accumulates with multiple dosing	Alprazolam: associated with less sedation but has a high incidence of interdosing anxiety
Clonazepam (Klonopin®) *long-acting*	Hepatic metabolism via CYP3A4; half-life is up 20–50 hours; fast onset with quick relief	

DSM-IV criteria for diagnosis of a phobia include persistent fear brought on by a specific object or situation (specific phobia) or related to social settings (social phobia), with an immediate anxiety response resulting from exposure to the situation. The patient must have insight and acknowledge that the fear is excessive, and thus they avoid the situation(s) if at all possible. The duration of the phobic fear must be at least 6 months if the person is under 18.

Treatment of specific phobias typically includes systematic desensitization and behavioral or cognitive–behavioral psychotherapies. Pharmacologic therapy has not been found to be particularly effective except for the brief use of benzodiazepines during predictable periods, such as airplane flights. Typical treatment involves relaxation training, usually coupled with visualization of the phobic stimulus, followed by progressive desensitization through repeated controlled exposure to the phobic cue (Ebert et al., 2000). Desensitization can effectively result in extinction of the anxiety response. A cognitive–behavioral approach can further add by managing the catastrophic thoughts associated with exposure to the situation.

A common phobia is agoraphobia, the fear of public places. It often develops secondary to panic attacks and the apprehension about having subsequent, unexpected attacks in public places. Up to 75 % of patients with agoraphobia have coexisting panic disorder. Most physicians diagnose panic disorder specifying whether it is panic disorder with or without agoraphobia. Patients with agoraphobia have anxiety about being in places where escape may be difficult, typically riding in a bus or train, or being in a crowd. They try to avoid such situations or only do so in the company of a trusted friend or loved one. Fortunately, agoraphobia usually resolves with treatment of the coexisting panic disorder.

Case Vignette 22.3.1 Lars Zdon

Lars Zdon, a 25-year-old male presents to you at the HMO primary care office where you work. His chief complaint is "I do this weird stuff." He describes several years of repetitive habits that cause him a great deal of distress. His daily routine includes shutting and locking the door of his house six times each morning and each night to be sure it is locked. He also washes his hands five or six times before each meal and after shaking someone's hands to be sure that they are clean. He admits that sometimes he cannot sleep at night because he is not sure if he locked his car door, so he gets dressed, walks to the garage, and checks it several times. He is sick and tired of these habits, but can't seem to get rid of them.

Please proceed with the problem-based approach!

Patients with obsessive-compulsive disorder (OCD) may be overwhelmed by obsessions, which are recurrent intrusive thoughts, as well as compulsions: the conscious, repetitive behaviors related to those thoughts. The obsessions and compulsions of these patients typically include repetitive behaviors (i.e., hand washing, checking) or mental acts (i.e., praying, counting). Patients with OCD generally have a sense that something terrible may occur if a particular ritual is not performed. If they resist performing a ritual, such as checking or cleaning, they may experience severe anxiety or an uncomfortable, nagging feeling of incompleteness (Rasmussen and Eisen, 1994). In addition to such rituals, patients with OCD often present with persistent intrusive thoughts that they try to suppress. Obsessions and compulsions can lead to extreme slowness or thoroughness and doubts that lead to reassurance-seeking rituals. Patients with OCD commonly seek care from physicians other than psychiatrists. In one study, 20 % of patients who visited a dermatology clinic had OCD, of which only 3 % had been previously diagnosed (Fineberg et al., 2003).

Obsessive-compulsive disorder has a prevalence of 2–3 % and occurs equally in males and females (Jenike, 2004). This anxiety disorder is among the four most common mental disorders, the others being phobias (most common), substance-induced disorders, and major depression. Childhood-onset OCD is more common in males and more likely to be linked genetically with attention-deficit hyperactivity disorder (ADHD) and Tourette's syndrome (Rasmussen and Eisen, 1994). The mean age at the onset of OCD ranges from 22 to 36 years; only 15 % of patients are older than 35 years when they develop OCD (Jenike, 2004). Men and women are equally affected.

In children OCD may present as a manifestation of pediatric autoimmune neuropsychiatric disorders associated with streptococcal infections (PANDAS). PANDAS may be similar in mechanism to other non-suppurative post-group A beta hemolytic streptococcal (GABHS) complications such a rheumatic fever. The working criteria for a diagnosis of PANDAS are: (1) presence of OCD and/or tic disorder; (2) pediatric onset; (3) abrupt onset and episodic course of symptom severity; (4) association with GABHS infections; and (5) association with neurological abnormalities (Murphy and Pichichero, 2002). Some studies have shown a dramatic resolution of OCD, anxiety, or tic symptoms within 14 days after appropriate treatment for GABHS infection (Murphy and Pichichero, 2002).

Obsessive-compulsive disorder tends to be underdiagnosed and undertreated for two reasons: (1) patients may be secretive or lack insight about their illness and (2) many health care providers are not familiar with the symptoms or are not trained in providing treatment (Jenike, 2004). The differential diagnosis for OCD includes generalized anxiety disorder, panic disorder, phobias, obsessive-compulsive personality disorder, and hypochondriasis (Rasmussen and Eisen, 1994). However, few of these diagnoses have associated rituals. The complex tics sometimes seen in patients with Tourette's syndrome may be difficult to distinguish from the compulsions seen in OCD, and some symptoms may overlap. Currently, impulse control disorders, such as compulsive gambling, eating disorders, and paraphilic disorders are not considered to be part of obsessive-compulsive disorder (Rasmussen and Eisen, 1994).

Case Vignette 22.3.2 Continuation

Mr. Zdon's past medical history is negative for major illnesses. He may have had frequent "strep throats" as a child.

Family history: He recalls that his mom was very particular about checking to make sure all house doors and windows were locked. She also prayed frequently throughout the day. No one in the family was ever diagnosed with mental illness, and no one has chronic medical illnesses.

Social history: Mr. Zdon lost some friends recently because they think he is "weird." He has missed multiple days at work in order to clean his house meticulously. He drinks alcohol on social occasions, but denies any other drug use.

His physical exam is unremarkable.

 Please proceed with the problem-based approach!

OCD likely has a genetic basis, as seen in twin studies and in studies of first-degree relatives of patients with OCD (Rasmussen and Eisen, 1994). There is no definitive understanding of the pathophysiology. Studies have shown a relationship between serotonin regulation and the pathophysiology of OCD; however, strong evidence is lacking. There may be a reduced serotonergic input into the fronto-subcortical circuits in OCD, which diminishes inhibitory regulation of serotonin on these circuits (Hasselbalch et al., 2007). The pathophysiology and treatment of OCD are summarized in Fig. 22.3.

The DSM-IV criteria for OCD emphasize that the obsessions/compulsions cannot be due to a direct physiologic effect of a substance, and that they must interfere with a person's normal routine or social activities. Therefore, social history is essential in these patients.

Case Vignette 22.3.3 Conclusion

Mr. Zdon acknowledges he is a little "obsessed" with cleaning his hands and locking his doors, but he cannot seem to suppress those thoughts. If he doesn't continue his ritual, he is preoccupied for the rest of the day thinking his hands are dirty and that everything he touches, including his food, is unsanitary. As a result he often throws out food and sometimes has to prepare three meals in order to eat one. He also worries that someone will break into his house while he is at work if he does not give into his need to repetitively lock the front door. You think back to your third year clerkships and remember that there is obsessive-compulsive disorder and also obsessive-compulsive personality disorder. You cannot remember much about the treatment, and you refer him to a psychiatrist for assessment and treatment.

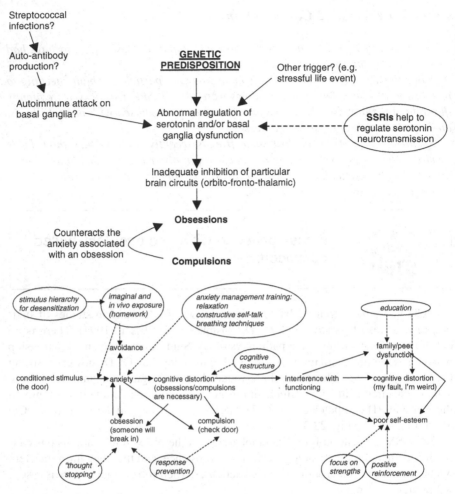

Fig. 22.3 Mechanistic diagram showing the pathophysiology of OCD, from both a neurobiologic (upper diagram) and psychosocial (lower diagram) perspective

Obsessive-compulsive personality disorder describes a person that is excessively preoccupied with details, lists, and organization. This type of person is inflexible and does not perceive the problem, meaning they have no insight (please refer to Chap. 24). Alternatively, people with OCD have insight and acknowledge the thoughts are a product of their mind. They are also aware that their obsessions and compulsions are unreasonable and excessive, and try to suppress the thoughts (as seen in this case), but are often unsuccessful (Sadock et al., 2005).

Treatment for OCD and obsessive-compulsive personality disorder differ, and a careful interview allows for an accurate diagnosis and treatment planning. A combination of pharmacotherapy and behavioral therapy is regarded as the optimal treatment for OCD, although mild OCD symptoms respond very well to behavioral treatment alone. First-line pharmacologic treatment of OCD includes serotonin-reuptake inhibitor drugs, including clomipramine, paroxetine, sertraline, fluoxetine, and citalopram. The daily dose usually needs to be higher for OCD than for depression, and the clinical response in OCD may be delayed for up to 12 weeks (Denys, 2006).

Psychotherapy typically consists of an exposure and response prevention, sometimes in combination with cognitive–behavioral therapy. Exposure and response prevention starts with the patient's complete list of obsessions, compulsions, and things he or she avoids arranged in a hierarchy from least to most anxiety provoking. The therapist introduces the least anxiety-provoking stimulus through imagery and repeatedly exposes the patient to it until the situation produces minimal anxiety (i.e., habituation). Exposure progresses to greater challenges, such as touching something "dirty" or listening to recordings of obsessive thoughts, accompanied by prevention of the ritual response (Jenike, 2004). Like pharmacotherapy, psychotherapy has been found to produce metabolic changes in the brain (seen on positron emission tomography) that correlate with clinical improvement (Schwartz et al., 1996).

Obsessive-compulsive disorder is a chronic disorder. Even with effective treatment, OCD rarely remits, but symptoms do diminish so that patients can work, raise a family, and have an active social life (Jenike, 2004). While many patients experience moderate symptoms, OCD can potentially be a severe and disabling illness. Response to pharmacotherapy in OCD is moderate and a subgroup of OCD patients remain significantly impaired (Sadock et al., 2005). When a patient achieves a good treatment response with medication, the anti-obsessional medication should continue for 12–18 months before attempting to discontinue medication (Denys, 2006).

Review Questions

1. What is the difference between PTSD and acute stress disorder?
2. What medications are used for treatment of PTSD?
3. Is panic disorder more common in females or males?
4. How long do panic attacks typically last?
5. Name five symptoms associated with panic attacks.
6. Name two classes of medications used for panic disorder.
7. What does the acronym PANDAS stand for?
8. What distinguishes OCD from obsessive-compulsive personality disorder?

References

Albers LJ, Hahn RK, Reist C, *Handbook of Psychiatric Drugs*, 2005 edition. CCS Publishing; 2005.
American Psychiatric Association. *Diagnostic and Statistical Manual of Mental Disorders,* 4th ed. Text revision. Washington, DC: American Psychiatric Press; 2000.

Bremner JD. "Traumatic stress: effects on the brain." *Dialog Clin Neurosci* 2006;8(4):445–461.

Denys D. "Pharmacotherapy of obsessive-compulsive disorder and obsessive-compulsive spectrum disorders." *Psychiatr Clin North Am* 2006;29(2):553–584, xi.

Ebert MH, Loosen PT, Nurcombe B. *Current Diagnosis & Treatment in Psychiatry.* McGraw-Hill; 2000. Chapter 22: Anxiety Disorders.

Fineberg NA, O'Doherty C, Rajagopal S, Reddy K, Banks A, Gale TM. "How common is obsessive-compulsive disorder in a dermatology outpatient clinic?" *J Clin Psychiatry* 2003;64:152–155.

Hasselbalch SG et al. "Reduced midbrain-pons serotonin transporter binding in patients with obsessive-compulsive disorder." *Acta Psychiatr Scand* 2007;115(5):388–394.

Jenike MA. "Clinical practice. Obsessive-compulsive disorder." *N Engl J Med* 2004;350(3): 259–265.

Kandel ER, Schwartz JH, Jessell TM. *Principles of Neural Science,* 4th ed. McGraw Hill; 2000. Chapter 61: Disorders of Mood: Depression, Mania, and Anxiety disorders.

Moore DP, Jefferson JW. *Handbook of Medical Psychiatry*, 2nd ed. Mosby; 2004. Chapter 83: Panic Disorder, Chapter 88: Posttraumatic Stress Disorder and Chapter 89: Generalized Anxiety Disorder.

Murphy ML, Pichichero ME. "Prospective identification and treatment of children with pediatric autoimmune neuropsychiatric disorder associated with group A streptococcal infection (PANDAS)." *Arch Pediatr Adolesc Med* 2002;156(4):356–361.

Olff M, Langeland W, Draijer N, Gersons BP. "Gender differences in posttraumatic stress disorder." *Psychol Bull* 2007;133(2):183–204.

Pelkonen M, Marttunen M, Henriksson M, Lönnqvist J. "Adolescent adjustment disorder: precipitant stressors and distress symptoms of 89 outpatients." *Eur Psychiatry* 2006;Dec 19.

Rasmussen SA, Eisen JL. "The epidemiology and differential diagnosis of obsessive compulsive disorder." *J Clin Psychiatry* 1994;55(Suppl 10):5–14.

Sadock BJ et al. *Kaplan and Sadock's Comprehensive Textbook of Psychiatry,* 8th ed. Lippincott Williams & Wilkins; 2005. Volume I, Section 14: Anxiety Disorders.

Schwartz JM, Stoessel PW, Baxter LR Jr, Martin KM, Phelps ME. "Systematic changes in cerebral glucose metabolic rate after successful behavior modification treatment of obsessive-compulsive disorder." *Arch Gen Psychiatry* 1996;53(2):109–113.

Chapter 23
Somatoform Disorders

Jonah Shull and Catherine McCarthy

In all areas of medicine, one of the most challenging classes of disorders to diagnose and treat are somatoform disorders. Somatoform disorders comprise a spectrum of illnesses in which psychological problems manifest as physical symptoms and complaints. Patients with these conditions are most commonly present to a primary care physician or an emergency room; psychiatry usually only becomes involved late in the medical history. Somatization disorder, conversion disorder, hypochondriasis, body dysmorphic disorder, and pain disorder all belong to this diagnostic class. It is important for all physicians to be aware of these conditions; early diagnosis can save the patient from unneeded procedures and save the physician from frustration.

At the end of this chapter, the reader will be able to

1. Apply the DSM-IV-TR criteria for somatoform and factitious disorders to clinical vignettes
2. Identify the elements of a complex medical history that are suggestive of a somatoform or factitious disorder
3. Describe treatment strategies for patients with somatoform or factitious disorders

Case Vignette 23.1.1 Presenting Situation: Janelle Patterson

At 9 p.m. on Christmas Eve, Janelle Patterson, a 29-year-old married white woman, presents to the emergency department where you are on duty. Her chief complaint is bilateral leg paralysis. Mrs. Patterson states she had no previous health problems. She lives with her husband and two children (2 and 4 years old). Mrs. Patterson was preparing Christmas dinner when she decided to sit down. When she tried to get up she could not use her legs. The patient then called her husband, and he came to her aid. He brought her to the emergency department for further evaluation. The patient was concerned that her house would not be ready for Christmas and that she was expecting company later in the day.

J. Shull,
Fellow, Child Psychiatry
University of Nevada School of Medicine

A. Guerrero, M. Piasecki (eds.), *Problem-Based Behavioral Science and Psychiatry*,
© Springer Science+Business Media, LLC 2008

Please proceed with the problem-based approach!

Case Vignette 23.1.2 Continuation

Mrs. Patterson denies any significant past medical history. She had two healthy pregnancies and normal vaginal deliveries. She sees her primary care physician yearly for physical exams which had always been normal.

She denies any past psychiatric history and appears a bit put off with this area of questioning. She had never been hospitalized in a psychiatric hospital. She had never attempted suicide. She had never been diagnosed with a psychiatric illness.

Mrs. Patterson states that she drinks a glass of wine a couple of times of year on social occasions. She denied any drinking in recent history as well as the use of illicit drugs. She does not use any tobacco products.

Social History: Mrs. Patterson has two older brothers who are healthy. She was raised by both parents, and she described her childhood as good. As early as 6 years of age she was expected to help with household chores because both her parents worked demanding jobs. Starting at the age of 15 she was responsible for making dinner for her older brothers, including planning meals, preparing them, and cleaning up afterward. Mrs. Patterson graduated high school, and had various jobs as a waitress and housekeeper in the local hotel industry. She is currently not working, and is happy to stay at home with her young children. She describes herself as happily married; she feels safe in her marriage and denies any abuse. She had been married for 5 years. Her husband is a long-distance truck driver, and Mrs. Patterson is alone with her children for up to a week at a time.

Please proceed with the problem-based approach!

Case Vignette 23.1.3 Continuation

Mrs. Patterson's physical exam reveals: Vitals: HR 72, BP 110/70, respiratory rate: 14, temp 98.4.

General: Mrs. Patterson is lying in her hospital bed. She has good hygiene and appears to be comfortable and in no distress.

Neurological: Mrs. Patterson has bilateral leg paralysis. She cannot voluntarily move her legs when asked by the examiner or bear any weight when asked to stand. Mrs. Patterson also lacks pinprick sensation to her waist, but has full sensation above her waist. Mrs. Patterson's patellar and Achilles reflexes were 2+ bilaterally. Passive movement of her legs by the examiner reveals a ratchet-like weakness. The rest of Mrs. Patterson's physical exam is normal.

Mental Status Exam: Mrs. Patterson is quite calm with regards to her paralysis and seems more concerned about her husband being able to finish dinner. She sits up during the interview. She describes her mood as "worried." Her affect is bright and seemed incongruent with her current physical symptoms. Mrs. Patterson denies any thoughts of suicide or hurting anyone else. She denies auditory hallucinations, paranoid thoughts. She exhibits no signs of delusional systems. Mrs. Patterson is alert and oriented and has no significant gaps in short, immediate, or long-term memory. She seems to have average intelligence, and she has no deficits in concentration or attention. Judgment and insight both appear good.

CBC and Chemistry Panel were all within normal limits.

MRI of brain was within normal limits.

Please proceed with the problem-based approach!

Case Vignette 23.1.4 Conclusion

Mrs. Patterson is admitted to the hospital for observation. In the hospital, Mrs. Patterson receives lorazepam (2 mg by mouth) to treat hypothesized underlying anxiety. She is praised when she tries to move her legs, and strongly encouraged when any sign of progress is made. No physical cause for the paralysis is identified. Mrs. Patterson has some toe movements before leaving the hospital, but is discharged with a wheel chair.

Over the next few weeks, her husband took some time off work and he was able to help her with all the household chores. Mrs. Patterson slowly regained function of her legs. Several months later in a follow-up at her family doctor, she had a normal neurological exam.

Learning Issues

Mrs. Patterson's case highlights several common aspects of conversion disorder, which is a disorder in which a patient presents with atypical neurological symptoms and no other physical findings. The incidence of conversion disorder is reported in the DMS-IV-TR to range from 11 to 800 cases per 100,000 and the male to female ratio is 2:1. Though it can be diagnosed at any age, it is most common in adolescents and young adults. Mrs. Patterson also represented a typical presentation because she had specific stressors, family and holidays, and a lack of support in her social environment. This stress manifested itself as paralysis. As a result of this, her husband took time off work and helped her; her psychological needs were met. Slowly, her symptoms of conversion disorder resolved on their own with conservative management.

Of course, in practice, conversion disorder can be much harder to recognize. First, conversion disorder manifests itself as one or more symptoms of deficits affect voluntary motor or sensory function. This deficit suggests a neurological or other general medical condition. Also, psychological factors have to somehow be connected with these symptoms. As with Mrs. Patterson, these symptoms cannot be intentionally feigned (APA, 2000). In addition to a complete medical work-up, it is important to have a thorough social history of a patient you suspect of having conversion disorder. However, it is a rule-out diagnosis. In this vignette, medical tests ruled-out that Mrs. Patterson did not have a stroke, tumor, or other obvious condition that would result in paralysis. It is important not to miss a potentially treatable medical condition when suspecting conversion disorder, such as multiple sclerosis or intracranial mass.

Unfortunately, not much is known about the mechanism of action of conversion disorder or how to treat it. Physicians should avoid communicating a judgmental attitude with patients who are suspected to have this condition or to tell them it's "just in their head." This would be frustrating to the patient who really experiences the symptoms they are describing. It is best to treat underlying anxiety and address the believed psychological stress that precipitated this episode. Anxiolytics are often used in combination with strong encouragement and supportive therapy. Ninety to 100 percent of conversion disorder patients have their symptoms resolved within a month, and up to 75 % of these patients never have a second episode (Kaplan and Sadock).

Case Vignette 23.2.1 Presenting Situation: Marianne Gunderson

You are a psychiatrist on the consult-liaison service of a teaching hospital. You were asked to evaluate Marianne Gunderson, a 46-year-old woman with seven previous hospital admissions over the last 3 years. Ms. Gunderson was admitted to the hospital last night for intractable back pain that could not be managed as an outpatient. Ms. Gunderson has gone to the emergency department 10 times over the past 3 months, and the ER staff decided to admit her for further evaluation. Ms. Gunderson was friendly but slightly annoyed when she realized a psychiatrist was sent to see her. "What– you people think this is all in my head?"

Please proceed with the problem-based approach!

Case Vignette 23.2.2 Continuation

After building rapport, Ms. Gunderson is willing to discuss her history, "So you can understand I'm not crazy."

Ms. Gunderson is single and lives with her mother and father. Both of her parents are elderly but in fairly good health. For as long as she can remember, Ms. Gunderson has been in poor health. As a teenager, she remembered having to go to the school nurse and her family doctor for severe abdominal pain on a regular basis. Though they could never find a cause of her pain, she missed many days of school and barely graduated high school.

She has worked at various locations as a cashier and an administrative assistant. However, she feels that her multiple illnesses have held her back and made working difficult. During her twenties, the patient experienced excessive menstrual bleeding. At the age of 31, she had a total hysterectomy. Since then, Ms. Gunderson has had four more surgeries in an effort to reduce adhesions and decrease chronic abdominal pain. She states none of the surgeries have really helped her and "new symptoms come up all the time."

Ms. Gunderson states that things really got bad in her thirties after she was rear ended by a car at a stop light. The car was only going around 5 mph but must have hit her "just right." She states that she had some "scans" that showed some disc degeneration. Ms. Gunderson also complains of numbness and tingling in her hands. Since then she has had two back surgeries. She was 41 when she received her last back surgery. Ms. Gunderson states the pain over the last year has been really bad and resists medications. She expects to "go under the knife again."

When asked about her living situation, Ms. Gunderson states she is the only daughter and has always lived with her parents because of her health problems. She feels her parents are very understanding and supportive. Ms. Gunderson has never been in a relationship. She states she just never has had any desire to have sex and so she figured there was not much point in having a boyfriend.

Currently, Ms. Gunderson complains of severe back pain that is not being relieved by narcotics. She states she also has abdominal pain that is diffuse. She also has been having severe headaches that could "kill a horse." She reports general aches and pains in all her joints which is a little better with ibuprofen. More recently, she has noticed a difficulty with her balance. She said, "I just don't feel right when I'm walking, like my balance is off."

Please proceed with the problem-based approach!

Case Vignette 23.2.3 Continuation

Physical Exam

   Ms Gunderson's Physical Exam reveals:

   Vitals: BP 115/68, HR 72, RR 24, temp 98.6, pulse oximetry 98% on room air.

   General: Ms. Gunderson is lying in hospital bed and appeared to be in discomfort. She is breathing slightly fast, and in mild discomfort.

   Head: She complains of some sinus tenderness

   EENT: normal limits

   Cardiovascular: normal limits

   Respiratory: Slightly tachypnic, however, lungs were clear to auscultation bilaterally.

   Abdominal exam: She is obese. Several scars from abdominal surgeries are visible. Ms. Gunderson complains of diffuse abdominal tenderness on palpation. Abdominal exam is otherwise unremarkable.

   Back: Scars from past surgeries. She reports diffuse tenderness when spinus processes were palpated and more severe tenderness when her lower back was palpated.

   Neurological: Normal reflexes. Normal strength bilaterally. Gait was normal.

Mental Status Examination

   General Appearance: Ms. Gunderson is a 46-year-old woman who looks her stated age. She is lying in a hospital bed wearing hospital gown. Her hygiene is fair. Her hair was unkempt; however, she was not malodorous and her nails were well groomed. She appears to be in discomfort.

   Attitude: Initially, Ms. Gunderson is guarded and angry that a psychiatric consult was requested. However, she becomes conversational during the course of the interview. She answers most questions but is short or evasive when psychological themes are asked.

   Speech: Normal tone, volume, rate, and rhythm.

   Thought process: Logical and goal-directed.

   Thought content: Ms. Gunderson denies suicidal or homicidal ideation. She cannot believe "you would even ask me that." She denies auditory or visual hallucinations and has no paranoid ideation. There is no evidence of delusional systems.

> *Cognition: She is alert and oriented with a 30/30 on her Mini Mental*
> *Status Exam. She has normal attention and concentration.*
> *Insight: poor*
> *Judgment: fair*

Case Vignette 23.2.4 Conclusion

After you complete the psychiatry assessment, you meet with Ms. Gunderson's hospital team to discuss your findings. Everyone was in agreement that Mrs. Gunderson had somatization disorder. For patients with this condition, it is important to have a single physician as a primary caretaker and you recommend that Mrs. Gunderson see her primary care doctor once a month. The monthly visit should be brief, but include a physical exam to address Ms. Gunderson's complaints. The goal of the primary care physician is to keep Ms. Gunderson from having unnecessary surgery as it would only complicate her condition. At the request of the inpatient team, you contact the primary care doctor and inform her of your findings and recommendations.

Over the following year, Ms. Gunderson follows-up with her primary care physician. Slowly, her doctor counsels her on the links between the mind and physical complaints. After several discussions with her doctor, Ms. Gunderson agrees to see a psychiatrist. She states she had "nothing else to lose," and she knows her primary doctor does not think she was crazy. Though she continues to have chronic pain and other somatic complaints, Ms. Gunderson does not have any back or abdominal surgeries over the next few years. Once Ms. Gunderson developed rapport with an outpatient psychiatrist, she required less frequent visits with her primary care provider.

Learning Issues

Ms. Gunderson provides an example of somatization disorder, previously known as Briquet's syndrome and hysteria. By definition, the physical complaints of somatization disorder begin before age 30. Therefore, a suspicion of this disorder requires a thorough medical and surgical history. Some of the complaints that the patient may have exhibited in the past may have resolved by the time of presentation. In addition to the age of onset, the diagnosis requires four pain symptoms, two gastrointestinal symptoms, one sexual symptom, and one pseudoneurological symptom. For patients with somatization disorder, it is important to prevent the patient from undergoing surgery or other procedures without significant physical or objective evidence of correctable pathology. Patients with this condition tend to be annoyed at the suggestions of seeing a psychiatrist since this appears to invalidate their experience of illness. It is important to be respectful of the strong belief these patients have in their symptoms. The primary care physician is usually in a critical role and needs to maintain rapport with the patient. If a patient with somatization disorder decides to seek another provider, then he or she could undergo further unnecessary and potentially risky tests and procedures. Frequent contact with primary care providers, initially as often as twice a week and later increased to monthly appears to be the best means to prevent unnecessary trips to the emergency department and unwarranted procedures. A related goal of the primary care physician is to increase rapport with the somatization disorder patient in order for the patient to agree to a psychiatric evaluation and treatment. If this transition is done well it will aid in initiating good rapport with her outpatient psychiatrist.

Somatization disorder is more common in women than in men: women outnumber men 5–20 fold. It is unknown why this difference exists, but some have proposed that there is a tendency among physicians to more readily diagnose women with this condition. Prevalence is estimated to be 0.2–2 % of women and 0.2 % of men in the general population although these may be underestimates (Kaplan and Sadock).

Like other somatoform disorders, the etiology of somatization disorder is unknown. Also, based on its criteria, it is not a condition that can really be diagnosed until after patients have exhibited significant complaints and morbidity. In this case, Ms. Gunderson had several surgeries before a diagnosis of somatization disorder was considered. Research is needed to determine an underlying cause and diagnostic tools.

Case Vignette 23.3.1 Presenting Situation: Janice Woodford

It is a cold, snowy morning in January the first time Ms. Woodford presents at the Family Medical Care office where you are in the last 6 months of residency. Many of the morning's patients had canceled due to the weather. Ms. Woodford has a list of nonspecific complaints to review with the doctor. She starts going over the list with the nurse, who initially listened patiently while she collected vital signs. The nurse was new to the practice, and she liked it when the patients had a single chief complaint, such as a sore throat. Feeling somewhat overwhelmed and uncertain, our nurse politely informs Ms. Woodford that she would send the doctor right in to see her, because it seems that she had a lot of important things to discuss with you.

You ask what you could do for her. She produces her crumpled up list and calmly stated that she had a lot of things to discuss. She begins with a complaint about headaches, which she has regularly, she said, for many years. She mentions that she faints frequently, when the headaches get bad. She even had a stroke. That was when she was 39, which was only 4 years ago. For more information about the history of a stroke you ask "Was it from a clot or from a bleed?" She does not know and her details are vague. She begins to talk about knee pain and bloody noses. You persist with information about the headaches "How often do you faint? Do you have any warning signs?" Ms. Woodford stated that she "faints all the time," and seems determined to move down her list. You attempt to structure the interview, but Ms. Woodford resists this and proceeds to the next item on her list. There is no emphasis given to major incidents like syncope or stroke, in comparison to the more minor complaints, such as her nosebleed or knee pain. To Ms. Woodford they seem equivalent, yet not necessarily worrisome; more like a routine laundry list of nuisances.

Please proceed with the problem-based approach!

You look at your watch as you reached up to scratch your head and note with surprise that you had already gone 5 minutes over the allotted 15-minute office visit. "There are some tests I want to order," you explain and write an order for blood tests, an EKG, and an echocardiogram. Ms. Woodford feels cut short, finding herself in the hallway with her referrals and her check-out slip. She does not mind having the tests done and willingly agrees to sign consents to release information from other doctors she has seen. There was not a whole lot else she had to do that day anyway, and it was still snowing lightly when she got outside to her car.

Please proceed with the problem-based approach!

Case Vignette 23.3.2 Continuation

You meet with Ms. Woodford for a follow-up visit the following Tuesday. She seems pleased with all of her test results, although somewhat puzzled. It was reassuring that the lab values were all normal and that the EKG and echocardiogram did not show any problems, but she wonders "What should we do about the fainting?" You arrange for a tilt table test, to see if that would replicate her symptoms. You are still waiting for old hospital records, and that he was sure that they would arrive by the next appointment.

The next week Ms. Woodford's cardiologist calls you to discuss the results of the tilt table test. He sounds perplexed. Normally, if a patient has a drop in blood pressure on the tilt table, they may faint or experience syncope. She had an episode of syncope but her measured vital signs remained normal. This was not consistent, the cardiologist explained. The cardiologist explains that he performed a bit of "detective work" while Ms. Woodford was "passed out." He lifted her limp arm above her head and then let go of her hand, positioned exactly over head.

Her hand fell, but somehow managed to miss her face. The cardiologist is suspicious of this clinical picture and recommends that Ms. Woodford be evaluated by a psychiatrist.

Please proceed with the problem-based approach!

Case Vignette 23.3.3 Continuation

Almost 2 years passed before Ms. Woodford has appointment at your office. Records never arrived from the office of the psychiatrist. A new, junior physician, Dr. Tanner, sees her and did not see the old chart. Ms. Woodford does not complain of fainting or headaches nor did she mention her history of a stroke. Her complaints center mostly on problems of bleeding. Apparently her period last month had not stopped and she has been bleeding for the last 5 weeks. The young, bright-eyed doctor suggests an endometrial biopsy to rule out uterine cancer. He explains the process to her with great patience and she agrees without raising any questions. The procedure is uncomplicated and she schedules to return the following week for her results.

At her next visit the following week, Dr. Tanner is delighted to share the good news of a normal pathology result. Ms. Woodford shakes her head understandingly and then begins to describe new complaints: her gums had been bleeding when she brushed her teeth, and she had been having bloody noses. There were bruises on her left arm and on her back and stomach. She even had a bruise on her cheek. She had no idea how she obtained any of these bruises. Her doctor shows his concern. Had someone been abusing her? Ms. Woodford adamantly denies abuse of any sort, ever. Dr. Tanner pondered over the bleeding, the bruising, and thinking leukemia he sends her to the lab for a blood count that day. The following week, again, Dr. Tanner is relieved to have good news to share with his patient. The blood count was normal with no evidence of leukemia. After a moment he begins to worry that she may have a bleeding disorder despite her normal blood counts. Ms. Woodford assures him that there are no bleeding problems in her family. She did not drink alcohol or have a history of liver problems.

Please proceed with the problem-based approach!

Case Vignette 23.3.4 Conclusion

During Ms. Woodford's next visit she reports blood in her urine and in her stool. Dr. Tanner tells her that one of her blood tests was abnormal. He asked her if she takes blood thinners, such as Coumadin® (warfarin) and she reports she does not. Then Dr. Tanner grows more and more perplexed. He repeats the abnormal blood-clotting test to confirm the accuracy and the result is the same. He wonders if someone is poisoning her and proceeds with a very detailed family and social history. She is a single mother, divorced, raising a teenaged son. Her relationship with her ex-husband is amicable. Her son has been in some trouble recently, but nothing out of the ordinary for a 15-year-old boy. The rest of her details seemed routine and unremarkable.

The next time Dr. Tanner sees Ms. Woodford she is in the emergency room. The previous evening Ms. Woodford began bleeding profusely after a bowel movement. The laboratory data showed that her blood-clotting time was dangerously elevated. Blood transfusions stabilize her and she is admitted to the hospital for observation. On her second day in the hospital her blood test for the chemical brodifacoum is elevated. Brodifacoum tests for levels of rat poison is similar to warfarin, a common blood thinner. Now Dr. Tanner understands why his confusing patient was bleeding and bruising. Rather than feeling pleased about solving the mystery, he now has a bigger puzzle to solve. He decides to ask the police for protection while she was in the hospital because he fears for her life. The teenage son was the number one suspect in his mind. He softly tells her what the blood test meant and that she had high level of rat poison in her system. She is oddly indifferent and does not seem concerned. Dr. Tanner is stunned. Ms. Woodford remains pleasant. The next thought that he had seemed too impossible to even consider. Could she be taking the rat poison herself? She would have had to have ingested at least 46-ounce boxes to achieve her current blood level. He asks her directly and she denies it. He suggests that the psychiatric team visit with her in the hospital. She remained pleasant and was almost too cooperative. He made the call. The next morning Ms. Woodford cannot be found. She has left the hospital.

 Please proceed with the problem-based approach!

Learning Issues

It is important to differentiate between symptoms that are produced intentionally and those that are not intentionally produced. In somatoform disorders the medical symptoms are not voluntarily or intentionally produced. In factitious disorders the symptoms are voluntarily produced. Ms. Woodford voluntarily produced her symp-

Table 23.1 Distinctions between somatoform disorders, factitious disorders, and malingering

Disorder	Production of symptoms	Gain from symptoms
Somatoform	Involuntary	Subconscious
Factitious	Voluntary	Sick role—no external gain
Malingering	Voluntary	External gain (financial, litigation, etc.)

toms by ingesting rat poison. This is a distinction from the first two cases. In the first case of conversion disorder the paralysis was involuntarily produced. Similarly, in the second case of somatization disorder, the patient had an array of symptoms that were not intentionally produced.

Factitious disorders involve mental or physical symptoms which the patient voluntarily produces without the gain of external incentives. It is important for the clinician to make the distinction between the malingering patient and the factitious patient. In malingering, the patient has the goal of gaining an external incentive. Incentives may include obtaining disability or sick leave. In factitious disorder there is no other goal than meeting a psychological need to assume the sick role (Table 23.1).

Factitious disorders have a broad range of clinical presentations. At one end of the spectrum, there may be only mild exaggeration of physical or mental symptoms. At the other end of the spectrum there may be extreme fabrication of mental or physical illness. This is called Munchausen syndrome. Patients may undergo repeated surgeries and travel from doctor to doctor. Munchausen syndrome patients often have extensive knowledge of medical terminology or have been employed previously in the medical profession. The presentation of abnormal bleeding and ingestion of rat poison is a common presentation of Munchausen syndrome.

In general, factitious disorders tend to occur more commonly in females. Munchausen syndrome, however, is more commonly reported to occur in men. The onset is generally in early adulthood, and frequently progresses to a pattern of vague symptoms and repeated hospitalizations. It is difficult to ascertain the true prevalence of factitious disorder as it is likely underdiagnosed due to the covert nature of the presentation. On the other hand, patients frequently travel to many hospitals and seek care from multiple doctors, which could cause overreporting of the illness. The consensus is that the prevalence in mental health centers may be as high as 1 % of consultations of mental health patients.

Review Questions

*(Please select the item which is **FALSE**)*

1. Individuals presenting with factitious disorder may

    (a) Be vague about their symptoms
    (b) Want to avoid jury duty

(c) Have a self-inflicted condition

(d) Have extensive knowledge of medical terminology

Patients diagnosed with Munchausen syndrome

(a) Are more often female

(b) May move from hospital to hospital

(c) May undergo multiple surgeries

(d) Are not seeking external gain

Answers

1. b, 2. a

Bibliography

Calabrese, L. (2003) Approach to the Patient with Multiple Physical Complaints. In T. Stern, J.B. Herman and P.B. Slavin (eds.), The MGH Guide to Psychiatry in Primary Care, 2nd edition, pp. 89–103.

Diagnostic and Statistical Manual of Mental Disorders Fourth Edition (DSM-IV-TR) (2000) American Psychiatric Press, Washington, DC.

Greenberg, Donna B. (2006) Somatization. UpToDate.com 2006.

Lipsitt, Don R. (2007) Factitious Disorder and Munchausen Syndrome. UpToDate.com 2007.

Loewenstein, M.J., Mackay, S., Purcell, S.D. (2000) Somatoform and Dissociative Disorders. In H.H. Goldman (ed.), Review of General Psychiatry, 5th edition, pp. 283–301.

Smith, Robert C. (2006) Primary Care Management of Medically Unexplained Symptoms. UpToDate.com 2006.

Sadock, Benjamin J., Sadock Virginia A. (2003). Kaplan and Sadock's Synapsis of Psychiatry: Behavioral Sciences, Clinical Psychiatry. 9th Edition. Lippincott Williams and Wilkins, pp. 643–675.

Chapter 24
Personality Disorders

Latha Pai, Melissa Piasecki, and M. Nathan Mason

Personality disorders are perhaps the most challenging psychiatric diagnoses as well as the most compelling. All health practitioners would do well to become facile with the identification and management of personality disorders. This may avoid unnecessary medical expenditures as well as other unsavory outcomes, such as litigation. What follows is a review of the personality disorders officially recognized by the current Diagnostic and Statistical Manual, Fourth Edition, Text Revision (DSM-IV-TR). Although the scientific database regarding personality disorders is growing, much remains to be discovered.

At the end of this chapter, the reader will be able to

1. Review the morbidity and mortality resulting from personality disorders
2. Diagnose a personality disorder according to DSM-IV-TR criteria
3. Discuss the treatment approaches for personality disorders

Case Vignette 24.1.1 Presenting Situation: Leslie Danforth

Leslie Danforth is a 24-year-old woman brought to your outpatient psychiatry clinic by her mother, who states she is frustrated by her daughter's behavior. Specifically, Leslie's mother is "fed up" by her daughter's inability to "get along" with people and hold a job long enough to live independently. Coming to see a psychiatrist is the "last resort."

Leslie's chief complaint is, "I am fed up with my mother trying to rule my life." During the introductions, the patient appears uncomfortable and looks around the interview room. She intermittently glances behind her. She finally requests that her chair be moved to a position where she can watch the door. Her mother is in tears.

 Please proceed with the problem-based approach!

L. Pai
Resident in Psychiatry, University of Nevada School of Medicine

A. Guerrero, M. Piasecki (eds.), *Problem-Based Behavioral Science and Psychiatry*,
© Springer Science+Business Media, LLC 2008

Case Vignette 24.1.2 Continuation

Leslie's mother tells you that her daughter lives with her because she has difficulty keeping a job. Leslie quickly interrupts her mother and asserts that her mother has always been against her, right from childhood and has favored all the other siblings over her. She adds (defensively) that it is never her fault when she leaves a job. Her bosses are always at fault. She has held a number of jobs as executive assistants and has been fired several times for going through confidential files and mails of colleagues. She reports that her peers would never be honest with her about the projects she would work on. She is confident that she was fired because she discovered too many "secrets" that would make her employer look bad.

Her mother states that her daughter has two broken engagements in the last 3 years. Again, Leslie quickly interrupts to state that both her fiancés were cheating on her and she could never marry someone she cannot trust. When questioned about how she knew of the infidelities, Leslie replies, "I do not need proof! I just know they were cheating on me!" She is able to carry out a conversation with logical and spontaneous speech. She denies the use of any drugs. She denies any auditory and visual hallucinations. She denies any history of a head injury.

 Please proceed with the problem-based approach!

Case Vignette 24.1.3 Conclusion

Leslie's lab tests (CBC, chemistry panel, thyroid panel) were all within normal limits from a general physical she had 3 months ago. Her urine drug screen is negative. You suggest that some of her experiences with relationships sound as if she might have gone through some difficult times. She agrees. You venture to offer a follow-up meeting to see if you can understand those times better and to see if there are any supports or services that you or the clinic might offer her. She agrees to a follow-up appointment in 2 weeks. She does not show up for this appointment and you never hear from her again.

 Please proceed with the problem-based approach!

Learning Issues

Personality disorders are chronic, maladaptive patterns of thinking and behaving. Usually the most problematic parts of personality disorders revolve around relationships with others. Many people who meet the criteria for a personality disorder do not view themselves as the source of their suffering. They are more likely to externalize the problems to other people.

The National Epidemiologic Survey on Alcohol and Related Conditions (NESARC) was a recent population-based study of over 40,000 Americans. It concluded that over 14 % of Americans suffer from at least one personality disorder (Grant, 2004). Due to their high prevalence in the general population, it is not surprising personality disorders are especially prevalent in those persons receiving outpatient or inpatient psychiatric care. At least 30 % of psychiatric outpatients suffer from at least one personality disorder (Koenigsberg, 1985). About 15 % of psychiatric hospitalizations are primarily motivated by problems related to a personality disorder, rather than an Axis I disorder (Loranger, 1990). About half of the remaining inpatients suffer from a comorbid Axis II disorder in addition to their primary Axis I disorder. For example, new personality disorders have recently been proposed, such as posttraumatic personality disorder (Classen et al., 2006).

The DSM-IV provides a means to diagnose personality disorders (American Psychiatric Association, 2000). The behavioral patterns associated with personality disorders affect the person in multiple areas and are inflexible. The problems they experience with friends are likely to be reflected in how they function with co-workers. Like all diagnoses, the diagnosis of a personality disorder is made when the symptoms rise to the level of clinical impairment or distress. The clinical findings of personality disorders are long term and there is no minimum time criterion as there is with other psychiatric diagnoses.

Most people with personality disorders exhibited the traits of the disorder in adolescence or earlier. Clinicians generally are reluctant to diagnose a personality disorder in someone under the age of 18. Such a diagnosis in someone under 18 requires the diagnostic criteria to be manifest for at least 1 year. One notable exception is that criterion B for antisocial personality disorder explicitly precludes the diagnosis being assigned to someone under the age of 18.

Personality disorders are coded Axis II disorders in multiaxial assessment. The disorders are grouped into three "clusters": Cluster A, odd or eccentric; Cluster B, dramatic or disruptive; and Cluster C, anxious or fearful. Co-morbidity among the personality disorders is common.

Cluster A

- Paranoid personality disorder
- Schizoid personality disorder
- Schizotypal personality disorder

Leslie Danforth's presentation is suggestive of paranoid personality disorder. The case information did not give enough information about her motives and thinking to meet full criteria so the diagnosis would reflect the limits of the database: paranoid personality traits or rule out paranoid personality disorder. DSM-IV-TR mentions this disorder may have a prevalence of 0.5–2.5 % in the general US population. More recently, the NESARC reported a prevalence rate of 3.8 % among males and 5.0 % among females in the United States for this disorder. A diagnosis of this personality disorder requires four or more of the following findings: (non-delusional) suspiciousness of harm, exploitation, or deception; preoccupation with unjustified doubts; reluctance to confide in others; tendency to read negative meanings into benign remarks and events; tendency to bear grudges; tendency to perceive attacks on one's character; and recurrent suspiciousness regarding fidelity of partner.

The personality disorders in Cluster A generally represent eccentric or odd behavioral patterns. Another disorder in this cluster is schizoid personality disorder. People with this disorder tend to avoid relationships outside of the immediate family. Approximately 3 % of the population would meet criteria for this personality disorder. The occupational choices of people with schizoid personality disorder (if they work outside the home) tend to be solitary, such as employment as night security guard. In order to diagnose an individual with schizoid personality disorder, there must be four or more of the following criteria, including: lack of desire of close relationships, tendency to engage in solitary activities, lack of interest in sex with another person, pleasure in only a few activities, lack of close friends/confidants outside of first degree relatives, indifference to praise or criticism, and emotional coldness.

The third personality disorder in Cluster A is schizotypal personality disorder. People with this disorder tend to have odd thoughts, behaviors, and speech. They may be noticeable because of their unusual appearance. Although schizotypal personality disorder superficially looks like a psychotic disorder, the odd beliefs are not full-blown delusions and there is no significant functional impairment (such as in most people with schizophrenia). Approximately 3 % of the population has this personality disorder. Epidemiologic studies suggest a link between schizotypal personality disorder and schizophrenia. Schizotypal personality disorder is more prevalent in families of schizophrenia probands than in the general population. Schizophrenia is more prevalent among the blood relatives of schizotypal personality disorder probands. There is an increased concordance for schizotypal personality disorder in identical twins compared to non-identical twins.

Several lines of evidence suggest a shared neurobiological basis with schizophrenia, including similarities in anatomy, neuropathology, neurophysiology, neurocognition, and upon gross physical examination. MRI studies show both conditions have associated increased cerebrospinal fluid, decreased temporal cortical volume, and gray matter, and decreased caudate volumes. Both have diminished interhemispheric connections and thalamic changes. Both schizotypal personality disorder and schizophrenia are associated with decreased metabolic activity of the temporal lobes although the finding is more pronounced in schizophrenia. Both have elevated cerebrospinal fluid levels of homovanillic acid, a major metabolite of dopamine.

Both have similar patterns of cognitive deficits, involving sustained attention, verbal learning, visual processing, and working memory. Both have reduced prepulse inhibition (PPI). PPI is an adaptation where the brain, probably the thalamus, helps a person filter out extraneous sensory data. Normally, a given stimulus will elicit a strong startle response. However, if the usual stimulus is preceded by a weaker stimulus (a so-called prestimulus or prepulse), then the startle response following the stimulus will be attenuated. Finally, on physical exam, people afflicted with schizotypal personality disorder or schizophrenia have aberrant eye tracking.

A diagnosis of schizotypal personality disorder requires five or more of the following criteria from the DSM-IV-TR: ideas of reference (non-delusional), odd beliefs or magical thinking, unusual perceptual experiences, odd thinking and speech, suspiciousness/paranoia, inappropriate affect, odd behavior, lack of close friends/confidants outside of first degree relatives, excessive social anxiety that does not decrease with familiarity and that tends to be associated with paranoia.

Proper diagnosis of Cluster A personality disorders is important, since each has a unique pattern of response to treatment. The current literature suggests psychotherapy or sociotherapy (support groups) offers no benefit to paranoid personality disorder. It is uncertain if psychotropic medications improve the longitudinal course of this disorder. However, if such a patient suffers an overtly psychotic decompensation, antipsychotic medications may have a role.

With schizotypal personality disorder, the literature again provides no support that psychotherapy is helpful. It is unclear if sociotherapy is beneficial. Some suggest that psychotropics may be modestly helpful in the longitudinal course of this disorder, although scientifically rigorous data are absent. For example, in 2004 Keshavan reported an open labeled study that suggested that olanzapine could decrease symptoms and improve overall functioning in schizotypal personality disorder. Finally, there is growing interest in non-neuroleptic psychotropics for the treatment of this disorder. In 2007, McClure reported the results of a parallel-design, double-blind, placebo-controlled trial. The alpha2A agonist guanfacine improved context processing in schizotypal patients.

Schizoid personality disorder has a treatment response profile which is unique among the personality disorders. Recent meta-analysis suggests that both psychotherapy and sociotherapy can decrease symptomatology in this disorder. However, pharmacotherapy offers no benefit.

Case Vignette 24.2.1 Presenting Situation: Brendan Ryles

Brendan Ryles is a 30-year-old man who is brought to the county hospital emergency department where you are on call. He is wearing handcuffs with a police escort from the county jail. His chief complaint is, "There was a misunderstanding when I was handling my business."

Mr. Ryles appears bruised and battered. He has several bleeding lacerations on his face and body. You also notice several healed scars. He appears agitated and angry and bellows: "Fix me!" At this point, the police escorts pull him back and request that he be patient.

Case Vignette 24.2.2 Continuation

You carefully clean and suture Mr. Ryles after appropriate anesthesia. While you are suturing he tells you in a conversational tone that he has been in prison for arson, armed robberies, and attempted murders.

Mr. Ryles says he grew up in a dysfunctional family where his father beat up his mother every day. He says he was suspended from junior high for fighting and never went back to school. He was put into foster care early on, and he says he has always gotten into trouble. He laughs as he recounts how he enjoyed making life miserable for his foster parents and was continuously moved from one care facility to another. Mr. Ryles finally ran away at age 14 after stealing money and some electronic items. He was arrested for this crime and put in a juvenile facility. He says he enjoys cheating people who are "too dumb not to cheat." Mr. Ryles reports that he drives even though he has a suspended driver's license for reckless driving and endangering others. His most recent accident involved a fatality that eventually led to his current incarceration.

Mr. Ryles has never been married and has four children with one on the way. He reports he got into a fight this time with two other inmates because they did not allow him to cut into the food line. He says he got angry and punched someone and this altercation evolved into to a fistfight with two or more people. When living "outside" Mr. Ryles drinks about a 6 pack every day and smokes about 1/1/2 pack a day. He says he has used multiple drugs including methamphetamine, PCP, marijuana, and pain medications.

Case Vignette 24.2.3 Conclusion

Mr. Ryles returned to jail. He received lock up orders to house in "Administrative Segregation" as a consequence for unprovoked violence. He eventually went to prison on a 10-year sentence.

Case Vignette 24.3.1 Presenting Situation: Sharon Young

While working as a resident on a university consult-liaison team, you are called to consult on a 22-year-old white woman admitted 2 days ago after overdosing on diphenhydramine and acetaminophen. Ms. Young is on the medical floor and is very reluctant to talk to "the shrinks." She appears irritable and states she doesn't think she is "crazy" or needs to see "a psychiatrist." With questioning, Ms. Young responds that she took a handful of each medication so she could kill herself. At this point in the interview she becomes quite upset, starts crying, and yells at you to leave her room and to leave her alone.

Case Vignette 24.3.2 Continuation

You leave the room and read through the patient's chart which was previously unavailable. You read that Ms. Young has had multiple visits to the ER for past suicidal thoughts and four attempts. The attempts were all medication overdoses at sublethal dosages. Ms. Young also has a history of self-inflicted superficial cuts to her forearms. The cutting and overdosing behaviors appear to coincide with a failed relationship or problems in school.

Ms. Young's past medication trials over the last 10 years include various antipsychotic medications and a large number of antidepressants. Her list of medications also included valproic acid for "mood stability" and a benzodiazepine for anxiety.

Case Vignette 24.3.3 Continuation

The next morning, Ms. Young is lying down in her bed flipping through the channels on the television. She had been crying and appears sullen with poor eye contact. When you question her about her mood, she looks at the floor and tells you she is not feeling good and is very depressed. You ask about her suicide attempt, and Ms. Young begins crying, explaining that her boyfriend had left her for someone else. She said she had tried so hard and wonders, "How could he ever leave me? How can he do this to me? After everything we have been through together!" She said he told her that he could not tolerate her behavior or her mood swings. She confronted him about an affair and cut her wrist telling him that he needs to stop talking to his other girlfriend. That is when he stormed out of the apartment. She then took the pills and hoped her boyfriend would feel bad about the way he treated her and come back. She reports that talking about that night makes her think about hurting herself.

Case Vignette 24.3.4 Conclusion

You arrange an "intake" appointment for Ms. Young at the community mental health center. You describe the "DBT" (dialectical behavior therapy) program as "made to order" for her. Ms. Young attends the intake appointment and reluctantly agrees to enroll in the DBT program. She attends almost all of the individual and group sessions and becomes increasingly interested in learning new behaviors and ways of coping with her emotions.

Learning Issues: Cluster B Personality Disorders

Patients with Cluster B personality diagnoses tend to have more contact with medical professionals than those from other clusters because of the associated high-risk behaviors which lead to medical consequences. Genetic factors contribute to the finding that borderline and antisocial personality disorders sometimes run in family pedigrees.

Cluster B: Dramatic or Disruptive

- Antisocial personality disorder
- Borderline personality disorder
- Histrionic personality disorder
- Narcissistic personality disorder

Antisocial Personality Disorder

Antisocial personality disorder (ASPD) is strongly associated with criminal behavior. However, an absence of criminal convictions does not rule out the diagnosis. Also strongly associated with this disorder are the psychoactive substance use disorders. Mr. Ryles presents with a history that is highly suggestive of the diagnosis. The diagnosis of ASPD requires three or more of the following DSM-IV-TR criteria: failure to conform to social norms and laws, deceitfulness, impulsivity, irritability and aggressiveness, disregard for safety, irresponsibility, and lack of remorse. DSM-IV-TR mentions this disorder may have a prevalence of 3 % in males and 1 % in females in the general US population. NESARC reports the prevalence to be 3.63 % overall in the United States (5.5 % among males and 1.9 % among females).

Scientists are beginning to unravel the biology of ASPD and related social phenomena. Recently, a group reported the results of fMRI studies of the brains of people who matched behavioral responses with hypothetical vignettes under study conditions. Available responses either entailed abiding by consensus social norms or violating them. Some vignettes entailed circumstances where serious rule violations may have been punished, whereas other stories suggested there was no possibility of punishment. That is, study participants were asked to ponder what they would do, if only they could "get away with it." These types of thoughts were consistently mapped to a few brain regions (Spitzer et al., 2007). This supports a recent model which suggests that dysfunction of brain structures (amydala, part of the frontal lobe) would impair one's ability to associate cause and effect, especially regarding punishment for specific behaviors.

As opposed to all other personality disorders, the individual diagnosed with ASP must be at least 18 years of age. Antisocial personality disorder is unique among the personality disorders because it has a requirement of a preceding childhood disorder: conduct disorder before age 15 (see Chap. 19).

Antisocial personality disorder has a unique treatment response profile. Current meta-analysis suggests psychotherapies or pharmacotherapies have nothing to offer persons with antisocial personality disorder. However, select sociotherapies may be modestly helpful.

Borderline Personality Disorder

Sharon Young's case illustrates some of the difficulties facing patients with borderline personality disorder: chaotic relationships, episodes of depressive feelings, self-harm, and poor skills in solving problems. DSM-IV-TR estimates about 2 % of Americans suffer from this condition. About 10 % of patients with this disorder eventually die by suicide. Borderline personality disorder patients may have brief periods of psychosis, usually paranoid beliefs, during extreme stress. Non-lethal self-harm can be prominent in borderline personality disorder and is called "parasuicidal" behavior to distinguish it from true suicidal intent.

Biological research in borderline personality disorder has found abnormalities in REM sleep cycles and endocrine abnormalities (cortisol and thyroid). Recent neuroimaging studies suggest that patients with this disorder process neutral visual information (such as photos of neutral facial expressions) as though they were threats.

In order to diagnose an individual with borderline personality disorder, he or she must report at least five of the following DSM-IV-TR criteria: frantic effort (to the point of self-injurious behavior) to avoid abandonment, a pattern of intense and unstable relationships alternating between extremes of idealization and devaluation, identity disturbance, impulsivity, recurrent self-injurious behavior, affective instability, chronic feelings of emptiness, inappropriate intense anger, transient paranoid ideation or severe dissociative symptoms.

Patients with borderline personality disorder are best treated in outpatient programs that offer dialectical behavioral therapy (DBT). This therapy treats patients individually and in groups and focuses on building skills and finding ways to manage intensely uncomfortable emotions without self-harm (Koerner and Linehan, 2000). There is some evidence that medications such as antidepressants or the newer antipsychotics have benefits, especially in the short term.

An important diagnosis to consider in patients with dramatic and destructive behaviors is bipolar disorder. The mood instability for borderline personality is short term—minutes to hours—and tends to be a reaction to an interpersonal event. Bipolar patients have elevations and depressions of mood that are persistent (a minimum of 1 week for mania) and distinct (an obvious difference from baseline) (see Chap. 22).

Histrionic Personality Disorder

Patients with histrionic personality disorder are often dramatic in their appearance and behavior. In the general medical setting, a histrionic patient may engage medical professionals with a charming (or even seductive) manner and entertaining or implausible descriptions of symptoms. Patients with histrionic personality disorder may display suggestibility and present with the symptoms of illnesses featured in the media. There is a considerable overlap between this personality disorder and somatization disorder as well as conversion disorder (see Chap. 24). Roughly 2 % of the general population meets criteria for histrionic personality disorder. The diagnosis of histrionic personality disorder requires five or more of the following DSM-IV-TR criteria: discomfort in situations where not the center of attention, inappropriate seductive or provocative interactions with others, rapidly shifting and shallow emotions, use of physical appearance to draw attention to self, impressionistic speech, self-dramatization, suggestibility, tendency to consider relationships to be more intimate than what they are in reality. Meta-analysis suggests psychotherapy can be significantly helpful for this disorder but sociotherapy or psychopharmacology has no role.

Narcissistic Personality Disorder

People with this personality disorder are likely to be demanding and dissatisfied patients. The disorder includes distorted beliefs about self-importance which can lead to inappropriate anger when confronted with the mundane realities of medical care such as waiting for appointments and completing redundant paperwork. Rejection, whether real or perceived, is another potential source of inappropriate anger. In order to diagnose an individual with narcissistic personality disorder, at least five or more of the following must be present: grandiose self-importance; preoccupations with fantasies of success, power, brilliance, beauty, or love; belief that one is unique and only understandable by other special people; need for excessive admiration; sense of entitlement; personal exploitativeness; lack of empathy; envy or belief that others are envious of self; arrogance. This personality disorder shares the same profile as histrionic personality disorder: psychotherapy can be quite helpful but sociotherapy or medication has no role.

Case Vignette 24.4.1 Presenting Situation: Carol Jennings

Ms. Jennings is a 34-year-old woman referred to you by her Ob/Gyn for marital and work problems. Her chief complaint is, "I made an appointment because my doctor told me to." She is the general manager of a local manufacturing company. Before she sits down in your office chair, she pulls a sanitizing wipe from her purse and wipes the chair. When she is seated comfortably on the chair, she looks at her watch and starts talking.

 Please proceed with the problem-based approach!

Case Vignette 24.4.2 Continuation

Ms. Jennings describes her job as a source of both great pride and frustration. She describes her career path as a "pursuit of perfection" and views herself as "very disciplined." She is annoyed if the employees under her supervision do not keep their desks or calendars well organized. She tries to help out with suggestions and offers of help to stay late with them to arrange their desks. She is planning on installing a mandatory time management system on the company server. She says she instead gets curt remarks from ungrateful people who tell her she is driving them "nuts" with her micro-management. She shakes her head in disbelief that anyone would make a choice to be inefficient.

 Please proceed with the problem-based approach!

Case Vignette 24.4.3 Continuation

Ms. Jennings describes her personal life as "married with one son." She says that her husband is a great guy if only he would listen to her. A recent fight was over his repeated requests for an extended (10-day) family vacation as part of a family reunion. She told him why this is impossible for her. Ms. Jennings keeps her 12-year-old son on a "strict leash." She feels her home would be a mess if both her husband and son were given too much responsibility. She has made it easy for them by placing a recyclable and a trash can in strategic places in each room and describes how her laundry room has special baskets for formal clothes, casual clothes, sportswear, etc. Ms. Jennings has conflict with her son over his wardrobe. She fails to understand why he refuses to wear perfectly good clothes that still fit and insists on spending money for new school clothes.

 Please proceed with the problem-based approach!

Case Vignette 24.4.4 Conclusion

Ms. Jennings repeatedly questions why she was in your office paying a large co-pay instead of with her colleagues at work or her husband. She demonstrated no insight into her role in the problems at work and home and declined to "waste time and money" on therapy appointments.

Cluster C: Anxious

- Avoidant personality disorder
- Dependant personality disorder
- Obsessive-compulsive disorder

Diagnosis of Cluster C Personality Disorders

Obsessive-Compulsive Personality Disorder

Carol Jennings displays many behaviors and attitudes consistent with obsessive-compulsive personality disorder. According to NESARC, this is the most common personality disorder, occurring in 7.9 % of all Americans. She attempts to impose her values of organization and time management on others and has little insight into how this creates conflicts. Her family and employees likely find her rigid and controlling.

The diagnosis of obsessive-compulsive personality disorder (OCPD) is distinct from the similarly named obsessive-compulsive disorder (OCD). Although both disorders may include preoccupation with order as well as anxiety, patients with OCD recognize their preoccupations as problematic and dysfunctional (see Chap. 23).

The criteria for OCPD include four or more of the following: excessive preoccupation with details, rules, or organization; perfectionism that interferes with task completion; excessive devotion to productivity to the exclusion of leisure and not out of economic necessity; overconscientiousness and inflexibility; inability to discard objects, including those without sentimental value; reluctance to delegate; miserliness; and rigidity/stubbornness.

Avoidant Personality Disorder

Patients with avoidant personality disorder are shy and sensitive. This personality disorder occurs in about 2.3 % of Americans. A fear of criticism and rejection may dissuade them from seeking personal and professional goals. This disorder is distinct from schizoid personality disorder (Cluster A), in which there is no desire for relationships (as opposed to shyness and sensitivity in spite of the desire for relationships). Avoidant personality disorder demonstrates a unique pattern of response to treatment. Such patients can enjoy a robust response to psychotherapy and a modest response to sociotherapy, but it is unclear if they benefit from medications.

The diagnosis of avoidant personality disorder requires four or more of the following DSM-IV-TR criteria: avoidance of job-related activities that involve interpersonal contact, because of fears of disapproval; unwillingness to become involved with people unless certain of being liked; restraint with intimate relationships because of fear of being ridiculed; preoccupation with criticism or rejection in social situations; inhibition in interpersonal situations because of self-perceived inadequacy; self-perception of being unappealing or inferior; reluctance to take risks that may lead to embarrassment.

Dependent Personality Disorder

Dependent personality disorder occurs in 0.4 % of males and 0.6 % of females in the United States. The hallmark of this disorder is an inability to assert an independent choice. Passive and developmentally immature behaviors can lead to parents caring for an adult child well after same-age peers have left home and started their own families. The treatments for avoidant personality disorder include insight-oriented therapy, behavioral therapy, assertiveness training, family therapy, and group therapy. High levels of separation anxiety or panic attacks may benefit from serotonergic antidepressants.

The diagnosis of dependant personality disorders requires five or more of the following DSM-IV-TR criteria: difficulty making everyday decisions without excessive guidance; need for others to assume responsibility for major areas of one's life; difficulty expressing disagreement out of unrealistic fear of loss of support; difficulty doing things on one's own because of lack of confidence; tendency to go take excessive measures to secure nurturance and support from others; discomfort or helplessness when alone; tendency to seek another relationship as a source of care and support when one relationship ends; and unrealistic preoccupation with fears of being left along to take care of oneself.

Review Questions

For questions 1–5, please match the following illness with its associated clinical presentation.

(a) Histrionic personality disorder
(b) Schizotypal personality disorder
(c) Avoidant personality disorder
(d) Dependent personality disorder
(e) None of the above

1. Family history often includes relatives with schizophrenia
2. Inappropriate provocative interactions with others
3. Inability to assert an independent choice
4. Delusional beliefs
5. Significant anxiety in social situations, notwithstanding desire for social relationships

Answers

1. b, 2. a, 3. d, 4. e, 5. c

References

American Psychiatric Association (2000). Diagnostic and Statistical Manual of Mental Disorders, 4th edition, Text Revision. Washington, DC: American Psychiatric Association.

Classen, C.C., Pain, C., Field, N.P., Woods, P. (2006). Posttraumatic personality disorder: a reformulation of complex posttraumatic stress disorder and borderline personality disorder. Psych Clin North Am 29(1): 87–112.

Grant, B.F., Hasin, D.S., Stinson, F.S., Dawson, D.A., Chou, S.P., Ruan, W.J., Pickering, R.P. (2004). Prevalence, correlates, and disability of personality disorders in the United States: results from the national epidemiologic survey on alcohol and related conditions. J Clin Psychiatry 65(7): 948–58.

Keshavan, M., Shad, M., Soloff, P., Schooler, N. (2004). Efficacy and tolerability of olanzapine in the treatment of schizotypal personality disorder. Schizophr Res 71(1): 97–101.

Koenigsberg, H.W., Kaplan, R.D., Gilmore, M.M., Cooper, A.M. (1985). The relationship between syndrome and personality disorder in DSM-III: experience with 2,462 patients. Am J Psychiatry 142(2): 207–12.

Koerner, K., Linehan, M.M. (2000). Research on dialectical behavior therapy for patients with borderline personality disorder. Psychiatr Clin North Am 23(1): 151–67.

Loranger, A.W. (1990).The impact of DSM-III on diagnostic practice in a university hospital. A comparison of DSM-II and DSM-III in 10,914 patients. Arch Gen Psychiatry 47(7): 672–5.

McClure, M.M., Barch, D.M., Romero, M.J., Minzenberg, M.J., Triebwasser, J., Harvey, P.D., Siever, L.J. (2007). The effects of guanfacine on context processing abnormalities in schizotypal personality disorder. Biol Psychiatry 61(10): 1157–60.

Spitzer, M., Fischbacher, U., Hermberger, B., Gron, G., Fehr, E. (2007). The neural signature of social norm compliance. Neuron 56(1): 185–96.

Chapter 25
Cognitive Disorders

Russ S. Muramatsu and Junji Takeshita

We hope you are continuing to enjoy learning about the different categories of psychiatric diagnoses! This chapter covers disorders that affect medically vulnerable and elderly patients, and that highlight the close connection between body, brain, and behavior.

At the end of this chapter the reader will be able to

1. Understand the concepts of cognition and memory and recognize when there is a change from baseline status
2. Compare and contrast normal age-associated forgetfulness, mild cognitive impairment, dementia, delirium, and depression
3. Present a differential diagnosis for dementia and delirium
4. Explain a comprehensive approach to evaluating a suspected cognitive disorder using a combination of history of illness, screening scales, and laboratory and imaging tests
5. Discuss the treatment of cognitive disorders with a focus on dementia of the Alzheimer's type and delirium

Case Vignette 25.1.1 Presenting Situation: Eli Thompson

Mr. Thompson is a 76-year-old man with a history of hypertension and diabetes. He "retired" 2 years ago from his full-time work of 35 years as a commercial house painter and has lived alone for the last year since his wife passed away from a hemorrhagic stroke. With hard work and dedication he advanced through the ranks of his job and eventually succeeded in starting his own company with 10 full-time employees. Over the years he spent more time getting new "jobs" rather than painting himself. He has always been quite proud of his accomplishments.

Over the last year, his adult son and daughter have become increasingly concerned with some of his behavior, and in the last 2 months have begun to

R.S. Muramatsu,
Fellow in Geriatric Psychiatry University of Hawai'i John A. Burns School of Medicine

A. Guerrero, M. Piasecki (eds.), *Problem-Based Behavioral Science and Psychiatry*,
© Springer Science+Business Media, LLC 2008

seriously question whether he can continue to live alone. His children noticed that he occasionally forgets the names of his grandchildren. Additionally, he is frustrated that he "can't do things like the old days," and he would say, "My memory is not like it was before." Most concerning is that he seems to be having problems with his medications. They noticed sometimes he forgets to take them and sometimes he takes the wrong ones or the wrong amount. As Mr. Thompson's primary care provider, you see him in your office with his daughter.

Please proceed with the problem-based approach!

At this point, the primary concern voiced both by Mr. Thompson and his family is a change in his cognition and memory. Before going any further, it is important to understand what is meant by cognition and memory. The term cognition (Latin: *cognoscere*, "to know") is used in several ways to describe the processes such as memory, attention, perception, action, problem solving, and mental imagery. Merriam-Webster Dictionary defines memory as: (a) the power or process of reproducing or recalling what has been learned and retained especially through associative mechanisms; (b) the store of things learned and retained from an organism's activity or experience as evidenced by modification of structure or behavior or by recall and recognition (Merriam-Webster, 2004).

There is a large array of bio-psycho-social factors that could potentially affect someone's cognition and memory. For example, almost every disorder in the DSM-IV-TR could likely affect cognition and memory in one way or another. Patients with schizophrenia typically have cognitive problems as well as a thought disorder. In this chapter we will limit our discussion primarily to the disorders classified under cognitive disorders, emphasizing dementia and delirium. The DSM-IV-TR (American Psychiatric Association, 2000) classifies delirium, dementia, and amnestic and other cognitive disorders as a group of disorders which features, "a significant impairment of cognition or memory that represents a marked deterioration from a previous level of function" (see Table 25.1).

Once a cognitive problem is suspected, the first step is to obtain a good, accurate history from the patient, family, and caregivers. The focus of the history is on the chronology of the cognitive changes including onset, course, progression, and associated symptoms. A complete "data set" is the most efficient way to narrow down the differential diagnosis from which eventually you will hopefully attain the best diagnosis. Mr. Thompson, for example, had a noticeable change in his behavior and cognition about 1 year ago, which coincided with the death of his wife. You might consider a diagnosis of a depressive disorder that is presenting with memory and concentration problems. On the other hand, a history of onset of cognitive problems as a young adult might suggest acute lead toxicity from exposure to lead-based paint.

Table 25.1 Delirium, dementia, and amnestic and other cognitive disorders

Delirium
  Delirium due to a general medical condition
  Substance intoxication delirium
  Substance withdrawal delirium
  Delirium due to multiple etiologies
  Delirium NOS
Dementia
  Dementia of the Alzheimer's type
  Vascular dementia
  Dementia due to a general medical condition
  Substance-induced persisting dementia
  Dementia due to multiple etiologies
  Dementia NOS
Amnesia
  Amnestic disorder due to a general medical condition
  Substance-induced persisting amnestic disorder
  Amnestic disorder NOS
Other
  Cognitive disorder NOS

Identifying Mr. Thompson's baseline level of cognition and functioning is helpful to figure out how quickly the problems are progressing and how severe they are. It also has some role in predicting performance on testing and prognosis. While Mr. Thompson's formal educational level was only a high school diploma, he demonstrated an above average intellect and resourcefulness as a successful business owner.

Upon closer inspection, you might suspect that his problems with cognition started even earlier. Often, family members only recognize a problem when the symptoms have become obvious. Looking back, there are sometimes subtle clues that indicate the process started much earlier. In Mr. Thompson's case you might wonder why he retired 2 years ago. Could he have had early dementia? Was he

Table 25.2 Cognitive disorder continuum

	Normal memory	Normal age-related decline	Mild cognitive impairment	Dementia
Memory deficits	None	Trace, may be transient	Mild, may be reversible	Moderate to severe, typically non-reversible
Other cognitive deficits	None	None	Possible	Definite
Level of function	Independent	Independent	Independent	Dependent

having difficulty keeping track of his business? Could this be just part of "normal" aging in a 74-year-old (Feldman and Jacova, 2005)? Table 25.2 lists other possibilities.

Case Vignette 25.1.2 Continuation

Further history reveals that Mr. Thompson has no personal history of depression or other psychiatric conditions. He has never used tobacco or any illicit drugs. He has been treated with an anti-hypertensive and oral hypoglycemic medication for the last 10 years. He has no family history of dementia or other neuro-psychiatric disorders. He denies any other symptoms or problems including problems with movement, falls, or hallucinations.

While he admits that he still misses his wife, he feels he is over his acute grief and hasn't become tearful or overwhelmingly sad for 6 months or more. In fact, other than sleep problems he does not endorse any other symptoms of depression including suicidality. He spends his time reading and working in his yard. His favorite past time, however, since his early twenties, was to "kick back" with his friends after a hard day's work and enjoy a "few" beers.

 Please proceed with the problem-based approach!

Here we get additional information that could be used to help with continued evaluation of what type or types of cognitive disorders we are dealing with. Notice we have not yet generated a differential diagnosis. We will do this after we have finished narrowing the problem down to a specific disorder class.

At this point a diagnosis of depression, although important to consider and differentiate from dementia, is low on the list of potential diagnoses. Alcohol intoxication or withdrawal delirium is a possibility given Mr. Thompson's alcohol use history. However, there is no evidence for a delirium at this time as his level of consciousness has been stable without fluctuation. His cognitive deficits seem more significant than just "normal" aging. The most likely diagnosis is an early stage dementia. Table 25.3 reviews differentiating factors between depression, dementia, and delirium (Arnold, 2004; Potter and Steffens, 2007) (see Table 25.3).

Although there are many different "dementias" as defined in the DSM-IV-TR all share common characteristics, including: memory impairment and at least one other cognitive disturbance (e.g., aphasia, apraxia, agnosia, executive functioning disturbance) that cause functional impairment; that represent a decline from previous functioning, and that do not exclusively occur during a delirium.

It is important to realize that dementia includes features beyond just a memory problem (a memory problem alone is an amnestic disorder). Now that we are pretty

Table 25.3 Differentiating the "3 Ds"

	Dementia	Depression	Delirium
Precipitating event	Uncommon (depends on type)	Sometimes May have a psychosocial stressor	Present Usually a change in medical condition or medications
Age of onset	Uncommon below age 60	Any age	Any age
Rate of onset	Insidious Months to years	Moderately acute Weeks to months	Acute Hours to days
Fluctuations	Stable throughout the day. May be worse at night ("sundowning")	Hourly to daily Worse in morning	Minutes to hourly Worse at night
Course	Progressive decline	Resolves with treatment, may reoccur or be chronic	Resolves with treatment
Duration	Lifetime (for non-reversible causes)	Moderate Weeks to months	Short Hours to weeks
Consciousness	Intact	Intact	Altered
Memory complaints	May be denied by patient	Common	None
Memory performance	Worse than self-assessment Does not improve with cues Normal effort	Better than self-assessment Improves with retrieval cues Decreased effort "don't know"	Usually no self-assessment Does not improve with cues Variable effort
Family history	Often non-contributory	Common to have a family history of mood disorders	Generally non-contributory
Personal history	Possible risk factors may be present	Common to have a history of stressors	Generally non-contributory

sure that we are dealing with a dementia, we must now review all of the potential etiologies. Giving a diagnosis of "dementia" is akin to giving a diagnosis of "fever," which is present in a variety of illnesses. In Mr. Thompson's case, certain potential etiologies include alcohol, lead exposure, and vascular events (see Table 25.4). There are also a few that need to be screened for with laboratory tests and brain imaging.

Case Vignette 25.1.3 Continuation

Mr. Thompson's Mini Mental State Examination testing reveals a score of 26 out of 30. He missed 3 points on orientation and 1 point on recall. His clock-drawing test

Table 25.4 Etiologies of dementia

Category	Example
Degenerative	Dementia of the Alzheimer's type, Parkinson's disease
Vascular	Multiple infarcts
Myelinoclastic	Multiple sclerosis
Inflammatory	Systemic lupus erythematosus
Infectious	Syphilis, AIDS
Toxic	Alcohol-related
Metabolic	Hepatic encephalopathy
Traumatic	Subdural hematoma
Neoplastic	Meningioma
Hydrocephalic	Normal pressure hydrocephalus
Psychiatric	Schizophrenia, dementia

Adapted from Gray and Cummings (1996)

was without errors, although he was somewhat slow in completing it. Throughout the testing, Mr. Thompson seemed motivated to perform well. Laboratory results were as follows: non-reactive RPR, low normal vitamin B12 level, normal folate level, normal TSH level, and normal chemistries and CBC. Heavy metal screening including lead is normal. You had debated testing for HIV but decided against it. A non-contrast CT scan of the brain is significant only for some mild cortical atrophy and "periventricular white matter changes."

 Please proceed with the problem-based approach!

The Mini Mental State Examination (MMSE), not to be confused with a Mental Status Examination (MSE), is a 30-point screening test for dementia that can be used in the clinical setting. It is perhaps the most utilized and recognized cognitive screening test (Folstein et al., 1975). Each question tests a specific area of cognition, for example, memory, language, and visual–spatial orientation, which can be correlated with the functioning of a specific area in the brain. The lower the score, the more severe the cognitive problem.

There are several important points to remember. The MMSE is purely a screening test; it does not diagnose dementia. Further cognitive testing is necessary in combination with history and labs, to confirm a diagnosis of dementia. There are several reported limitations with the MMSE. For example, the questions overemphasize memory and underemphasize or do not even test for executive functioning. Performance on the MMSE is affected by culture and educational level. Someone who has more "educational reserves" may continue to score high on the MMSE while having significant change in cognitive ability from baseline. Even problems with vision or hearing must be taken into account as they could affect performance.

Table 25.5 Laboratory and imaging evaluation for dementia

ROUTINE	NON-ROUTINE
CBC	Syphilis screening
Glucose	Lumbar puncture
Serum electrolytes	EEG
BUN/creatinine	Genetic testing for DLB or CJD
Serum B12 levels	APOE genotyping for DAT
Thyroid function tests	SPECT
Liver function tests	Linear or volumetric MR or CT
Computed tomography (CT) imaging	PET
Magnetic resonance imaging (MRI)	
NOT ENOUGH EVIDENCE	
Other genetic markers for AD	
CSF or other biomarkers for AD	
Tau mutations for FTD	
AD gene mutations in FTD	

Adapted from Kawas (2003) and Knopman et al. (2001)

The MMSE score can be used to categorize the severity of the cognitive deficit. The true value of the test, however, is to track performance over time, and thereby be able to evaluate the progression of disease or success of treatment. In general, a score > 26 is considered normal; 20–26 suggests mild dementia; 10–19 suggests moderate dementia; and <10 suggests severe dementia. On average, without treatment, people with dementia will lose 2–4 points each year.

The Clock-Drawing Test is another screening test for dementia. Patients are presented with a circle drawn on a piece of paper. They are told, "This circle represents a clock face." They are then asked to, "Fill in the numbers to look like a clock and then set the time to 10 minutes past 11." Shulman [2000] indicates that the cognitive skill necessary for completion of this task include: (1) comprehension, (2) planning, (3) visual memory and reconstruction, (4) visual-spatial abilities, (5) motor programming and execution, (6) numerical knowledge, (7) abstract thinking, (8) inhibition of the tendency to be pulled by perceptual features of the stimulus, and (9) concentration and frustration tolerance. It can be used similarly as the MMSE to track changes over time.

Standard laboratory and imaging test for dementia are shown in Table 25.5. Heavy metal screening is typically not done but ordered in this case as the patient was a painter. The most likely diagnosis for Mr. Thompson at this point is dementia of Alzheimer's type. A definitive diagnosis can only be made at autopsy.

Case Vignette 25.1.4 Continuation

Two weeks later, you receive a call from Mr. Thompson's daughter who is distraught. She tells you that she is at her father's house and just now found him lying on the

floor moaning in pain. You tell her to call 911. In the emergency room, an x-ray reveals that Mr. Thompson has fractured his hip. His daughter tells her brother on the phone, "See I told him to get rid of that ugly living room area rug . . . I knew he would trip on that one day . . ." Mr. Thompson was admitted to the orthopedic service and you see him the next day to manage his general medical problems.

Upon greeting him in his hospital room, you realize that he is not himself. He thinks he is at home and shares with you how people were outside his window last night trying to break into his house to steal his money. He is unable to give the correct date, month, or year for that matter. Looking at the nursing notes, you learn that he had been severely agitated and combative with staff requiring him to be physically restrained during the night. An electrocardiogram reveals some tachycardia but normal QTc. You believe that his tachycardia is due to agitation rather than alcohol withdrawal and decide to give an antipsychotic rather than a benzodiazepine. You are concerned about QTc as antipsychotics can prolong QTc. After the addition of a very low dose of antipsychotic medication his confusion improves and eventually it is tapered off. One-week post-surgery Mr. Thompson is ready for discharge.

Please proceed with the problem-based approach!

Mr. Thompson had another, more dramatic change in his cognition and memory. His confusion is much worse and there are new symptoms of delusions and hallucinations. The time course of worsening symptoms and onset of new symptoms are too sudden to be consistent with progression of the dementia. Also, it is too much of a coincidence that this presentation coincides with the hip fracture, hospitalization, and surgery. Notice again the importance of understanding the chronology of symptoms in narrowing the differential diagnosis.

An acute delirium best explains Mr. Thompson's presentation. Possible etiologies include alcohol, pain medications, or the surgery itself. Like with dementia, there are many different causes of delirium (see Table 25.6). Irrespective of etiology, delirium as defined in the DSM-IV-TR includes the following characteristics: disturbance of consciousness and attention; a change in cognition (e.g., memory, orientation, language) or development of perceptual disturbance not accounted for by dementia; and acute onset with fluctuating course.

Delirium can be categorized into hyperactive and hypoactive delirium. Physicians are far more likely to be called by nursing staff for the former (as was the case for Mr. Thompson). While the exact pathophysiology underlying delirium is not known, one hypothesis is that there is a decreased level of acetylcholine and an increased level of dopamine present. The pharmacologic treatment of delirium and agitation is for the most part with low doses of typical antipsychotic medications (American Psychiatric Association, 2006; Meagher, 2001). The one major exception

Table 25.6 Etiologies of delirium: "I WATCH DEATH"

Category	Example
Infectious	Encephalitis
Withdrawal from drugs	Alcohol
Acute metabolic disorder	Electrolyte disturbance
Trauma	Closed-head injury
CNS pathology	Seizure
Hypoxia	Hypotension
Deficiencies in vitamins	Thiamine
Endocrinopathies	Hyper/hypoglycemia
Acute vascular insults	Stroke
Toxins or drugs	Medications
Heavy metals	Lead

Adapted from Wise and Trzepacz (1996)

to this is the presence of alcohol or sedative hypnotic withdrawal, which should be primarily treated with benzodiazepines. In Mr. Thompson's case, haloperidol was used with good success.

Case Vignette 25.1.5 Continuation

Mr. Thompson is admitted to a nursing home for rehabilitation. His children have the long-term plan to sell his house and move him into an assisted living facility. On repeat Mini Mental State Examination testing he scores 23 out of 30. Mr. Thompson has great difficulty settling into his new environment. He is unhappy about sharing a room with another person. He is irritable toward both the staff and his family and ask everyone "Why can't I go home?" The physical therapist expressed concerns that he wasn't progressing as fast as she thought he should in therapy. When asked about his progress, he replies, "Don't ask me . . . how should I know . . . I don't even know why I'm here really . . . "

Mr. Thompson's score on the Geriatric Depression Scale is 9 out of 15, highly suspicious for the presence of a depression. Mr. Thompson denies feeling depressed, but is willing to take an antidepressant medication, "Go ahead . . . whatever you think . . . you're the doctor." You prescribe low dose of an SSRI and spend time listening to his concerns. Two weeks later, Mr. Thompson seems to be in a little better mood; his family also noticed a small change. By 4 weeks, his mood had changed considerably. He is no longer so irritable and is even beginning to like his living environment. At the end of 8 weeks, he has made so much progress in therapy that the treatment team began planning for discharge back to the community.

Please proceed with the problem-based approach!

Again Mr. Thompson has had a change in his cognitive functioning as seen by his MMSE score and clinical presentation. Dementia, delirium, and depression are, as usual, the primary differential considerations. As before, the progression is abrupt. Delirium is not likely, although residual cognitive deficits post-delirium is possible problem. The most likely problem at this point, however, is depression. In elderly patients, depression after nursing home placement is not uncommon and may present with atypical symptoms.

Elderly patients commonly have many physical illnesses and symptoms which overlap with neurovegetative symptoms like changes in weight, sleep, or fatigue. Focusing on the other symptoms of depression like suicidal thoughts, feelings of guilt, or feelings of hopelessness can be more helpful. It is also important to realize that depression is not an inevitable and untreatable outcome of either aging or nursing home placement.

The Geriatric Depression Scale is a screening test for depression in the elderly patients. There are two versions of the scale: a 30-point version and a shorter 15-point version (Brink et al., 1982; Sheikh and Yesavage, 1986). The questions differentiate depression from depression-like symptoms from other physical illnesses. The higher the score the more likely the patient is depressed.

Please refer to Chap. 21 for more specific information on Major Depressive Disorder. Depression and dementia can occur totally independent of each other. They can both occur at the same time in a person but be independent of each other. Dementia can be associated with and or be a cause of depression. Depression is a risk factor for dementia, may be a prodrome to dementia, causes cognitive deficits itself, and worsens the physical and functional symptoms of dementia (Potter, 2007). Screening for depression is a recommended part of routine workup for dementia (Knopman et al., 2001).

Case Vignette 25.1.6 Conclusion

A year-and-a-half later, Mr. Thompson shows up in your outpatient clinic with his daughter. "I'm living by myself now," he says smiling, although you know from his daughter that he is in an assisted living facility and requires hired caregivers to assist with daily activities such as medication management. His Mini Mental State Examination today indicates a score of 20/30, and there is no indication of depression or acute confusion. You spend the rest of the time talking to Mr. Thompson and his daughter educating them on the course of illness and what to expect in the future.

 Please proceed with the problem-based approach!

With the delirium and depression resolved, Mr. Thompson's underlying dementia continues to slowly progress, as indicated by his declining MMSE score. As part of the treatment plan you discuss the use of medications such as acetylcholinesterase inhibitors and N-methyl-D-aspartate (NMDA) antagonists with Mr. Thompson and his daughter.

The primary pathophysiologic process underlying dementia of Alzheimer's type is the production of abnormal proteins in the brain and the subsequent development of beta-amyloid plaques and neurofibrillary tangles. These abnormalities correlate with neuronal dysfunction and ultimately degeneration of a cluster of neurons that produce acetylcholine (nucleus basalis of Meynert). This decreases the production of the neurotransmitter acetylcholine, which is thought to play a role in cognition. Acetylcholinesterase inhibitors, like donepezil, while not affecting the underlying pathophysiology or reversing dementing diseases, helps limit the degradation of the existing acetylcholine and therefore slows down the effects of the disease. Acetylcholinesterase inhibitors are typically more effective in the early phase of

Table 25.7 General stages of dementia

Mild (early-stage)	Memory loss and/or other cognitive deficits are noticeable
	Can compensate and may continue to function independently
Moderate (mid-stage)	Memory and other cognitive deficits worsen
	Accompanied by personality and physical changes
	More dependent on others
Severe (late-stage)	Deterioration of the personality
	Loss of control of bodily functions
	Total dependence on others

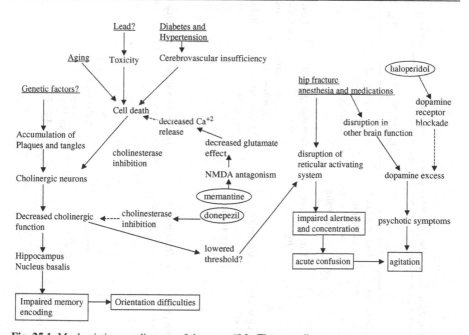

Fig. 25.1 Mechanistic case diagram of the case, "Mr. Thompson"

Table 25.8 Bio-psycho-social formulation of the case, "Mr. Thompson"

	Biological		Psychological		Social	
	Factor	Intervention	Factor	Intervention	Factor	Intervention
Predisposing factors	History of heavy alcohol use and exposure of lead paint	Stopped drinking and no longer painting	Death of his wife 1 year ago	None	Less immediate social support after wife's death	None
	Diabetes and hypertension	Oral hypoglycemic and anti-hypertensive medications	Loss of his job due to retirement	None		
Precipitating factors	Cognitive decline and memory problems	Comprehensive evaluation	Role transition from independent to dependent	Individual counseling	Inappropriate level of care	Hospital and then nursing home admission
					Inadequate environment	Education of family
Perpetuating factors	Delirium and depression	Haloperidol to treat delirium	Dealing with loss and change	Medication and supportive therapy	Need for increased care and supervision	Change in living enviroment
		SSRI to treat depression				
	Worsening dementia	Acetycholinesterase inhibitors and NMDA antagonists				Education of family

Alzheimer's dementia. N-methyl-D-aspartate (NMDA) antagonists like memantine work on a different neurotransmitter, glutamate. Glutamate is involved in the release of calcium from neurons. Too much calcium causes death of the cell and memantine interferes with this process.

Table 25.7 describes the stages of dementia of the Alzheimer's type and the common progression of the illness. Dividing the disease into stages can help families plan for the future. Realize, however, that no two patients are alike; the type of symptoms and rate of progression may differ. People with dementia of the Alzheimer's type live for an average of 10 years after the diagnosis and most die from complications such as pneumonia and decubitus ulcers.

We close with a summary diagram (Fig. 25.1) and bio-psycho-social-cultural-spiritual formulation (Table 25.8) of Mr. Thompson's case.

Review Questions

1. In evaluating a patient with cognitive deficits which of the following is most useful:

   (a) Obtaining serum anticholinergic level
   (b) Administering the Geriatric Depression Scale (GDS)
   (c) Getting an adequate history
   (d) Checking Mini Mental State Examination (MMSE)
   (e) Ordering a computed tomography (CT) of head

2. The Mini Mental State Examination (MMSE) is most useful for which of the following:

   (a) Diagnosing dementia
   (b) Evaluating frontal lobe functioning
   (c) Determining progression of cognitive deficits
   (d) Screening tool for mania
   (e) Evaluating which patients should be on a acetylcholinesterase inhibitor

3. Delirium is differentiated from dementia by which of the following feature:

   (a) Fluctuation in consciousness
   (b) Severity of cognitive deficits
   (c) Relationship with psychosocial stressors
   (d) Improved cognitive examination with cues
   (e) Family history

4. Memantine helps with cognition through the following mechanism:

   (a) Acetylcholine
   (b) Dopamine
   (c) Norepinephrine
   (d) Serotonin
   (e) N-methyl-D-aspartate (NMDA)

Answers

1. c, 2. c, 3. a (The hallmark of delirium is fluctuation in consciousness), 4. e

References

American Psychiatric Association (2000). *Diagnostic and Statistical Manual of Mental Disorders DSM-IV-TR Fourth Edition.*
American Psychiatric Association (2006). APA Practice Guideline for the treatment of patients with delirium. In *American Psychiatric Association Practice Guidelines for the Treatment of Psychiatric Disorders: Compendium 2006.*
Arnold E (2004). Sorting out the 3 D's: delirium, dementia, depression. *Nursing*, 34: 36–42.
Brink TL, Yesavage JA, Lum O, Heersema P, Adey MB, Rose TL (1982). Screening tests for geriatric depression. *Clinical Gerontologist*, 1: 37–44.
Feldman HH, Jacova C (2005). Mild cognitive impairment. *American Journal of Geriatric Psychiatry*, 13: 645–655.
Folstein MF, Folstein SE McHugh PR (1975). Mini Mental State: a practical method for grading the cognitive state of patients for the clinician. *Journal of Psychiatric Research*, 12: 189–198.
Gray KF, Cummings JL (1996). Dementia. In *Textbook of Consultation-Liaison Psychiatry* (pp. 268). Washington, DC: Rundell/Wise.
Kawas CH (2003). Early Alzheimer's disease. *New England Journal of Medicine*, 349: 1056–1063.
Knopman DS, DeKosky ST, Cummings JL et al. (2001). Diagnosis of dementia (an evidence based review): report of the Quality Standards Subcommittee of the American Academy of Neurology. *Neurology*, 56: 1143–1153.
Meagher DJ (2001). Delirium: optimizing management. *British Medical Journal*, 322: 144–149.
Potter GG, Steffens DC (2007). Contribution of depression to cognitive impairment and dementia in older adults. *The Neurologist*, 13: 105–117.
Sheikh JI, Yesavage JA (1986). Geriatric Depression Scale (GDS): recent evidence and development of a shorter version. In *Clinical Gerontology: A Guide to Assessment and Intervention* (pp. 165–173). New York: The Haworth Press.
Shulman KI (2000). Clock-drawing: is it the ideal cognitive screening test? *International Journal of Geriatric Psychiatry*, 15: 548–561.
Wise MG, Trzepacz PT (1996). Delirium (confusional states). In *Textbook of Consultation-Liaison Psychiatry* (pp. 268). Washington, DC: Rundell/Wise.

Chapter 26
Sleep Disorders

Ole J. Thienhaus and Nathanael W. Cardon

Introduction

Complaints of poor sleep or insomnia are among the most common reasons why patients consult their primary care physician. The diagnosis of insomnia, however, is non-specific and easily confused with parasomnias and hypersomnias. So the clinician must fully assess the sleep problem and rule out a primary or underlying condition (Taylor et al., 2007) before treating sleeplessness symptomatically with a hypnotic (medication to induce sleep). The three cases in this chapter illustrate insomnia as well as less common sleep disorders.

At the end of this chapter, the reader will be able to

1. Discuss a differential diagnosis for symptoms of insomnia
2. Identify the behaviors associated with parasomnias
3. Develop a plan for assessment of daytime hypersomnia

Case Vignette 26.1.1 Presenting Situation: Maria Thompson

Maria Thompson is a 36-year-old married woman who is the mother of two pre-teen boys. She comes to your primary care office with the complaint of "not sleeping." Until a few years ago, she never noticed any sleeping problems although she describes herself as a light sleeper at all times. Now, her insomnia causes her to toss and turn for at least 2 hours. She grows increasingly worried about not getting enough sleep, before she finally drops off. During the night, she wakes up for no reason at all, or because of a trivial noise or minimal urge to use the bathroom. Then she cannot go back to sleep as she thinks about the difficult problems in her home.

Please proceed with the problem-based approach!

O.J. Thienhaus
Professor and Chair of Psychiatry, University of Nevada School of Medicine

A. Guerrero, M. Piasecki (eds.), *Problem-Based Behavioral Science and Psychiatry*,
© Springer Science+Business Media, LLC 2008

Insomnia

Epidemiology: Insomnia, defined as any combination of symptoms, including difficulty falling asleep, frequent waking, and early morning awakening is one of the most common complaints among primary care patients. It is estimated to affect 60 million Americans each year, affecting about 40 % of women and 30 % of men. The prevalence of insomnia increases with age.

Differential Diagnosis: The clinical examination and history are the most critical elements directing the clinician toward a differential diagnosis. Difficulty sleeping (insomnia/dyssomnia) should be distinguished from excessive sleepiness (hypersomnia). Physical, psychological, and other underlying causes should also be considered and ruled out. The type of insomnia (e.g., difficulty falling asleep as opposed to early morning wakening) can be determined by specific, clarifying questions. Alcohol or sedative use, smoking, and mood disorders can cause insomnia and inquiries about them are part of a careful history. Possible underlying medical problems such as endocrine disorders can be identified on physical examination and targeted laboratory tests. A sleep study is the ideal way to objectively measure the quality of a patient's sleep and monitor for physiologic events disturbing sleep, discussed further in the cases below.

Case Vignette 26.1.2 Continued

Mrs. Thompson has already tried to adjust her sleep time, at the suggestion of a magazine article, and goes to bed at least an hour after her husband. When she wakes up and has a hard time going back to sleep, she often finishes out the night on the living room couch so as not to disturb her husband. She is awake early in the morning, but feels exhausted and worn out. "Often it's hard to get up and started on the day." Coffee helps, but by noon, she is ready "to crawl back into bed," if only she felt she actually could get back to sleep. The patient believes that her two boys have begun to worry about her. Her husband is at times solicitous about her health and at other times irritated with her perceived "laziness." He wonders "if we'll ever have sex again."

A few months ago another physician checked Mrs. Thompson's thyroid status (which was normal), and prescribed sleeping pills. First, she tried hydroxyzine, then zolpidem. Later, she tried a low dose of trazodone. Mrs. Thompson says that all these medications "made me even more tired" but none helped her sleep through the night.

Please proceed with the problem-based approach!

At this point, Mrs. Thompson's case should raise some eyebrows because she is not responding to prescribed sleep medications. She seems to distinguish her problem not as being lack of tiredness, but that of not falling asleep, as if something else is keeping her aroused. Consider the history and further questioning below:

Case Vignette 26.1.3 Continued

History: Mrs. Thompson says that she has always been in good health. The two childbirths were the only times she was in the hospital. After the second baby, she had "the blues" for a while, but got over it after a few weeks. She denies any family history of psychiatric illness. Her mother, who died of cervical cancer at age 41, had also been having sleeping problems, but Mrs. Thompson thinks this was related to the cancer.

Mrs. Thompson does not drink alcohol and has never used illicit drugs. She takes no medications. She appeared somewhat tense at the beginning of the interview, and when asked about her feeling "at a dead end" she suddenly bursts into tears. She is worried about her failures as a wife and mother. She has been withdrawing from activities she could and should be spending with her family. Mrs. Thompson used to enjoy running a book-club with neighborhood friends, but, after her second son was born, gave up on that, at first because she was too busy taking care of the baby, later because she did not feel like doing it.

Mental Status Examination: Mrs. Thompson is alert and fully oriented. Her affect is dejected, tearful, and weary, but she responds to your supportive comments and maintains stable eye contact. She describes her mood as "worried." There is no evidence of cognitive impairment, thought disorder, or perceptual disorder. She denies feeling suicidal.

Please proceed with the problem-based approach!

Mrs. Thompson's tearful affect, sense of failure, and anhedonia (lack of pleasure), suggest that the original complaint of insomnia is likely a symptom of a major depressive episode. As with other common, general symptoms such as fatigue and weight loss, insomnia should not be reduced to a purely symptom-based diagnostic label. The original treatments geared toward sleep were ineffective because they did not address the primary cause of Mrs. Thompson's insomnia.

Case Vignette 26.1.4 Conclusion

After further questioning, you discover that Mrs. Thompson meets criteria of Major Depressive Disorder with five out of nine criteria in the DSM-IV-TR lasting longer than 2 months. After discussion of several treatment options, she agrees to a trial with an antidepressant and a limited supply of a benzodiazepine. In addition, she appreciates that the latter medicine may only have a limited role in her improvement and that psychological interventions, family therapy, and supportive counseling regarding stress management and coping could be most important for her recovery. She agrees to schedule an appointment with a local therapist covered on her insurance plan. You see Mrs. Thompson weekly for a month, and then schedule a 3-month follow-up appointment. She reports improvement in mood, sleep, and energy and has started to see the therapist.

Treatment: Treatment of insomnia targets underlying primary pathology whenever it is present. For example, successful treatment of a depressive disorder will improve related sleep problems. In primary insomnia or when coexisting diagnoses have only an aggravating effect, the clinical target is the insomnia (Morgenthaler et al., 2006). First-line interventions include sleep hygiene and the practice of relaxation techniques (see chapter 4). Sleep medications can assist these interventions and build a positive reward experience. Hypnotic medications exert their effects in one of three neurotransmitter systems: The histamine receptors such as diphenhydramine and hydroxyzine (most over-the-counter sleep aids), the GABA receptors (benzodiazepines and "Z-drugs"), or the melatonin receptors (ramelteon). In short-term situations where insomnia results from a time-limited stress exposure (e.g., during a hospital stay), pharmacologic intervention can be justified as the first choice of treatment (Morin et al., 2007). Long-term use of sleep medications remains controversial because of the potential for abuse and dependence with most hypnotics (Taylor et al., 2006). Ramelteon and eszopiclone, a Z-drug, have been shown to maintain long-term effectiveness for insomnia with minimal risk of dependence.

Case Vignette 26.2.1 Vickie Sippets

Vickie is a 17-year-old high-school student seen in clinic with her parents. Her mother explains she and her husband are worried about their daughter who started sleepwalking about 6 weeks earlier. At first Vickie's parents thought she was waking up to use the bathroom, and was so groggy she would not respond. When it happened nearly every night they led her back to her room and woke her up. Several minutes into the interview, Vickie speaks for the first time, and tells you she was quite puzzled and could not explain how she ended up out of bed.

Please proceed with the problem-based approach!

Parasomnias

Epidemiology: Parasomnias are less common than insomnias and mostly affect children and young adults. Somnambulism (sleep walking disorder) is by far the most prevalent parasomnia with an estimated prevalence of 5–15 % among children in the United States.

Differential: Vickie's presentation suggests somnambulism (Lee-Chiong, 2005). Somnambulism is a primary sleep disorder that may require treatment. Other possibilities need to be considered, and the differential diagnosis includes a seizure disorder with psychomotor phenomena (partial complex seizures), and a factitious disorder (Eisensehr and Schmidt, 2005). In a factitious disorder, the patient assumes a sick role in order to obtain gratification of certain psychological needs of which he or she is not consciously aware (see chapter 29).

Case Vignette 26.2.2 Continued

History: Vickie and her mother report that there is no past history of any psychiatric problems. Her performance in school is above average, and she enjoys sports. She broke up with a boyfriend about a year earlier and has not been dating since. She denies any use of drugs or alcohol. She has not been sexually active and has taken a voluntary vow to remain celibate until married. Vickie hopes to study psychology in college.

You ask Vickie's parents to step out for a moment, and then ask Vickie further questions about her personal life. She continues to endorse her same convictions and history that she is confused about what is going on, and that she has not taken any alcohol or drugs.

Mental Status Examination: Vickie is a young woman in no acute distress. She appears age-appropriate in her development and intellectual function. There is no evidence of psychosis or cognitive impairment.

Please proceed with the problem-based approach!

Diagnosis: The key to diagnosis in sleep disorders is an electrophysiological evaluation known as a polysomnograph, or sleep study (Szelenberger et al., 2005). During the assessment, an electroencephalogram (EEG) records wave patterns from non-REM sleep (stages 1–4), and REM (rapid eye movement) (Table 26.1). Concurrently, muscle activity, respiratory rate, heart rate, and pulse oximetry are measured during periods of sleep and wakefulness. A sleep study with polysomnographic EEG data should show, in the case of somnambulism, an onset of motor phenomena coinciding with deep non-REM sleep (stages 3 and 4, also called delta sleep) earlier in

Table 26.1 Sleep stages

Sleep stage	EEG findings	Clinical findings
Stage I	Low voltage, fast waves	Light sleep, easily aroused
Stage II	Sleep spindles and K complexes	Easily awakened; metabolism slows
Stages III and IV	Slow delta waves	Deep sleep, no muscle movement, difficult to awaken. Sleep stage for sleep walking, enuresis, and night terrors
Rapid eye movement (REM)	Highly active, with small and irregular waves similar to waking state	Four to five distinct periods in 90 minutes cycles during night of sleep, increased in the last one-third of the night; dreams occur

the night, with REM sleep toward morning (Guilleminault et al., 2006). In order to diagnose a partial complex seizure disorder (also called temporal lobe epilepsy or psychomotor seizure disorder), a sleep-deprived EEG uses nasopharyngeal leads to detect abnormal electrical activity in deep brain structures. When a patient had an abnormal EEG, neurologists will further evaluate for the cause of the abnormal activity and will treat the patient with antiseizure medications. If a sleep EEG study does not offer a clear diagnosis, psychological testing may be useful to determine if personality factors would make the patient more likely to communicate her distress by developing physical symptoms.

Case Vignette 26.2.3 Conclusion

Vickie's sleep studies support a working diagnosis of somnambulism. When Vickie and her parents return, you explain to them that sleepwalking is a fairly common occurrence in children and young adults, and usually resolves spontaneously. Because she is not awake during motor activities there is a possibility that Vickie could harm herself. It is therefore important to make her environment safer, e.g., by blocking staircases and locking away knives. You further explain that the incidence of somnambulism may increase with anxiety, stress, and unresolved conflicts, such as her break-up with the boyfriend. Her parents accept this with some hesitancy, but agree after further reassurance that they can return if the problem worsens or does not go away.

Treatment: With somnambulism, the first intervention is educational. Occasionally, a clinician will reduce the frequency of somnambulism by temporarily prescribing a benzodiazepine or other tranquilizers which would be considered if Vickie's problem worsened or did not go away.

Case Vignette 26.3.1 Randolph Jegniff

Mr. Randolph Jegniff, an obese, 30-year-old recently married man comes to your primary care clinic at his wife's suggestion. He reports that during their recent honeymoon his wife noticed that "the little naps I take" occur frequently and without any warning: "She'd be driving the car, and talking to me, and suddenly, I was gone." His wife told him that he "looked funny" when he fell asleep "like I had collapsed." Sometimes, he would briefly just "slump down like he'd been hit on the head" and she wondered if he'd gone asleep again, except he seemed to be alert, and straightened up again after a few seconds.

Please proceed with the problem-based approach!

Hypersomnias

Differential and Epidemiology: The facts in the case above suggest a hypersomnia, and specifically the possibility of narcolepsy with cataplexy (abrupt loss of muscle tone) (Dauvilliers et al., 2007). Other possibilities include sleep apnea, a petit mal seizure disorder, as well as a problem adjusting flexibly to alternating sleep–wake times [sometimes called "shift worker syndrome" (Ohayon et al., 2002)].

Narcolepsy has prevalence rates of less than 10 %, and is rarer than parasomnias or insomnias (Longstreth et al., 2007). Untreated, it has the potential for serious functional impairment but has an excellent prognosis with treatment response. Sleep apnea is another relatively common hypersomnia. It is estimated to be as prevalent as 9–24 % in men aged 30–60, 4–9 % for women of the same age (Rowley, 2006). Sleep apnea may lead to a host of related symptoms, including cognitive and mood problems. A rare cause of hypersomnia is Kleine–Levin syndrome. This is a primary hypersomnia affecting adolescents with sleep attacks that can last for 2 days, with periods of irritability, hyper-sexuality, and confusion.

Case Vignette 26.3.2 Continued

History: Mr. Jegniff works as a post-doctoral student at the near-by college. He denies any medical problems. He admits to an occasional glass of wine, but no recreational drugs since his late teenage years when he had occasionally smoked marijuana. He characterizes himself as a light sleeper who needs "lots of naps during the day." Mr. Jegniff remembers a few embarrassing occasions when he briefly fell asleep while teaching classes. At those times, he considered such episodes "a wake-up call" to try and get more sleep during the night. With further questioning

Mr. Jegniff and his wife concur that he does not have trouble snoring at night, waking up to catch his breath, or periods of simply not breathing for several seconds.

Physical/Mental status examination: 30-year-old obese male with a 15-inch neck circumference, oral pharyngeal cavity appears clear and unobstructed. No other abnormal findings.

 Please proceed with the problem-based approach!

Diagnosis: The key to differential diagnostic understanding with narcolepsy is a sleep study with polysomnographic EEG data. This examination will provide data regarding latency of sleep onset which is reduced in narcolepsy to 5 minutes or less from a normal average of 20 minutes. Sleep EEGs may also show brief intrusions of REM sleep during "twilight" periods. This abnormal REM activity is responsible for the sleep paralysis and hypnogogic (falling asleep) and hypnopompic (waking up) hallucinations associated with narcolepsy. The decreased latency of sleep onset in narcolepsy is accompanied by electromyographic findings suggestive of cataplexy. The EEG would also be helpful in the diagnosis of sleep apnea as well as a petit mal seizure disorder. With Mr. Jegniff, a larger neck circumference, crowded pharynx, and history of snoring would support the diagnosis of obstructive sleep apnea. A history of periodic respiratory cessation, followed by waking or other catching of breath, would support investigation of a much less common central sleep apnea.

Case Vignette 26.3.3 Conclusion

Mr. Jegniff is scheduled for a sleep study which comes back strongly suggestive of narcolepsy. His treatment begins conservatively with a well-designed sleep hygiene schedule. Mr. Jegniff needs to go to bed at approximately the same time every night, avoid sleep-delaying activities or stimulants, sleep in the same room, get up at about the same time, etc. You explain that this will reduce the frequency of sleep attacks and minimize functional impairment due to narcolepsy, and that this is why his symptoms worsened with the vacation. In addition, he is prescribed modafinil (Provigil®) to increase his daytime alertness, especially after he demonstrates desire to regain the confidence to drive.

Treatment: Once diagnosed, patients must start taking precautions to avoid complications. For instance, a person with untreated narcolepsy should not drive. The condition itself is otherwise benign, and, with treatment, there are usually no limitations on patient functioning. The vulnerability must be kept in mind; however, when a patient with a history of narcolepsy undertakes intercontinental travel or starts variable shift work, patient, family, and physician ought to prepare for a possible relapse.

Narcolepsy appears to be the result of deficient hypocretin production in the brain. In the research laboratory, CSF levels of the neurotransmitter hypocretin are low or non-existent in narcolepsy (Seigel and Boehmer, 2006). Modafinil is a compound that seems to stimulate hypocretin secretion (Seigel and Boehmer, 2006). Traditionally, stimulants such as methylphenidate have been used as well. In addition, tricyclic antidepressants can reduce the incidence of cataplexy. Sodium oxybate (the same compound as the club drug GHB) is a medication that reduces the number of cataplexy attacks in patients with narcolepsy.

Sleep apnea often improves with weight loss, although many patients require positive pressure oxygen during the night to maintain normal blood oxygenation levels. Some patients have surgery known as uvulopalatopharyngoplasty (UPPP) on their soft palates to remove soft tissue and improve nighttime airflow (Rowley, 2006).

Table 26.2 Dysomnias

	Diagnostic features	Special features
Dysomnias		
Primary insomnia	One month or more of poor sleep	Rule out substances, mood disorders, pain, environmental causes
Primary hypersomnia	One month or more of excessive sleep	Rule out substances, endocrine, mood, and causes
Hypersomnias		
Narcolepsy	Cataplexy, hallucinations, sleep paralysis, and sleep attacks	Sleep study
Obstructive sleep apnea	Interruptions of breathing during the night, periods of low blood oxygenation	Excessive soft tissue in oropharynx. Desaturation of blood triggers brief awakenings for breathing
Central sleep apnea	Interruptions of breathing during the night, periods of low blood oxygenation	Dysfunction of thalamus due to neurological disorder
Circadian rhythm sleep disorder	Mismatch of sleep – wake cycle and environment	Includes shift work, jet lag,
Nocturnal myoclonus	Jerking movements of legs while sleeping	May have symptoms during the day as well
Restless leg syndrome	Uncomfortable leg sensations that interfere with sleep	
Kleine–Levin Syndrome	Periodic hypersomnia with episodic increases in appetite and sexual activity	Affects mainly adolescent males

Table 26.3 Parasomnias

Parasomnias	Diagnostic features	Special features
Sleepwalking	Repeated episodes of walking during sleep, difficult to wake	Amnesia for episode
Sleep terror	Awakenings related to intense fear state	Patient not alert, no recall of a dream, awakens with a scream, usually early in sleep cycle
Nightmare disorder	Awakenings related to vivid nightmares	Patient is alert upon awakening

Table 26.4 Related sleep diagnoses

Nocturnal bruxism	Teeth clenching and grinding during the night	May require mouth guard to protect teeth
Nocturnal enuresis	Bed wetting after age 6	Primary: no history of nocturnal bladder control
		Secondary: previous bladder control
Sleep hyperhidrosis	Night sweats	May be related to menopause, some serious illnesses

Review Questions

1. The most common form of insomnia is

    (a) Insomnia due to major depressive disorder
    (b) Insomnia due to hyperthyroidism
    (c) Restless leg syndrome
    (d) Primary insomnia
    (e) Shift worker syndrome

2. In the differential diagnosis of somnambulism, factitious disorder can be detected

    (a) By psychological evaluation
    (b) By a specific EEG pattern
    (c) By polygraph test
    (d) By waking up the patient
    (e) By examination of the CSF

3. In the treatment of narcolepsy, the most important element is

    (a) Modafinil in the morning
    (b) Cognitive behavioral therapy
    (c) Sleep hygiene
    (d) Aversive conditioning
    (e) Methylphenidate

4. In the diagnostic assessment of persons with insomnia, which factor is not usually of importance?

    (a) Total sleeping time
    (b) Daytime sleepiness
    (c) Sleep onset latency
    (d) Coexisting psychiatric problems
    (e) Socioeconomic class

Answers

1. d, 2. a, 3. c, 4. e

Appendix Populated Table

Table 26.5 Maria Thompson

What are the facts?	What are your hypotheses?	What do you want to know next?	What specific information would you like to get?
36-year-old woman, married, mother of two pre-teens	Overwhelmed with perceived family obligations?	What does "overwhelmed" mean?	Which times in child-raising present with particular demands on parents?
	Stress can lead to abnormalities in cortisol regulation/PHA feedback	When did she notice that having two kids was more demanding?	
Complaint of insomnia	Primary versus secondary insomnia?	Any lifestyle facets to explain poor sleep?	Has a sleep study been done to objectify the complaints?
Light sleeper at all times	Predisposition for sleep disorder?	Were there any periods when she did NOT have sleep problems?	To determine which sleep stage is affected?
Tosses and turns for at least 2 hours	Increased sleep latency due to situational factors?	Any subjective factors preventing her from going to sleep?	
Throughout the night she wakes up	Interrupted sleep as a symptom of MDD	Are there any other signs and symptoms of a mood disorder?	Would a dexamethasone suppression test be useful?
Cannot go back to sleep	Early morning wakening as a symptom of MDD	Any PMH suggestive of endocrine abnormalities, manic or hypomanic episodes, substance abuse?	Is psychological testing going to help in order to determine deficits in self-confidence?
Worried	Concerns about problems and adequacy could point toward a mood disorder		
Troubling problems she has not been able to resolve		Lab: TFTs, LFTs	

References

Dauvilliers Y, Arnulf I, Mignot E: Narcolepsy with cataplexy. Lancet 2007;369:499–511.

Eisensehr I, Schmidt D: Epilepsie und Schlafstörungen. MMW Fortschr Med 2005;147(Spec. No. 2):54–57.

Guilleminault C, Kirisoglu C, da Rosa AC, Lopes C, Chan A: Sleepwalking, a disorder of NREM sleep instability. Sleep Med 2006;7:163–170.

Lee-Chiong TL Jr: Parasomnias and other sleep-related movement disorders. Prim Care 2005;32:415–434.

Longstreth WT Jr, Koepsell TD, Ton TG, Hendrickson AF, van Belle G: The epidemiology of narcolepsy. Sleep 2007:30:13–26.

Morgenthaler T, Kramer M, Alessi C, Friedman L, Boehlecke B, Brown T, Coleman J, Kapur V, Lee-Chiong T, Owens J, Pancer J, Swick T, American Academy of Sleep Medicine: Practice parameters for the psychological and behavioral treatment of insomnia: an update. An American Academy of Sleep Medicine Report. Sleep 2006;29:1415–1419.

Morin AK, Jarvis CI, Lynch AM: Therapeutic options for sleep-maintenance and sleep-onset insomnia. Pharmacotherapy 2007;27:89–110.

Ohayon MM, Lemoine P, Arnaud-Briant V, Dreyfus M: Prevalence and consequences of sleep disorders in a shift worker population. J Psychosom Res 2002;53:577–583.

Rowley, J. Obstructive Sleep Apnea–Hypopnea Syndrome. EMedicine.com. http://www.emedicine. com/med/topic2697.htm. Nov. 2006.

Siegel JM, Boehmer LN: Narcolepsy and the hypocretin system—where motion meets emotion. Nat Clin Pract Neurol 2006;2:548–556.

Szelenberger W, Niemcewicz S, Dabrowska AJ: Sleepwalking and night terrors: psychopathological and psychophysiological correlates. Int Rev Psychiatry 2005;17:263–270.

Taylor DJ, Mallory LJ, Lichstein KL, Durrence HH, Riedel BW, Bush AJ: Comorbidity of chronic insomnia with medical problems. Sleep 2007;30:213–218.

Taylor JR, Vazquez CM, Campbell KM: Pharmacologic management of chronic insomnia. South Med J 2006;99:1373–1377.

Chapter 27
Eating Disorders

Hy Gia Park and Cathy K. Bell

Eating disorders and obesity are problems that dramatically impact psychological and medical well-being. These disorders carry some of the highest mortality rates in psychiatry.

At the end of this chapter, the reader will be able to

1. Describe the medical approach to a patient presenting with an eating disorder
2. Compare the epidemiology, pathophysiology, DSM-IV-TR diagnostic criteria, clinical course, treatment, and prognosis for anorexia nervosa and bulimia nervosa
3. Discuss how to evaluate and manage a patient with obesity

Case Vignette 27.1.1 Presenting Situation: Olga Mathias

Olga Mathias is a 15-year-old female in the 9th grade at a local private school. Her concerned parents brought her to the emergency room for "weakness and almost passing out while getting out of bed this afternoon." Olga concurs with her mother's story but thinks that her mother is completely blowing this situation out of proportion. "It's really not that big of a deal. My mom is such a control freak. She just has to get involved in every part of my life! Can I go home now?" she shouts angrily.

History obtained from Olga reveals that she has not eaten for the past 2 days prior to this near-syncopal episode. "You'd be stressed too if you maintained a 4.25 GPA! I also have an upcoming gymnastics competition but since I'm here I can't really expect to win, can I?" she says in a strained tone. Her mother chimes in, "See, she really has just not been herself since starting high school. She is always sad or irritable, sleeps in late, spends a lot of time by herself, and exercises constantly. If she shows up for meals, she'll often open a can of kidney beans, eat very little of it but drinks ten glasses of water and spends most of her time cutting up the food into tiny pieces and moving the pieces around her plate. She'll use an entire roll of paper towels in two days because she uses them to cover her plate and hide food."

H.G. Park
Fourth-year Medical Student, University of Hawai'i John A. Burns School of Medicine

A. Guerrero, M. Piasecki (eds.), *Problem-Based Behavioral Science and Psychiatry*,

Her parents note that she's probably lost about 40 lbs in the last 4 months. Olga admits that she hasn't had her period for at least the past 6 months.

Please proceed with the problem-based approach!

At this point, an eating disorder is an obvious diagnosis. Eating disorders are a complex set of illnesses that encompass a wide spectrum of abnormal eating patterns and can occur in all stages of life, from infancy to the elderly. The disturbances in eating behavior involve the manner, type, quantity, and rate of consumption of food. These disorders have a number of co-occurring psychiatric and medical conditions. The diagnoses of specific eating disorders are established in the *Diagnostic and Statistical Manual of Mental Disorders*, Fourth Edition, Text Revision (DSM-IV-TR) (see Table 27.1).

The two main eating disorders are anorexia nervosa (AN) and bulimia nervosa (BN). Both conditions are characterized by a preoccupation with and excessive self-critique of weight and body shape.

Anorexia nervosa and bulimia nervosa are considered diseases of the industrialized world (particularly the United States, Canada, Europe, Australia, New Zealand, Japan, and South Africa) (APA, 2000). Women are more commonly afflicted; the male–female prevalence ratio ranges from 1:6 to 1:20 (APA, 2006; Halmi, 2007). The lifetime prevalence of AN and BN in women is estimated to be 0.3 and 1 %, respectively. Anorexia nervosa and BN generally develop during adolescence. The

Table 27.1 Eating disorders recognized in the DSM-IV-TR

Name of disorder	Description of disorder
Pica	Persistent eating of nonnutritive substances, such as clay, lead, feces, hair, etc.
Rumination disorder	Repeated regurgitation and rechewing of food after feeding
Feeding disorder of infancy or early childhood	Persistent failure to eat adequately as evidenced by significant failure to gain weight or weight loss
Anorexia nervosa (subtypes: restricting versus binge eating/purging)	Persistent low body weight accompanied by intense fear of weight gain and becoming fat, disturbed body image, and amenorrhea for at least three menstrual cycles
Bulimia nervosa	Recurrent episodes (at least twice per week for 3 months) of binge eating and inappropriate compensatory methods (including self-induced vomiting, laxative use, fasting, and excessive exercise) to avoid weight gain; and absence of anorexia nervosa
Eating disorder not otherwise specified	Disorders of eating that do not meet the criteria for any specific eating disorder

majority of AN patients develop the disorder between ages 13 and 20 (Halmi, 2007). Peak age of onset for bulimia nervosa is 18 years (Mehler, 2003).

Although Olga probably has an eating disorder, there are other diagnoses to consider:

- General medical conditions (usually not associated with excessive worry about weight or body image)
- Major depressive disorder (usually not associated with desire to lose weight or fear of gaining weight)
- Psychotic disorders (there may be fear that food has been poisoned as part of paranoid ideation; however, there is usually no impairment in body image, desire to lose weight, or fear of gaining weight. Also, these patients tend to have bizarre thinking and behavior about things other than food)
- Social phobia (usually not restricted to reluctance to eat in public)
- Obsessive-compulsive disorder (obsessions occur in other areas besides food, weight, and body image; food rituals are not intended for weight loss)

So, further evaluation is needed.

Case Vignette 27.1.2 Continuation

You meet with Olga and her family to gather more information. Her parents report that she began changing her eating habits about 2 years ago. She would diet often, only eat salads for dinner, spend a lot of time in front of the mirror, complain that she was too fat, and wear baggy clothes. When asked, Olga reports that her ideal body weight is 80 lbs, and she thinks that her thighs and abdomen are too big. She states that she wakes up at 6 a.m. every morning to run 4 miles. She admits to occasional binge eating (donuts, cookies) and purging by vomiting. Olga continues to insist that she feels fine and that she wants to go home.

Olga is reluctant at first to be examined but eventually obliges with much coaxing. She appears thin and pale, with dark sunken eyes. She is dressed in a loose-fitting t-shirt and baggy jeans. Her vital signs are: temperature 97.1 °F, pulse 52 per min, blood pressure 84/64, respiratory rate 16 per min, weight 88.6 lbs, height 63 in., body mass index (BMI) 15.7. The remainder of the physical examination is remarkable for: lanugo (soft, downy hair on her chest and arms), thinning hair, slight peripheral edema, and loss of subcutaneous fat. The mental status examination reveals poor cooperation and eye contact, rapid and loud speech, angry and tearful affect, poor concentration, and poor insight and judgment. Her laboratory findings are: Hb 8.2; MCV 90; leukocyte count 3,500; serum Na^+ 130; serum glucose 55.

Olga's parents admit their unwilling child to the inpatient psychiatric unit where she remains for the next 3 months. During the course of her hospitalization, she participates in treatment, which includes a cardiac evaluation, weight restoration through gradual refeeding, psychoeducation as well as individual and family psychotherapies. Olga grows increasingly irritable and repeatedly asks to be discharged. "I don't need doctors, nurses, psychiatrists, and dietitians. I'm totally fine so let me go home!" After her weight has been restored to near her ideal weight, Olga starts taking the medication fluoxetine. Two weeks later, she is discharged home on the condition that she has weekly follow-up visits with her pediatrician, a nutritionist, and a therapist.

Please proceed with the problem-based approach!

Based on Olga's presentation the criteria for anorexia nervosa are met and the most appropriate diagnosis would be anorexia nervosa, binge-eating/purging type. Of note, AN has a worse prognosis than BN.

One of the trademarks of AN is impaired insight into the nature of their illness. Patients are often brought in for medical attention by loved ones. Although accurate histories are not easily obtained from patients, their accounts, along with collateral sources of information (e.g., family members, friends, and teachers), paint pictures of a preoccupation with food, weight, calories, and physical appearance. Patients with AN develop rituals around the consumption of food such as eating slowly, cutting food into small pieces, rearranging the food on the plate, and even hiding food in clothing. Other elements that reflect a preoccupation with weight are strict exercise routines, constant weighing on scales, repeated checking in mirrors, purging behavior including excessive use of laxatives, and social withdrawal. Adolescents with anorexia nervosa will have delayed psychosocial development and adults will report decreased libido (Halmi, 2007).

Histories of patients with BN, on the other hand, will reveal an abnormal eating pattern of binge eating and fasting. During binges, there is a sense of loss of control as patients with BN may consume large volumes of high caloric food in a short time. Often the binges are terminated by interruption, fatigue, abdominal discomfort, or vomiting or feelings of depression, guilt, and disgust. Because of their fear of weight gain, patients will fast for long periods of time in between the binges. Additionally,

Table 27.2 Common signs and symptoms of eating disorders

Anorexia nervosa	Bulimia nervosa
Loss of subcutaneous fat tissue	Normal weight or overweight
Orthostatic hypotension	Dental enamel erosions[a]
Bradycardia	Erosions on the dorsum of the hands (Russell's sign)[a]
Amenorrhea	Enlargement of the salivary glands[a]
Alopecia	Gastroesophageal reflux[a]
Lanugo-like body hair	Dyspepsia[a]
Hypothermia	Metabolic hypokalemic alkalosis[a]

[a]*Can be seen in both binge/purge subtype of anorexia nervosa and purging subtype of bulimia nervosa*

these patients tend to eat in secrecy and have an impaired ability to sense satiety after meals (APA, 2000; Halmi, 2007).

Patients suffering from eating disorders will present clinically with a wide range of symptoms. Those with less severe illness may have nonspecific complaints, such as fatigue, dizziness, or lack of energy. Patients with AN will often wear loose-fitting clothes in an attempt to hide their emaciated bodies. In order to conceal their true weight, patients with AN may fluid load, put weights in their pockets, or wear multiple layers of clothing before stepping on a scale. Additional signs and symptoms of patients with AN and BN are presented in Table 27.2. Eating disorders are associated with a variety of abnormal laboratory findings, represented in Table 27.3 (APA, 2000, 2006; Halmi, 2007; Yager and Andersen, 2005).

Table 27.3 Common laboratory findings in eating disorders

Anorexia nervosa	Bulimia nervosa
Chemistry Decreased K^+, Na^+, Cl^-, Mg^{2+}, P^{3+}, and Zn^{2+} Metabolic alkalosis Elevated serum amylase, blood urea nitrogen (BUN), cholesterol Abnormal liver function test	*Chemistry* Decreased K^+, Na^+, Cl^-, Mg^{2+}, P^{3+} Metabolic alkalosis (with vomiting)/acidosis (with laxative abuse) Elevated serum amylase
Hematologic Anemia Leucopenia Decreased serum ferritin, B12, folate, and niacin (in severe cases)	*Urinalysis* Increased urine-specific gravity and osmolality *EKG*
Endocrine Low estrogen Low testosterone (in males) Low-normal T_4; low T_3 Prepubertal patterns of luteinizing hormone (LH), follicle stimulating hormone (FSH) secretion Increased serum cortisol	Prolonged QT and PR intervals Depressed ST segment Widened QRS complex *Brain imaging*
EKG Bradycardia or arrhythmia QTc prolongation Increased PR interval First-degree heart block ST-T wave abnormalities	Cortical atrophy Enlarged ventricles Decreased gray and white matter *DEXA*
Brain Imaging Enlarged ventricles Decreased gray and white matter	Osteopenia Osteoporosis
Dual-energy X-ray absorptiometry (DEXA) Osteopenia Osteoporosis	

Table 27.4 Complications from eating disorders

Central nervous system	Cognitive impairment; anxious, depressed, irritable mood; seizures; peripheral neuropathy
Skin	Xerosis; lanugo-like body hair; hair loss; acne; carotenoderma (yellowish skin); acrocyanosis (bluish hands or feet); purpura; stomatitis; nail abnormalities
Cardiovascular	Cardiomyopathy and cardiac failure secondary to ipecac abuse; arrhythmias; congestive heart failure; cardiac arrest
Pulmonary	Pneumomediastinum
Gastrointestinal	Benign parotid hyperplasia; gastric dilatation; esophageal or gastric rupture; delayed gastric emptying; impaired sense of hunger and satiety; delayed small bowel transit time; pancreatitis; necrotizing colitis; constipation
Musculoskeletal	Muscle wasting; peripheral myopathy; arrested skeletal growth; osteopenia and osteoporosis leading to pathologic fractures
Hematologic	Thrombocytopenia; clotting factor abnormalities
Endocrine and metabolic	Severe electrolyte abnormalities; vitamin deficiency; thyroid dysfunction
Renal	Renal failure
Reproductive	Infertility; miscarriages; pregnancy complications

Medical complications from eating disorders are primarily a consequence of starvation and weight loss in AN and the form and frequency of purging behavior in BN. As shown in Table 27.4, the resulting complications from both these disorders affect multiple organ systems of the body (APA, 2006; Halmi, 2007; Mitchell and Crow, 2006).

There are few randomized clinical trials that evaluate treatments for eating disorders. This is in part due to the intrinsic difficulties associated with studying this population which is resistant to treatment and has high drop-out rates and incomplete hospitalization courses. As a result we lack a standard of care for treating patients with eating disorders.

Treatment of AN requires a multidimensional treatment approach with medical management, psychoeducation, psychotherapy, and medication. The treatment team includes a primary care physician, a dietitian, nurses and a psychiatrist, psychologist, or therapist trained in treating patients with eating disorders (APA, 2006; Yager and Andersen, 2005). The treatment setting is typically determined by the severity of the illness. Options include outpatient care, day programs, residential programs, general psychiatric units, specialized eating disorder inpatient units, and medical intensive care units. Treatment on an outpatient basis is best reserved for patients who have had the illness for less than 6 months, with no binging or purging and active family involvement (APA, 2006).

Medical management of patients with AN is complex due to the effects of starvation and the medical interventions themselves. Physicians must closely monitor vital signs, intakes and outputs, electrolyte status, cardiopulmonary and gastrointestinal function, and physical activity Weight restoration through refeeding with adequate calories is the first intervention taken since it facilitates the success of other interventions in the treatment plan. Refeeding reduces apathy, lethargy, and obsessions related to food and body image. Weight gain of one to three pounds weekly in the inpatient setting and a half to two pounds weekly in the outpatient setting is typical. Refeeding syndrome occurs in approximately 6 % of patients and includes abdominal pain, bloating, and peripheral edema or more serious complications such as cardiopulmonary, neurological, and neuromuscular dysfunction (Yager and Andersen, 2005).

Behavioral treatments are an essential component for treating AN. These interventions include individual and family psychotherapy, nutritional counseling, and group therapies. They are often employed despite minimal evidence-based support for their use.

Although it is not a primary treatment modality, fluoxetine appears to decrease relapse episodes and depressive symptoms and helps to maintain weight gain in weight-restored patients. Atypical antipsychotics, such as olanzapine and risperidone, may help with weight gain, decrease obsessional and distorted thoughts, decrease anxiety, and even improve insight.

Bulimia Nervosa

The primary objectives in the treatment of BN are to treat the associated medical complications and to break the binge–purge cycles with medications and psychotherapy. Medical management of complications addresses oral and dental care, associated gastrointestinal illnesses, bone health, and electrolyte and acid–base imbalances (e.g., hypokalemic metabolic alkalosis) (Mehler, 2003). Psychiatric management of BN typically involves cognitive behavioral therapy (CBT) as first-line treatment since it is one of the few treatments that has consistently been shown to be effective in randomized controlled trials, especially if administered by a trained professional (Halmi, 2007). Cognitive behavioral therapy can be used in group or individual settings and aims to challenge the core beliefs that drive the illness and break the circle of destructive thoughts, feelings, and binge–purge behaviors.

Antidepressants can be effective adjuvant interventions in reducing the severity of bulimic symptoms, including binge eating and purging behaviors, obsessive thoughts related to food, weight, and body shape, relapse rates, and symptoms of depression and anxiety. Fluoxetine is the only Food and Drug Administration (FDA)-approved pharmacologic agent for the treatment of BN. Bupropion is specifically contraindicated for patients with eating disorders. The combination of antidepressants and CBT appears to be most effective in reducing the frequency of binging and purging (Mehler, 2003). Eating disorder support groups and Twelve Step programs such as Overeaters Anonymous may also be helpful during treatment and relapse prevention (APA, 2006).

Knowing the chronic nature of anorexia nervosa, we wonder how well Olga will follow up with outpatient therapy.

Case Vignette 27.1.3 Continued

Olga stops going to her appointments after only 2 weeks after discharge. In the course of 1 year, Olga is reluctantly brought in to the emergency room on two occasions for syncopal episodes. Each time, she unwillingly is admitted for medical stabilization, weight restoration, and psychosocial support, but she does not adhere to treatment after discharge. Olga is angry at her parents for forcing her into treatment. Her parents are beside themselves, blaming themselves for her condition, and feeling helpless as they watch her spiral into a skeletal version of her former self. They decide to send her to an intensive residential program for eating disorders despite Olga's resistance. One year later, a very emaciated and angry Olga is brought in again to the emergency room by her parents for "heart problems" from binge–purge behaviors.

 Please proceed with the problem-based approach!

In general, follow-up studies conducted 6 years after disease onset show that eating disorders develop into chronic illnesses with high rates of mortality. Among patients with AN approximately 25 % of patients recover, 25 % show no change in their condition, and the remainder of patients show some slight improvement. The prognosis for patients with BN similarly shows that half of these patients have residual features even after treatment. The high rates of morbidity from these diseases correlate to high mortality rates; compared to all other psychiatric disorders, eating disorders have the highest death rates. The long-term mortality rate for BN is between 0 and 3 % (Halmi, 2007) and the rate for AN is approximately 20 % (Robergeau et al., 2006). Death most often results from suicide or the effects of starvation (APA 2006); 25–35 % of patients with BN attempt suicide, as opposed to 3–20 % of patients with anorexia nervosa (Franko and Keel, 2006), but the rate of death from suicide is higher among patients with AN.

Several factors are prognostic predictors in eating disorders. For example, a shorter duration of illness and onset between the ages of 12 and 18 are associated with better outcomes (Halmi, 2007). On the other hand, lower body weights at diagnosis, vomiting, binge eating, alcohol and substance abuse, depression, and chronic illness carry a poor prognosis.

How did this bright, athletic teenager develop an eating disorder, and how will you effectively manage her treatment?

There is a strong genetic link in eating disorders. The risk of AN and BN is increased among first-degree biological relatives of individuals with these disorders as well as in families with depression, substance abuse, and obesity (APA, 2000, 2006). Investigators have identified genes that may be linked to eating disorders. Two genes on chromosome 1 called the opioid delta receptor (OPRD1) and

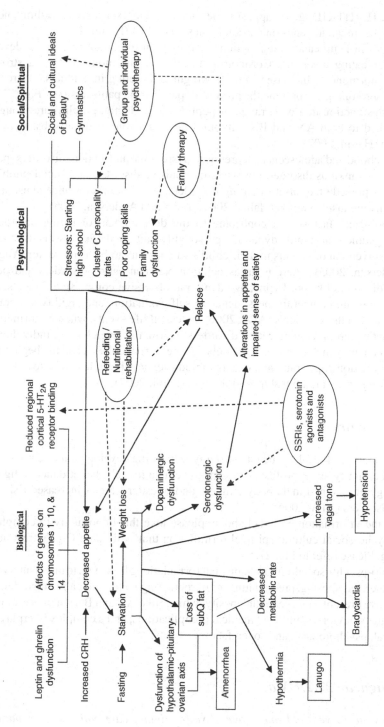

Fig. 27.1 Bio-psycho-social-cultural-spiritual formulation of case vignette, "Olga"

serotonin 1D (HTR1D) genes appear to be linked to anorexia nervosa. Bulimia nervosa may be linked to genes on chromosomes 10 and 14 (Halmi, 2007).

Changes in neuroendocrine functions also play an important role in the development of eating disorders. Corticotrophin-releasing hormone (CRH), a strong anorectic hormone, is increased in underweight and dieting individuals. Dysregulation of serotonergic, norepinephrine, and dopaminergic pathways (see Fig. 27.1) and the dysfunction in a wide range of peptides (e.g., leptin, ghrelin) are thought to be linked to both AN and BN, although the exact role of these substances is unknown (Halmi, 2007).

In childhood and adolescence, depression, dysthymia, and anxiety disorders (particularly overanxious disorder, obsessive-compulsive disorder, and social phobia) sometimes precede the onset of eating disorders. Alcohol or substance abuse and impulsivity are also common (Halmi, 2007; Yager and Andersen, 2005).

Psychological factors that contribute to the development of eating disorders include dysfunctional family dynamics, personality traits, and life stressors. Over- or under-involvement of parents in their child's life appears to be a risk factor (Yager and Andersen, 2005). There is an association between eating disorders and personality disorders like borderline, avoidant, and obsessive-compulsive. Traits such as perfectionism, competitiveness, negative self-evaluation, and rigidity are commonly found in these patients (APA, 2006). Stressful life events, whether normative or traumatic, can precipitate eating disorders. Normative events in an individual's development may include the onset of puberty, the start of college, and the beginning of a new relationship. Traumatic events include sexual abuse, loss of a loved one, the breaking up of a relationship, and illness (Halmi, 2007).

Social Factors

Cultural and social ideals of beauty strongly impact the development of eating disorders. Certain types of professions, such as female models, ballet dancers, figure skaters, gymnasts, and male body builders and wrestlers, are at increased risk for eating disorders (APA, 2006).

With the information provided above, please take this opportunity to complete a bio-psycho-social-cultural-spiritual formulation that will guide Olga's treatment planning. Please refer to Fig. 27.1.

The bio-psycho-social-cultural-spiritual formulation allows you to target interventions at the predisposing, precipitating, or perpetuating factors for eating disorders

Next, we present a brief case on obesity, which (like AN and BN) involves abnormal eating behaviors, significant medical complications, and a complex interplay of biological, psychological, and social factors.

Case Vignette 27.2.1 Mac

"Mac" is the 13-year-old son of one of your primary care patients. Your patient asks you to evaluate Mac because "I think he must have some emotional problem,

because of his weight." He is 5 feet tall and weighs 180 pounds (BMI=35). His diet includes fast food, candy, soda (from the refrigerator), and typical school lunches.

 Please proceed with the problem-based approach!

In adults, overweight is defined as BMI of 25–29.9, while obesity is defined as BMI of 30.0 or more. In children and adolescents, overweight is defined as a BMI greater than or equal to the 95th percentile for age and sex. In the United States, the prevalence of overweight children is rising and is currently 10.3 % among 2–5 year olds, 15.8 % among 6–11 year olds, 16.1 % among 12–19 year olds, and 65.1 % among adults aged 20 years and above. The prevalence of obesity in adults is now 30.4 % (Hedley et al., 2004). The prevalence is higher in certain ethnic groups (including Pacific Islanders and other indigenous people exposed to Western diets). The risk of an obese child developing obesity (and associated cardiovascular and metabolic complications) increases with age. Early detection (through frequent monitoring of BMI during pediatric office visits) and intervention for obesity is part of routine pediatric practice.

Case Vignette 27.2.2 Continuation

Mac denies symptoms suggestive of a mood, anxiety, or binge-eating disorder.

Past medical and developmental history: Mother had a history of gestational diabetes mellitus. Birth weight was 9 pounds. He was exclusively bottle-fed. He has been greater than 95th percentile in weight since infancy.

Family history: Everyone on the father's side of the family is overweight, including the father. Mother has a history of depression. Grandmother has a history of dementia.

Social history: He is the only child at home. The other adults are the parents and grandmother. He has minimal access to outdoor activities. He watches 4 hours of TV per day. Father works two jobs. The mother cares for the grandmother.

Examination is significant for: nasal speech, nasal congestion, and fidgeting.

Labs: include a normal thyroid test.

The assessment of obesity requires screening for the general medical etiologies for (e.g., genetic and endocrine disorders) and complications of (e.g., diabetes, hypertension, hyperlipidemia, obstructive sleep apnea syndrome) obesity. It is also important to screen for potential psychiatric co-morbidities summarized in Table 27.5.

Table 27.5 Psychiatric co-morbidities that should be screened for when evaluating a patient with obesity

Psychiatric condition	Relationship with obesity
Binge-eating disorder (eating disorder not otherwise specified)	Increased caloric intake (without compensatory weight loss mechanisms) may lead to obesity
Major depressive disorder	Increased appetite may lead to increased caloric intake, which may, in turn, lead to obesity
Adjustment disorder	Obesity may lead to low self-esteem and social ostracism
Attention-deficit hyperactivity disorder	Inattention, impulsivity, and sub-optimal organizational skills may interfere with intended diets and activity schedules
Psychotic disorders, mood disorders, and other psychiatric conditions that require chronic medications	Medications may increase appetite and/or cause obesity through other mechanisms
Many psychiatric disorders	May interfere with judgment around food choices and/or ability to comply with weight loss regimens
	Associated poverty and untoward psychosocial circumstances may limit food choices and availability of healthy and safe activities

You need additional history in order to consider the biological, family, and societal factors that predispose to and perpetuate obesity. A diagram of the case of "Mac" is shown in Fig. 27.2 (Birch and Fisher, 1998; Kohl and Hobbs, 1998).

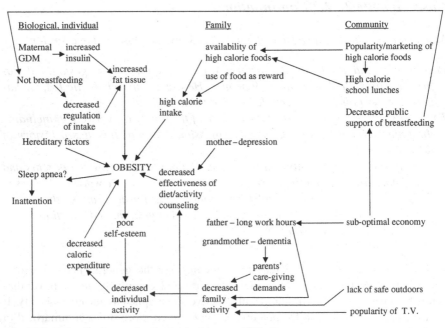

Fig. 27.2 Causative factors for obesity in the case of "Mac"

Table 27.6 Individual-level interventions for treating obesity

First-line interventions
Goal-setting (e.g., cessation of weight gain and/or modest weight loss) and monitoring of weight
Dietary counseling (e.g., regular meals, healthy meal choices)
Self-monitoring and anticipation of triggers for eating
Establishing healthful activity routines
Regular physician follow-up to monitor progress
Second-line interventions
Specialist referral
Consideration of medications:
Orlistat
Blocks intestinal absorption of fat
Multivitamin supplementation is recommended
Food and Drug Administration (FDA)-approved for patients older than 12 years
Sibutramine
Blocks reuptake of norepinephrine and serotonin
FDA-approved for patients older than 12 years
Third-line interventions
Bariatric surgery: for severe obesity (BMI>40) in adults and possibility in adolescents with complications

As "Mac" illustrates, treatment and prevention of obesity needs a comprehensive approach. In this specific case, treatment interventions may include: addressing any co-morbid sleep apnea and attentional difficulties, improving the family's capacity to adhere to diet and activity recommendations, and addressing potentially controllable community risk factors (such as unhealthy school lunches).

Options for treating obesity are summarized in Table 27.6 (adopted from Singhal et al., 2007):

Review Questions

1. Which of the following statements is TRUE about the epidemiology of eating disorders?

    (a) Anorexia nervosa is more common than bulimia nervosa.
    (b) The prevalence of anorexia nervosa is approximately 3 %.
    (c) The prevalence of anorexia nervosa is higher in developed countries.
    (d) Anorexia nervosa and bulimia nervosa typically have their onset during adulthood.
    (e) (b) and (c).

2. The first priority in the management of anorexia nervosa is

    (a) Initiation of a medication that reduces eating disordered behaviors, such as fluoxetine

(b) Medically supervised refeeding

(c) Initiation of a medication that promotes weight gain, such as olanzapine

(d) Exploration of childhood conflicts that have led to poor self-esteem and refusal of food

(e) None of the above

3. A 15-year-old female is brought to the pediatrician because she was caught "making herself vomit." She endorses recurrent episodes of binging and purging. She is also significantly underweight and fearful of becoming fat. She has not had any menstrual periods for the past 6 months. The most likely diagnosis is

(a) Bulimia nervosa

(b) Anorexia nervosa, binge-eating/purging type

(c) Anorexia nervosa, restricting type

(d) Eating disorder not otherwise specified

(e) Rumination disorder

4. A mother asks the pediatrician what can be done to insure that her 1-year-old baby will not develop the problems of obesity that the two older teenage sons have. All of the following would be helpful things to advise her EXCEPT

(a) Establishing regular family routines around meals

(b) Establishing regular family routines around physical activity

(c) Reducing exposure to television

(d) Bottle-feeding using commercially prepared formula

(e) Involving other family members in discussion about healthy diet and activity

5. Who are responsible for addressing the growing epidemic of obesity in the United States?

(a) Physicians

(b) Parents

(c) Lawmakers

(d) Food manufacturers

(e) All of the above, plus more

Answers

1. c, 2. b, 3. b, 4. d, 5. e

References

American Psychiatric Association (2000). *Diagnostic and Statistical Manual of Mental Disorders*, 4th ed., Trade Revision. Washington, DC: American Psychiatric Publishing.

American Psychiatric Association (2006). *Practice Guidelines for the Treatment of Patients with Eating Disorders*, 3rd ed. Washington, DC: American Psychiatric Publishing.

Birch, L.L., Fisher, J.O. (1998). Development of eating behaviors among children and adolescents. *Pediatrics* 101: 539–549.

Franko, D., Keel, P. (2006). Suicidality in eating disorders: Occurrence, correlators, and clinical implications. *Clin Psychol Rev* 26: 769–782.

Halmi, K.A. (2007). Anorexia nervosa and bulimia nervosa. In A. Martin and F.R. Volkmar (Eds.), *Lewis's Child and Adolescent Psychiatry* (pp. 592–602). Philadelphia: Lippincott Williams & Wilkins.

Hedley, A.A., Ogden, C.L., Johnson, C.L., Carroll, M.D., Curtin, L.R., Flegal, K.M. (2004). Prevalence of overweight and obesity among US children, adolescents, and adults, 1999–2002. *JAMA* 291: 2847–2850.

Kohl III, H.W., Hobbs, K.E. (1998). Development of physical activity behaviors among children and adolescents. *Pediatrics* 101: 549–554.

Mehler, P.S. (2003). Bulimia nervosa. *N Engl J Med* 349: 875–881.

Mitchell, J.E., Crow, S. (2006). Medical complications of anorexia nervosa and bulimia nervosa. *Curr Opin Psychiatry* 19: 438–443.

Robergeau, K., Joseph, J., Silber, T.J. (2006). Hospitalization of children and adolescents for eating disorders in the state of New York. *J Adolesc Health* 39: 806–810.

Singhal, V., Schwenk, W.F., Kumar, S. (2007). Evaluation and management of childhood and adolescent obesity. *Mayo Clin Proc* 82(10): 1258–1264.

Yager, J., Andersen, A.E. (2005). Anorexia nervosa. *N Engl J Med* 353: 1481–1488.

Chapter 28
Sexual Disorders

Crissa R. Draper, Nikhil Majumdar, William T. O'Donohue,
and Melissa Piasecki

Sexual disorders can be the source of great suffering to people, sometimes due to embarrassment, sometimes due to physical pain, sometimes due to missed positives (e.g., affiliation, intimacy pleasure), and sometimes due to illegality. Although medical research has produced some useful medical, and in some cases surgical, treatments, behavioral approaches are usually first line treatment due to their efficacy, safety, and cost.

At the end of this chapter, the reader will be able to

1. Identify sexual disorder in a primary care setting
2. Describe a first line of behavioral and medical intervention
3. Identify when referrals might be more appropriate

Case Vignette 28.1.1 Presenting Situation: Lewis Stevens

Mr. Stevens is a 28-year-old man who teaches 5th grade in the public school system. He comes to see you because of a "masturbation problem" at the primary care clinic where you work. He says he does not feel his masturbation activities are appropriate and would like help to decrease his libido. When asked about his history, he states that he has had a standing problem with alcohol abuse that has gotten worse in the last couple of years, which is about how long he has been working as a teacher. He also reports having been molested as a child. The client is hesitant to give any details about his presenting problem; he simply repeats that he would just like help with his masturbation problem. With continued questioning, the client eventually reveals that he generally masturbates three or four times per week.

C.R. Draper
Graduate Student in Psychology,
University of Nevada, Reno

A. Guerrero, M. Piasecki (eds.), *Problem-Based Behavioral Science and Psychiatry*,
© Springer Science+Business Media, LLC 2008

Please proceed with the problem-based approach!

The only thing that can be clear from the presentation so far is the lack of information. The presenting problem does not seem necessarily problematic, and the presenter clearly seems to be withholding information. Because his masturbation habit is not abnormal in frequency, further information should be sought about what is "inappropriate" or problematic about the behavior.

Case Vignette 28.1.2 Continuation

With prompting, the client admits that frequency is not the problem; he would like to never masturbate again—the content of his fantasies is the problem. He says that while he has never acted on his fantasies, during masturbation he fantasizes about early pubescent girls and views child pornography. He expresses concern that, while this fantasy has been present as long as he can remember, with the daily exposure to the 10-year-old girls in his class, the fantasies are more realistic and pervasive. He confides to you that he has become interested in a specific girl in his class and has started buying her gifts and wants to invite her for tutoring after class.

Please proceed with the problem-based approach!

Pedophilia as a sexual orientation is generally not considered curable. Although there have been no conclusive genetic studies performed on pedophiles as a population, some circumstantial evidence suggests one etiological possibility is an intrauterine neurohormonal process with lifelong effects (Quinsey, 2003). In recent years the treatment goal with pedophilic patients is not necessarily to remove all sexual urges, but instead to help the clients control pedophilic urges, keeping them as thoughts instead of actions. Daily interactions with children would make this more difficult. While it is a good sign that he has not yet acted on his urges (or at least admitted that he has), the fact that he has been forming a personal relationship with a specific girl is more troublesome, as this may be "grooming behavior" that can lead to physical contact.

The DSM-IV-TR states that, for a person to meet the diagnostic criteria for pedophilia, he (or she, although female pedophiles are far less common) must meet the following conditions: recurrent intense sexually arousing fantasies, sexual urges, or behaviors involving sexual activity with a prepubescent child or children; either acting upon these urges or experiencing significant distress or impairment as a result of urges or fantasies; time duration of at least 6 months; and age of at least 16 years and 5 years older than the child or children being fantasized about.

Characteristics of the paraphilias are summarized in Table 28.1.

Another consideration at this point is the issue of mandated reporting. Requirements differ from state to state, but in general, a report must be made when "the reporter, in his or her official capacity, *suspects* or *has reasons to believe* that a child has been abused," as well as when the reporter has access to definitive knowledge of such abuse (Child Welfare Information Gateway, 2005, italics added). As a mandated reporter in a primary care clinic you are only required to report your suspicions and are not required to take on an investigative role. In this case your patient has asserted that he has not acted on his urges, so there may not be anything to report. You need to report child molestation, not pedophilic urges. However, when treating a pedophile, the clinician must be sure to refer to local laws and other resources (local child protective services) regarding mandated reporting. Consulting with peers is often helpful.

Table 28.1 DSM-IV-TR paraphilias

All of the following disorders have the following criteria (DSM-IV-TR):

1. Over a period of at least 6 months, recurrent, intense sexually arousing fantasies, sexual urges, or behaviors involving these specific stimuli

2. The person has acted on these urges, or the sexual urges or fantasies cause marked distress or interpersonal difficulty

Name	Stimulus
Exhibitionism	Exposure of one's genitals to an unsuspecting stranger
Fetishism	Non-living objects (e.g., female undergarments, body)[a]
Frotteurism	Touching and rubbing against a non-consenting person
Sexual masochism	The act (real, not simulated) of being humiliated, beaten, bound, or otherwise made to suffer
Sexual sadism	The act (real, not simulated) in which the psychological or physical suffering (including humiliation) of the victim is sexually exciting to the person
Transvestic fetishism	Cross-dressing
Voyeurism	The act of observing an unsuspecting person who is naked, in the process of disrobing, or engaging in sexual activity
Paraphilia not otherwise specified	Examples include, but are not limited to, telephone scatologia (obscene phone calls), necrophilia (corpses), partialism (exclusive focus on part of body), zoophilia (animals), coprophilia (feces), klismaphilia (enemas), and urophilia (urine)

[a]Additional criteria: The fetish objects are not limited to articles of female clothing used in cross-dressing (as in transvestic fetishism) or devices designed for the purpose of tactile genital stimulation (e.g., a vibrator)

Case Vignette 28.1.3 Conclusion

*The first and foremost behavioral prescription for Mr. Stevens is to find a new job. Relapse prevention is the treatment with the most evidence for treating child molestation among pedophiles. A principle of this model is that pedophiles should eliminate contact with children for the rest of their lives, and this should be especially true for one-on-one contact. He finds a faculty position at the local community college teaching education. Additionally, he has agreed to have a trusted family member (in this case, his brother) put parental controls on his computer to block him from viewing child pornography. He reports that working with adults instead of children and staying away from pornography has helped diffuse his urges. Because he has not acted on the pedophilic urges, he is prescribed an SSRI instead of a more intensive treatment with testosterone-reducing medication to reduce his sexual desire and afford him more control over his urges. He is also referred to a sex-specific therapist, who begins a regimen of weekly cognitive behavioral therapy (CBT), and he is asked to purchase and work through the evidenced-based self-help book, **Sexual Addiction Workbook,** by Sbraga-Penix and O'Donohue. He finds that his fantasies do diminish, and he never acts on them.*

 Please proceed with the problem-based approach!

Removing exposure to children is the obvious and necessary first step in treating pedophilia. This may also include removing or reducing Internet access, if this is a common form of child exposure for the client. Testosterone-reducing prescriptions such as Depo-Provera have been found effective in treating pedophilia, theoretically due to the idea that the reduction of libido will increase the ability to control pedophilic urges. This extreme treatment, however, may not be necessary for a client who has been able to control these urges on his own, even with factors that might make this difficult (i.e., alcohol use and daily interactions with children). Serotonin-selective reuptake inhibitors (SSRIs) are less intrusive and have been found effective in reducing sex drive.

When assessing and treating pedophilia, it is important to note that minimization and denial are common, and therefore self-report should not be the only source of information. People with this disorder only tend to seek treatment when they get caught; therefore it is often possible to obtain collateral information from the legal sources, such as a parole officer. Objective assessments with instruments, such as the strain gauge or penile plethysmograph which indicate arousal from deviant stimuli, can add to the database whenever their use is feasible; however, these assessments can be difficult and expensive to administer.

It is essential to assess for immediate risk when assessing a patient with pedophilia. In the current example, the immediate risk would be to the children in his class. More often, child sexual abuse occurs within the home, and an immediate safety plan should be made if any children live in a home with the client. It is extremely rare for females to exhibit pedophilic or other paraphilic behaviors.

People with pedophilia require treatment with a specialist. Experts in this field use objective testing, such as plethysmography, and are often members of the Association for the Treatment of Sexual Abusers. For more information on how to select a qualified sex-specific therapist, refer to the *Stop Child Molestation Book* (Abel and Harlow, 2001). Pedophilic patients should continue to have a treatment relationship with a physician, so pharmacological treatment remains an option if needed. In this case, Mr. Stevens received medication to help with the urges and a referral to a sex-specific therapist for more intensive intervention. These therapists are sometimes also called sex therapists; however, "sex therapist" can also refer to a marriage or couples counselor. The naming conventions are not important, but finding a therapist who specializes in deviant sexual behavior is important.

Three classes of medication have shown benefit in the treatment of paraphilias such as pedophilia: SSRIs, antiandrogen hormones, and luteinizing hormone-releasing hormone (LHRH) agonists. There is evidence that the SSRI sertraline and the antiandrogen cyproterone acetate in particular may have the beneficial effect of decreasing deviant sexual behavior while not decreasing non-deviant sexual behavior. One expert author in the field has suggested an algorithm for treating paraphilias by starting all cases with CBT, a relapse-prevention program, and an SSRI. For moderate cases, titrated doses of oral antiandrogen may be used, while for more severe cases, antiandrogen may be given intramuscularly. Treatment for catastrophic cases includes a weekly high-dose LHRH agonist or antiandrogen injection to completely suppress all endogenous androgens and sex drive (Bradford, 2001).

Case Vignette 28.2.1 Presenting Situation: Joshua Templar

Joshua Templar is a 42-year-old man who comes to your family medicine clinic. He insists he is in need of Viagra® (sildenafil). Although he has not lost complete erectile function, he is often unable to maintain an erection during prolonged sexual encounters. He says this medication is the only thing that will help him "keep up" with his wife, who is 31 years old. He is not interested in discussing the problem in depth, and appears uncomfortable with the topic. You are not convinced that sildenafil is the best option for Mr. Templar, but he insists that he knows what he needs. He adds that when he was on vacation in Costa Rica last summer the waiters at the resort restaurants routinely provided him with sildenafil and that before he left he purchased a supply to use at home. His supply ran out a few months ago.

Please proceed with the problem-based approach!

Erectile dysfunction ("Male Erectile Disorder" in the DSM-IV-TR) can have both psychological and physiological causes. There is evidence that the majority of diagnosed cases have psychological rather than general medical causes (Skaer et al., 2001). More often than not, there is some interaction between the two pathways.

A simple way to test for organic causes is asking patients if they awake with an erection and, if they do, about the quality of the erection. If this information is not available another method of gaining this information is a nocturnal penile tumescence test. Men without organic erectile dysfunction will generally have erections with every cycle of REM sleep throughout the night, which is called nocturnal penile tumescence (NPT). Several assessment devices are available for NPT, including the stamp test and the strain gauge. A stamp test works by putting adhesive "stamps" (similar to postage stamps) around the penis before sleeping. If the sealed row of stamps is broken during the night, this would be evidence that organic functioning is intact. Similarly, the snap gauge consists of a sleeve that has several "snaps" down the shaft. The gauge is useful in that it assesses not only whether any tumescence was achieved, but also the length of the turgidity.

Mr. Templar's age raises some concern, as erectile dysfunction does not generally occur before the age of 50.

Case Vignette 28.2.2 Continuation

After repeated prodding during his intake, you establish that Mr. Templar is pre-diabetic and fairly sedentary and that he smokes about two packs of cigarettes a day. He is overweight with a body mass index of 34, and he has a family history of myocardial infarction at an early age. Additionally, he says that he and his wife get along and communicate well and have had a healthy sex life in the past. You suggest that he quit smoking, exercise regularly, and modify his diet. He seems unsatisfied with your recommendation but leaves the appointment without vocal protest. You schedule a follow-up appointment for 1 month later.

Please proceed with the problem-based approach!

Mr. Templar's cardiovascular risks call for further investigation and may account for the early age of onset of erectile dysfunction. Behavioral prescriptions should target cardiovascular risk factors, because smoking, high glucose levels, and sedentary habits are likely contributing factors, if not the primary cause, of erectile dysfunction.

Case Vignette 28.2.3 Conclusion

Mr. Templar returns 1 month later, smelling of smoke and appearing the same as he had appeared during the first visit. He reports that he has been trying to cut back on smoking and to eat better, but to no avail. He again asks you for the prescription for Viagra®. You relent and write a sildenafil prescription, but not without a conversation. You not only counsel Mr. Templar that you understand how difficult it can be to make health behavior changes, but also explain the potential risks of letting these behaviors persist. You also give him a pamphlet about erectile dysfunction and request that he read the whole thing. You insist that Mr. Templar schedule a follow-up appointment to monitor blood pressure and metabolic labs, either with yourself or with a general practitioner of his choice. You also refer the patient to a local dietician and give him information on an online smoking cessation program, such as quintet.com.

Sildenafil is effective in over 70 % of erectile dysfunction reports (Lyseng-Williamson and Wagstaff, 2002). Like related compounds tadalafil and vardenafil, it acts to indirectly increase levels of cyclic guanosine monophosphate (cGMP) in the corpus cavernosum of the penis. Cyclic GMP causes the penis to vasodilate and is normally increased by parasympathetic release of nitric oxide (NO). Sildenafil's direct action is to bind up the enzyme phosphodiesterase type 5, which would otherwise reduce levels of cGMP (Kerins et al., 2001). This process still depends on sexual stimulation to activate the NO/cGMP system and should not cause an erection without sexual arousal.

Since 1990, erectile dysfunction (ED) reporting and request for treatment has nearly doubled, as has the diagnosis of male erectile disorder. In turn, the pharmaceutical treatment has also dramatically increased. While these facts might suggest that ED reporting has been exaggerated since the introduction of sildenafil and related drugs, it may be that the significant increase simply sheds light on the magnitude of the problem and is not necessarily related to over-reporting since the introduction of medications (Skaer et al., 2001). With sildenafil's increase in use, however, care must be taken of its potentially dangerous hemodynamic side effects. This is especially true in combination with nitrate medications, which together can cause dramatic drops in blood pressure (Kerins et al., 2001).

Additionally, there is evidence to suggest that the benefits of prescribing medications for ED may outweigh the costs: "Sildenafil treatment significantly improves quality-of-life related to sexual function and general well being; potential healthcare savings may result as these effects trickle down" (Lyseng-Williamson and

Table 28.2 DSM-IV-TR sexual dysfunctions

Hypoactive sexual desire disorder[a]	Deficient or absent sexual fantasies and desire for sexual activity
Female sexual arousal disorder	Inability to attain or maintain physiologic arousal until completion of sexual activity
Male erectile disorder[a]	Recurring inability to achieve or maintain an erection until completion of the sexual activity
Female orgasmic disorder	Delay or absence of orgasm following normal excitement and sexual activity. (SSRI medications frequently cause secondary orgasmic disorders)
Male orgasmic disorder	Delay or absence of orgasm following normal excitement and sexual activity. (SSRI medications frequently cause secondary orgasmic disorders)
Premature ejaculation	Ejaculation with minimal sexual stimulation before or shortly after penetration and before the person wishes it
Dyspareunia[a]	Recurrent or persistent genital pain associated with sexual intercourse. Can be diagnosed in men or women but is most common in women
Sexual aversion disorder	Persistent or recurring aversion to or avoidance of sexual activity. Sexual topics may provoke extreme anxiety
Vaginismus	Recurrent or persistent involuntary spasm of the vaginal muscles that interferes with sexual intercourse. May be related to dyspareunia

[a]These disorders also have a separate disorder listed in the DSM-IV-TR when "due to medical condition."

Wagstaff, 2002). These authors suggest that sildenafil is a cost-effective option, since empirically based behavioral treatments (such as changes in diet and exercise) might not work in the general population.

One study also suggests that psycho-education combined with sildenafil works better than medication alone; and therefore, psycho-education should be provided along with sildenafil prescriptions (Bach et al., 2004).

Erectile dysfunction is one of the many sexual dysfunctions identified in the DSM-IV-TR and summarized in the Table 28.2.

Case Vignette 28.3.1 Presenting Situation: Tom Roberts

You are a private practice psychiatrist who specializes in gender identity disorders (GIDs). Tom Roberts is a 23-year-old male graduate student who came to see you because he is interested in gender reassignment surgery. He has done his Wikipedia research and would like to begin the process of becoming a woman by living as one for the required time. Mr. Roberts tells you that he has always felt uncomfortable as a man and, even as a child, always believed that he was "a girl inside." He is very excited about the opportunity to feel "normal," and wants to start the reassignment process right away.

Please proceed with the problem-based approach!

Transsexualism, while previously seen as a purely psychological process, has been increasingly understood in neurobiological terms thanks to modern research. Gender differences are well established in the shape and size of brain structure. The differences include the size and shape of cell body clusters, known as nuclei, in the hypothalamus of the brain and in the bed nucleus of the stria terminalis. Recent studies have found multiple male-to-female transsexuals with female bed nucleus characteristics and at least one case has been reported of a female-to-male transsexual with male dimorphic characteristics (Zhou et al., 1995; Kruijver et al., 2000).

Related research has shown that sex hormones have lifelong effects on the human brain. Recent studies demonstrate that cross-sex hormone treatment can alter the morphology of the total brain, particularly the hypothalamus, toward the average brain architecture of the opposite sex (Hulshoff et al., 2006). It is not yet clear how to weigh the relative contributions of genetics and hormonal exposure during pregnancy versus postnatal rearing (Crespi and Denver, 2005). Evidence for a purely hormonally derived differentiation is limited at best (Hrabovsky and Hutson, 2002).

Case Vignette 28.3.2 Continued

You explain to Mr. Roberts that gender reassignment is a long process and not necessarily an entirely positive journey. Mr. Roberts remains enthusiastic. You administer a number of psychological assessments and explain that there are many options he should keep in mind throughout the treatment. He must complete a 12-month period of hormonal treatment while living as a woman before surgery is an option. He could also choose to try hormone-only treatment or learning to adapt to gender identity disorder without any medical intervention. You also explain the risks of both the surgery and the hormonal treatment in great depth and note that one-third of male-to-female transsexuals are anorgasmic post-surgery.

Mr. Roberts is still optimistic about his treatment decision and does not demonstrate any signs or symptoms of a comorbid psychiatric disorder. You refer him to the rest of his gender reassignment treatment team: a surgeon, an endocrinologist, and a clinical psychologist—all with experience treating gender identity disorder. You provide written documents to the endocrinologist of your approval to begin hormonal treatment. After a few months of this treatment, he will be ready to begin his real-life experience of living completely as a woman for a full year.

Please proceed with the problem-based approach!

Some people find comfortable ways to deal with GID without the team intervention, either with or without psychotherapy. Another large section of the population finds that they can adapt well enough with only the first line hormonal treatment, such as estrogens (for feminization and decreased libido), antiandrogens (to decrease body hair and contribute to feminization), and progestogens (for breast development and psychological effects). While hormone treatment is obviously less intrusive and reversible, it poses potential adverse side effects, including blood clots, weight gain, emotional disorders, liver disease, gallstones, hypertension, and diabetes mellitus. The blots clots can be medically serious, with a possibility of fatality for those with cardiovascular disease (Meyer et al., 2001).

Depending on a psychiatrist's training, the roles of the endocrinologist and the psychotherapist can be wrapped into that of the psychiatrist. The role discussed in this case is only that of assessment. While it is not necessary in all cases, patients undergoing sexual reassignment surgery should receive psychotherapy throughout all phases of the treatment. This can help the client cope with the challenges of the new gender role and also address commonly comorbid disorders, including autogynephilia (arousal due to imagining oneself as a woman) and transvestism (arousal due to cross-dressing).

Case Vignette 28.3.3 Continued

Tom Roberts—now Adele Roberts—comes in for another assessment appointment after having completed the year-long real-life experience phase. She has been living as a woman for a year and has legally changed her name. She remained a student throughout the year, but was fired from her job. She reports this was discrimination against her transgender state. Ms. Roberts shows signs of a mild depression and has lost the enthusiasm that seemed so prominent a year ago. You wonder whether the experience has made her think about whether to progress to surgery for definitive treatment of gender identity disorder. She responds that she wants to complete the process to become a woman but is now dealing with large stressors due to this change. On top of losing her job, she lost health insurance. Her family members have significantly distanced themselves. These responses, combined with objective assessment measures and your overall clinical interview, reassure you that she is a viable candidate for reassignment surgery. At this point, you submit documentation to the surgeon that you believe the surgery is a feasible option for this client.

Please proceed with the problem-based approach!

The goal of this phase of assessment is to assure that the client is consolidating her gender identity. This would help confirm the hypothesis that her distress will be diminished with the surgery. Ms. Robert's reports of stress at this stage are not uncommon, and the "change of gender role and presentation can be an important factor in employment discrimination, divorce, marital problems, and the restriction or loss of visitation rights with children" (Meyer et al., 2001). Instead of focusing on the individual's adaptability to these understandable stressors, this stage of clinical interviewing instead focuses on the client's ability to function as an adult of the desired sex, including the ability to maintain a job or function in the capacity of a student. Documentation of this functionality should be provided by a third-party source.

In the case of a male-to-female transsexual such as Ms. Roberts, who is attracted solely to men, she would be considered a heterosexual male-to-female transsexual. It is generally accepted that transsexualism is neither dependent on nor related to sexual orientation, although the range of sexual orientation tends to be more diverse in transsexual populations (De Cuypere et al., 2004).

Case Vignette 28.3.4 Conclusion

Ms. Roberts returns 1 year after the surgery for a follow-up assessment. She is no longer experiencing any dysphoria about her gender, but is still adjusting to her new life. When asked if she has any questions, she reports that she has been avoiding her general practitioner because she is not sure what to expect or what evaluations she needs.

Please proceed with the problem-based approach!

Outcome research suggests that regrets concerning the decision to undergo reassignment surgery are fairly rare and that surgery commonly reduces or eliminates the gender dysphoria. On the other hand, "outbursts of regret" have been reported as well as development of borderline personality disorder. Generally, however, reported feelings of regret tend to focus on the functional result of the surgery and not on the treatment decision itself (Lawrence et al., 2005; Olsson and Möller, 2006; Smith et al., 2001). If the surgery successfully produced non-problematic genitals, the individuals remain largely satisfied. The majority of post-operative transsexuals express an increased satisfaction with their sex life and their new genitals. Female-to-male transsexuals tend to have more difficulty forming relationships after the surgery and sometimes experience pain during intercourse due to the erectile prosthesis.

As a gender specialist, it might be a good idea to inform the client of what she should learn to expect from her general practitioner, as a non-specialist may not be equipped to understand the health needs of a post-operative transsexual. Male-to-female transsexuals should be treated as females in their checkups, including mammograms. The prostate gland is not removed during the reconstructive surgery, however, and therefore the client should request regular prostate exams as well. Additionally, female-to-male patients should still seek annual papanicolaou examinations unless a complete hysterectomy had been performed (Sobralske, 2005).

Review Questions

1. How long must a person have recurrent sexual arousal from a specific stimulus to be diagnosed with a paraphilia?

    (a) 1 month
    (b) 6 months
    (c) 12 months
    (d) Any amount of time if the arousal is intense enough to require treatment

2. At what point is a doctor mandated to report on pedophilic child abuse?

    (a) When a patient states they have pedophilic urges
    (b) When a patient asks for medication to control pedophilic urges
    (c) When the doctor suspects or has reason to believe a child has been abused
    (d) None of the above

3. By what mechanism do sildenafil-like drugs benefit erection?

    (a) Directly on the parasympathetic nervous system
    (b) Indirectly on the parasympathetic nervous system
    (c) Directly on the corpus cavernosum vascular system
    (d) Indirectly on the corpus cavernosum vascular system

4. Before what age is erectile dysfunction generally considered unusual?

    (a) Before age 40
    (b) Before age 50
    (c) Before age 60
    (d) Before age 70

5. Which of these is a serious medical complication of hormone treatment therapy?

    (a) New onset diabetes insipidus
    (b) New onset schizophrenia

(c) Development of brain aneurysms

(d) Development of blood clots

6. What is the most common regret in transsexuals after sexual reassignment surgery?

(a) Regret with the functional result of the surgery, not the treatment decision itself

(b) Regret with the treatment decision itself, not the functional result of surgery

(c) Regret with having to maintain hormone therapy

(d) Regret with not being able to have children in the usual way of their reassigned gender

7. The most common cause of erectile dysfunction is

(a) Physiological

(b) Psychological

(c) Environmental

(d) A combination of biological and psychological factors

8. According to the Harry Benjamin Standards of Care, it is suggested that individuals seeking sexual reassignment surgery first live as a member of the opposite sex for

(a) 2 months

(b) 6 months

(c) 1 year

(d) 2 years

Answers

1. b, 2. c, 3. d, 4. b, 5. d, 6. a, 7. d, 8. c

References

Abel, G.G., Harlow, N. (2001). Stop Child Molestation Book: What Ordinary People Can Do in Their Everyday Lives to Save Three Million Children. Philadelphia, PA: Xlibris Corporation.

Bach, A.K., Barlow, D.H., Wincze, J.P. (2004). The enhancing effects of manualized treatment for erectile dysfunction among men using sildenafil: a preliminary investigation. Behavior Therapy 35:55–73.

Bradford, J.M. (2001). The neurobiology, neuropharmacology, and pharmacological treatment of the paraphilias and compulsive sexual behaviour. Canadian Journal of Psychiatry 46(1):26–34. Review. PMID: 11221487 [PubMed—indexed for MEDLINE].

Child Welfare Information Gateway (2005). Mandatory reporters of child abuse and neglect. State statutes series. http://www.childwelfare.gov/systemwide/laws_policies/statutes/manda.cfm. Accessed June 14, 2007.

Crespi, E.J., Denver, R.J. (2005). Ancient origins of human developmental plasticity. American Journal of Human Biology 17:44.

De Cuypere, G., T'Sjoen, G., Beerten, R., Selvaggi, G., De Sutter, P., Hoebeke, P., Monstrey, S., Vansteenwegen, A., Rubens, R. (2004). Sexual and physical health after sexual reassignment surgery. Archives of Sexual Behavior 24(6):679–690.

Hrabovsky, Z., Hutson, J.M. (2002) Androgen imprinting of the brain in animal models and humans with intersex disorders: review and recommendations. Journal of Urology 168:2142.

Hulshoff Pol, H.E., Cohen-Kettenis, P.T., Van Haren N.E.M., et al. (2006). Changing your sex changes your brain: influence of testosterone and estrogen on adult human brain structure. European Journal of Endocrinology 155:S107–S114.

Kerins, D., Robertson, R., Robertson, D. (2001). Chapter 32: Drugs used for the treatment of myocardial ischemia. In J.G. Hardman, L.E. Limbird (eds), Goodman & Gilman's The Pharmacological Basis of Therapeutics, 10th edn. San Francisco, CA: McGraw-Hill.

Kruijver, F.P., Zhou, J.N., Pool, C.W., et al. (2000) Male-to-female transsexuals have female neuron numbers in a limbic nucleus. The Journal of Clinical Endocrinology and Metabolism 85:2034.

Lawrence, A.A., Latty, E.M., Chivers, M.L., Bailey, J.M. (2005). Measurement of sexual arousal in postoperative male-to-female transsexuals using vaginal photoplethysmography. Archives of Sexual Behavior 43(2):135–145.

Lyseng-Williamson, K., Wagstaff, A.J. (2002). Management of Erectile Dysfunction: Defining the Role of Sildenafil. Disease Management & Health Outcomes 10(7):431–452.

Meyer III, W. (2001). The Harry Benjamin International Gender Dysphoria Association's standards of care for gender identity disorders, sixth version. Journal of Psychology & Human Sexuality 13(1):1–30.

Meyer III, W., Bockting, W., Cohen-Kettenis, P., Coleman, E., DiCeglie, D., Devor, H., Gooren, L., Joris Hage, J., Kirk, S., Kuiper, B., Laub, D., Lawrence, A., Menard, Y., Patton, J., Schaefer, L., Webb, A., Wheeler. C. (2001) The standards of care for gender identity disorders, sixth version. International Journal of Transgenderism 5(1). http://www.symposion.com/ijt/soc_2001/index.htm.

Olsson, S.E., Möller, A. (2006). Regret after Sex Reassignment Surgery in a Male-to-Female Transsexual: A Long-Term Follw-UP. Archives of Sexual Behavior, 35(4):501–506.

Quinsey, V.L. (2003). The etiology of anomalous sexual preferences in men. Annals of the New York Academy of Sciences 989:105–117; discussion 144–153. Review. PMID: 12839890 [PubMed—indexed for MEDLINE].

Skaer, T.L., Sclar, D.A., Robison, L.M., Galin, R.S. (2001). Trends in the rate of self-report and diagnosis of erectile dysfunction in the United States 1990–1998: was the introduction of sildenafil an influencing factor? Disease Management & Health Outcomes 9(1):33–41.

Sobralske, M. (2005). Primary care needs of patients who have undergone gender reassignment. Journal of the American Academy of Nurse Practitioners 17(4):133–138.

Smith, Y.L.S., van Goozen, S.H.M., Cohen-Kettenis, P.T. (2001). Adolescents with gender identity disorder who were accepted or rejected for sex reassignment surgery: a prospective follow-up study. Journal of American Academy of Child and Adolescent Psychiatry 40(4):472–481.

Zhou, J.N., Hofman, M.A., Gooren, L.J., Swaab, D.F. (1995). A sex difference in the human brain and its relation to transsexuality. Nature 378:68.

Chapter 29
Other Disorders

Anthony P.S. Guerrero

Welcome to the last chapter of this textbook! We sincerely hope that you have enjoyed this overview of the key topics in behavioral sciences and clinical psychiatry. To round out your learning, we will end with a glimpse into "other disorders" and hopefully review some of the other conditions and principles discussed elsewhere in this textbook.

At the end of this chapter, the reader will be able to

1. Discuss the approach to "other" psychiatric symptom clusters that do not automatically lead to diagnosis of the disorders heretofore discussed
2. Discuss the epidemiology, mechanisms, clinical presentation, clinical evaluation, differential diagnosis, and treatment of adjustment disorders, dissociative disorders, impulse control disorders, and psychological factors affecting general medical conditions

Case Vignette 29.1.1 Presenting Situation

Hauʻoli Smith is a 10-year-old female who is hospitalized for migraine headaches with significant pain and nausea requiring intravenous medications and fluid. Laboratory tests did not indicate any other medical problems besides the migraines. It was felt that her degree of pain is significantly more than what would be expected for this condition.

Nursing staff reported that Hauʻoli seemed to most be in pain when her mother and stepfather were in the room together. She otherwise would seem "fine." Additionally, it had been noted that there were recent family stressors, including marital conflict between the mother and stepfather and the birth of a new sibling, who is now 3 months old. The mother had reported that, particularly in the last few months, Hauʻoli has been crying more, arguing more, and complaining more of headaches. A psychiatric consultation was therefore requested to evaluate for

A.P.S. Guerrero
Associate Professor of Psychiatry and Pediatrics, Associate Chair for Education and Training, Department of Psychiatry, University of Hawaiʻi John A. Burns School of Medicine

A. Guerrero, M. Piasecki (eds.), *Problem-Based Behavioral Science and Psychiatry*,
© Springer Science+Business Media, LLC 2008

"adjustment difficulties," to rule out a psychological component to the headaches, and to provide "counseling" if indicated.

Please proceed with the problem-based approach!

At this point, a diagnosis of an adjustment disorder, while only one of several diagnostic possibilities (to be discussed further), is a reasonable one to consider. An adjustment disorder involves clinically significant (e.g., socially, academically, or occupationally impairing; or involving disproportionate distress) emotional/behavioral symptoms arising, within 3 months, from an identifiable stressor. As with many of the conditions you have learned thus far, these symptoms are not better explained by another Axis I or Axis II condition, including bereavement. Finally, these symptoms should not persist beyond 6 months following the termination of the stressor or its sequelae. According to the DSM-4TR, adjustment disorders should be further classified as being acute (lasting less than 6 months) or chronic (lasting 6 months or longer) and as being predominantly with depressed mood, anxiety, mixed anxiety and depressed mood, disturbance of conduct, mixed disturbance of emotions and conduct or unspecified.

Adjustment disorders are among the most common of the psychiatric disorders, with an apparently increased prevalence in general medical and psychiatric settings. As previously noted, in considering the diagnosis of an adjustment disorder, it is significantly important to consider other (though perhaps less common) differential possibilities. For the case above, reasonable diagnoses to consider would have included

- Major depression (e.g., with crying and irritability)
- Physical or sexual abuse of a child (e.g., with unexplained somatic symptoms, family stressors that are not yet clarified)
- Anxiety disorder (e.g., posttraumatic stress disorder, separation anxiety disorder)
- Mood disorder secondary to a general medical condition (e.g., intracranial pathology)
- Somatoform or pain disorder
- Malingering

The differential possibilities discussed above should stimulate us to recall the information we have learned in the previous chapters on Mood Disorders and Suicide (Chap. 21), Violence and Abuse (Chap. 7), Anxiety Disorders (Chap. 22), and Somatoform Disorders (Chap. 23)! Do you recall which of these conditions are relatively more common than the others?

Malingering is a condition that we discussed in Chap. 23. For review, according to the DSM-4TR, it involves "the *intentional* production of false or grossly exaggerated physical *or psychological* symptoms, motivated by *external incentives.*"

Table 29.1 Characteristics of malingering, factitious disorder, and other somatoform disorders

Disorder	Intentional production of symptoms	Motivation for behavior	Presentation of symptoms	Clinical findings
Malingering	Yes	External incentive (e.g., economic gain, avoiding legal responsibility, etc.) "secondary gain"	Often dramatic demonstrations of disability or symptoms	History may be internally inconsistent. Physical and/or mental status findings may be inconsistent with known presentations of illness or plausible physiological mechanisms
Factitious disorder	Yes	To assume the sick role "primary gain"		
Other somatoform disorders (e.g., somatization disorder, pain disorder, conversion disorder, etc.)	No	Not applicable	Often less dramatic demonstrations of disability or symptoms; indifference may be present	

Usually, malingering is considered when physical symptoms or complaints are present; however, psychological symptoms (including psychosis) can also be malingered. Malingering is differentiated from factitious disorder and many of the somatoform disorders (Chap. 23) by the characteristics summarized in Table 29.1.

Because it is not clear that this patient is intentionally producing these symptoms, additional evaluation is necessary.

Case Vignette 29.1.2 Continuation

You meet with Hauʻoli and family. While Hauʻoli is not worried that the headaches represent anything other than her migraines, the mother and stepfather report that they are somewhat concerned that these symptoms might indicate the presence of an "aneurysm," which the maternal great grandmother, who was close to the patient, died from 5 months ago. You encourage them to discuss this concern with the medical team.

The family notes that, in the past few months, there have, in fact been multiple stressors, including the birth of the patient's half-sister (who is the only other child in the family), loss of the stepfather's job, increased marital conflict—probably related to the financial pressures of the stepfather's job loss, and the beginning of a new academic year in a new school. Per the family's report, there are no previous behavioral concerns. She has had a history of migraines from an early age that was usually well controlled with prophylactic medication. There are also no other general medical problems, and there was no pattern of recurring somatic complaints other than the migraines. There is a strong family history of migraines, and the mother notes that her own migraines began during childhood.

In your individual interview with Hauʻoli, she admits that she has been feeling sad, "bummed out," and "a little worried" over all of the "money problems" their family has been having. She believes that her migraines may be worse whenever she feels stress. While she says that she likes the new baby, she "never really liked the idea of mom getting remarried." She recalls that in the previous marriage, "my real dad was always drunk, and he used to hit her, so that's why they got a divorce." While she reports being afraid whenever she witnessed violence, she denies any nightmares, flashbacks, or significant distress upon reexposure to reminders of previous trauma. She denies any past or present history of physical or sexual abuse. She denies excessive worry about her mother's safety, or anxiety upon separating from her family to attend school and other activities. While she has had poor appetite and sleep for the past 2 days, since the migraine difficulties began, she denies any previous sleep, appetite, or energy-level changes and denies any definite anhedonia or suicidal or homicidal ideations. While cooperative with your interview, she does appear uncomfortable, and she prefers to have the lights off. Vital signs are significant for mild tachycardia.

Based on the above presentation, various differential possibilities appear to have been ruled out. Of note, even though there may have been neurovegative symptoms to suggest depression (e.g., with sleep and appetite changes), these symptoms did not occur in the absence of the migraine headaches, and did not last for 2 weeks or longer.

With the other possibilities in the list above ruled out, the diagnosis of adjustment disorder, acute, with mixed anxiety and depressed mood, is most probable. In addition, it appears that there is an exacerbation of the migraine headaches in the context of the adjustment disorder, and it may therefore be appropriate to diagnose on Axis I: Specified Psychological Factor Affecting General Medical Condition, more specifically a *mental disorder affecting migraine headaches.* Diagnostic criteria for this Axis I diagnosis include the presence of a general medical condition and evidence that psychological factors adversely affected the general medical condition through either the physiological sequelae of the psychological factors (*which may be applicable in this case*) or interference of the psychological factors with prevention or treatment of the general medical condition. Specific descriptors for the "specified psychological factor" include "mental disorder" (*which this particular patient is also diagnosed with on Axis I*), "psychological symptoms," "personality traits or coping style," "maladaptive health behaviors," "stress-related physiological response," or "other or unspecified psychological factors."

Beyond just DSM-4TR diagnosis, this case illustrates the importance of bio-psycho-social formulation in insuring optimal treatment—as is often the case when managing adjustment disorders, either on its own or in the context of a general medical condition.

Please take this opportunity to do a bio-psycho-social formulation for this case.

Case Vignette 29.1.3 Conclusion

You work collaboratively with the pediatric team to optimize medical management of acute pain. You provide individual and family supportive counseling and psychoeducation, and you address the family's concern that someone might be thinking that this is "all in her head." You "prescribe" an expected course of recovery, while still allowing the patient to express the pain that likely goes along with her migraine headaches. You also consult with your team psychologist on relaxation and other behavioral techniques that might help with pain management. On outpatient follow-up, you provide individual and family psychotherapy, which proves to be very effective. You encourage the parents to spend individual time with the patient, even in the face of the demands of the new baby. Several months later, her headaches are under stable control, and there are no further hospitalizations.

As depicted in Table 29.2, with the construction of a bio-psycho-social formulation, it will be possible to target interventions to optimally manage all mechanisms leading to the adjustment disorder with impact on the general medical condition. In most situations, because of the acute and (by definition) environmentally influenced nature of adjustment disorders, time-limited psychotherapy that improves individual coping and addresses environmental contributors to the symptoms is usually what is indicated. Prognosis is generally favorable, depending on the nature, pervasiveness, and chronicity of the precipitating circumstances.

The case above presented a diagnostic challenge, in which many other Axis I conditions were considered. The following case presents a further diagnostic challenge.

Case Vignette 29.2.1 Presenting Situation

Mr. John Flame is a 25-year-old male who is brought into the emergency room by the police, who reported that he was "acting suspicious" around the scene of a fire. The police officer also told you that one of his colleagues recalled this gentleman from the scene of another fire several weeks earlier, and therefore was worried that this patient may be a "pyromaniac." They noticed that he was not making sense when initially questioned, but wondered whether or not he was faking his psychotic symptoms to avoid going to cell block.

Please proceed with the problem-based approach!

Pyromania belongs to a series of disorders in the DSM-4TR called "impulse control disorders." The disorders in this category and the general characteristics of the impulse control disorders are summarized in Table 29.3.

Table 29.2 Bio-psycho-social–cultural–spiritual formulation of the case vignette, "Hau'oli"

	Biological		Psychological		Social–Cultural–Spiritual	
	Factor	Intervention	Factor	Intervention	Factor	Intervention
Predisposing factors	Genetic predisposition to migraines	Continued migraine prophylaxis	Previous family transitions—parental divorce, witness to domestic violence	Individual counseling, safety education	Previous family transitions—parental divorce, witness to domestic violence	Family counseling to effectively manage conflicts
Precipitating factors	Acute migraine with pain	Medication management per pediatric team, relaxation and behavioral techniques to assist with pain management	Stressors: new baby, worry about parental conflict, new school	Individual counseling	Parental conflict affecting patient	Family counseling to effectively manage conflicts and to insure optimal parental support through other transitions
Perpetuating factors	Sensitization to pain	Effective treatment of acute pain, continued migraine prophylaxis	Pain being a route to receiving attention	Family counseling to insure regular attention to patient	Pain being a route to focusing attention on patient rather than other family conflicts	Family counseling to effectively manage conflicts

Table 29.3 Characteristics and treatments of the impulse control disorders

Impulse control disorder	Key characteristics	Possible treatments
Intermittent explosive disorder	Discrete episodes of aggressive and/or destructive behavior, out of proportion to precipitating psychosocial stressors (differentiated from seizure phenomena, which more commonly manifest as repetitive and/or purposeless behaviors)	Psychotherapy, anticonvulsants, lithium, antipsychotics, serotonin-selective reuptake inhibitors, propranolol
Kleptomania	Stealing objects that are not personally or monetarily valuable	Psychotherapy, serotonin-selective reuptake inhibitors
Pyromania	Purposeful, repetitive fire setting	Psychotherapy, insure safety
Pathological gambling	Persistent and recurrent maladaptive gambling	Psychotherapy, self-help groups, serotonin-selective reuptake inhibitors
Trichotillomania	Recurrent hair pulling	Psychotherapy, serotonin-selective reuptake inhibitors
Impulse control disorder not otherwise specified	Not meeting criteria for any other condition listed above	

General characteristics of the impulse control disorders

- Failure to resist impulses that lead to the behaviors described above
- Symptoms are not better explained by another disorder, including substance use disorders and general medical conditions
- (Implied) impairment in functioning

Therefore, before we conclude that this patient has either pyromania or another impulse control disorder, we should further analyze the differential possibilities, which for this case, should include

- Psychotic disorders (with disorganized thoughts and behavior)
- Mood disorders, including bipolar disorder, with psychotic features
- Substance use disorders, including substance intoxication and substance-induced psychotic disorders
- Psychotic disorder secondary to a general medical condition
- Malingering (to avoid arrest or incarceration, as suggested by the police officer in this case)

Once again, we are challenged to recall the various conditions from the previous chapters. Did you remember to never forget, in your list of differential possibilities, conditions secondary to either substance use or general medical conditions? ☺Like with the first case vignette, the possibility of malingering is once again raised. At this point, given that we have not yet explored the other differential possibilities, it would be clinically unsound (and potentially a reflection of the stigma of mental illness—do you remember Chap. 13?) to assume that this patient is malingering.

Case Vignette 29.2.2 Continuation

Mr. Flame states that he is a "highly intelligent and gifted grand master spirit." Notwithstanding his claim that he has been "specially chosen to chant away the fire demons and stop them from entering the mortal universe," he denies any recollection of having been near a fire recently, as he has "been in a spiritual trance." He denies any history of fire setting or particular excitement upon seeing fires. He gives the history of having been treated several times at a facility located in another state. You find the history difficult to obtain, because of his tangential thought processes, but you maintain your composure and ability to be empathic, as you recall from a textbook you once read (Chap. 17) that, often, a challenging interview often reflects the effects of the very illness that one should be attempting to treat. Besides the tangentiality, your mental status examination is significant for poor hygiene and bizarre dress, continuous speech that is difficult to interrupt, flat affect, religious preoccupations, auditory hallucinations, and proverb interpretations that are either very bizarre or very concrete. He performs adequately on basic tests of concentration and memory. You conclude to yourself that, if he were, in fact, malingering, he would need to be a very skilled and knowledgeable actor. He appears to be physically healthy, and screening laboratory studies, including a urine toxicology, are negative.

At this point, given the extensive psychopathology observed, it would seem that malingering and pyromania are less likely as possibilities. One new possibility that might be considered at this point is a dissociative disorder. Table 29.4 presents the general characteristics of the dissociative disorders.

Once again, without further collateral information, and with significant evidence for other psychiatric syndromes that could explain his symptoms, it is not clear that this patient meets the criteria for any of the dissociative disorders.

Case Vignette 29.2.3 Continuation

With his permission, you are able to gather collateral information from Mr. Flame's family and from his previous psychiatrist. They confirm that he has the diagnosis of bipolar disorder, Type I, and that he functions very well when he is stable on his medication, valproic acid. In fact, he is a well-respected research scholar who recently relocated in order to pursue doctoral-level studies. You admit him for further treatment, and he stabilizes very nicely on valproic acid and an atypical antipsychotic. He regrets that he allowed his medications to run out. He explains that, since his move, it was difficult to secure health insurance. He notes that many

Table 29.4 General characteristics of the dissociative disorders

Dissociative disorder	Key characteristics
Dissociative identify disorder (aka, multiple personality disorder)	More than one distinct identity or personality state that recurrently controls a person's behavior
Dissociative amnesia	Episodes of inability to recall important personal information (usually associated with traumatic events)
Dissociative fugue	Sudden travel away from home, inability to recall one's past, and confusion about personal identity
Depersonalization disorder	Recurrent feelings of detachment from one's mind or body
Dissociative disorder not otherwise specified	Dissociative symptoms not otherwise meeting criteria of any of the above disorders

Other characteristics of the dissociative disorders

- Symptoms are not better explained by another disorder psychiatric disorder (including psychotic and posttraumatic stress disorders), substance use disorders, and general medical conditions (particularly, transient global amnesia, which affects ability to learn new information)
- (Implied) impairment in functioning
- Relative preservation of other mental processes (e.g., ability to register new information, unlike in certain neurological conditions)

Treatment considerations for the dissociative disorders

- Psychotherapy and psychopharmacotherapy targeted toward comorbid conditions and/or specific impairments and symptoms
- Medication-assisted interviews (e.g., amobarbital or benzodiazepine) may assist in uncovering traumatic memories; however, it is not clear that psychotherapeutic interventions done while under the effect of medications may be effective

---

of the healthcare plans significantly restrict behavioral health and/or medication benefits. You ponder the lessons you learned in this case and you resolve to become an advocate for accessible mental health care for everyone.

Although this chapter may seem like the one that covers "miscellaneous" conditions, we believe that the conditions we have introduced in this chapter are excellent ones to discuss at the conclusion of this book for the following reasons. First, because adjustment disorders and psychological factors affecting medical conditions (both of which were illustrated in the first case) and impulse control and dissociative disorders (both of which were considered in the second case) typically are not associated with any one underlying neurobiological mechanism, they illustrate the importance of treatment planning according to (can you guess what?) the bio-psycho-social–cultural–spiritual matrix. Secondly, because these conditions tend to have lengthy lists of differential diagnoses, discussion of these conditions also illustrates the usefulness of the problem-based learning approach, which helps the clinician to thoughtfully consider other possibilities. Finally, these conditions illustrate the wide spectrum of psychiatric illnesses, ranging from the very common, potentially under-recognized, and generally self-limiting (e.g., adjustment disorders) to the relatively rare, potentially over-publicized by the media, and often chronic (e.g., impulse control disorders such as pyromania, dissociative disorders such as dissociative identity disorder). We hope that, like the clinician illustrated in the last vignette, you will become a physician who is knowledgeable about the scope of psychiatric illnesses and empathetically responsive to the behavioral health needs of patients.

Review Questions

1. Which of the following features would be *least* consistent with the diagnosis of an adjustment disorder:

   (a) Persistence of symptoms beyond 6 months, in response to a chronic, severe stressor
   (b) The presence of mixed anxiety and depressive symptoms
   (c) The presence of transient psychotic symptoms
   (d) Significant interference with functioning
   (e) None of the above

2. A high school student with bronchial asthma tends to have exacerbations of illness around significant stress. Prior to final exams, and also coinciding with cold weather, he suffers from a particularly severe attack, resulting in hospitalization in the intensive care unit and significant wheezing, respiratory distress, and hypoxia. The patient is a high-achieving student who regrets needing to have the exams rescheduled. From a psychiatric perspective, the most appropriate diagnosis would be

   (a) Psychological factors affecting general medical condition
   (b) Malingering
   (c) Factitious disorder
   (d) Conversion disorder
   (e) None of the above

For questions 2–4, please match the following illness with its associated clinical presentation

   (a) Dissociative fugue
   (b) Dissociative amnesia
   (c) Intermittent explosive disorder

3. Discrete episodes of aggressive and/or destructive behavior
4. Sudden travel away from home, inability to recall one's past
5. Episodes of inability to recall important personal information

Answers

1. c, 2. a, 3. c, 4. a, 5. b

Bibliography

American Psychiatric Association. (2000). *Diagnostic and statistical manual of mental disorders DSM-IV-TR* (4th ed., text revision). Washington, DC: Author.
Sadock B.J. and Sadock V.A. (2003). Kaplan and Sadock's Synopsis of Psychiatry: Behavioral Sciences/Clinical Psychiatry. 9th Edition. New York: Lippincott Williams & Wilkins.

Index

A

Abdomen
  injuries, 91
  pain, 107–108, 172, 322, 343
  trauma, 96, 100–101
Abel, G.G., 413
Ability to experience pleasure, loss
    of, 147
Abnormal brain activity, 6
Abnormal Involuntary Movement Scale
    (AIMS), 301
Abnormal mood and confusion, mechanisms
    behind, 5–6
Abstinence, 73
Abstraction, 239
Abstract thinking, 22
Abuse and neglect
  of adults, 90–95
  of children, *see* Child neglect and abuse
  effects on brain, 41
Abuser characteristics, in domestic
    violence, 92
Abuse victims
  reasons for staying in abusive
    relationship, 94
  steps to help, 93–94
  unable to break out of violence, 94
    patient-related reasons, 94
    physician-related reasons, 94
Abusive parents, characteristics, 97–98
Acamprosate, 280
Acceptance, 217
Accountability, 129
Acculturative stress, 190
Acetaminophen, 220, 242, 249, 358
Acetylcholinesterase inhibitors, 377–378
Acquired immunodeficiency syndrome
    (AIDS), 134, 173, 189, 319, 372

Action
  ethical assessment, 123
  stage in behavior change, 52
Active–passive model, of physician-patient
    relationship, 112
Actual physical abuse, 90
Acupuncture, 220
Acute bipolar mania, 322
Acute dystonia, 299
Acute stress disorder, 90, 326, 328
Adaptation and coping
  appraisal support, 80
  bio-psycho-social-cultural-spiritual
    conceptualization, 84–87
  case conceptualization, 80–81, 83, 86
  definition of, 78
  development influence, 84
  emotional support, 80
  factors influencing, 84
  fear and sadness correlates, 79–80
  gender influence, 84
  individual's and social network relationship
    role, 80
  informational support, 80
  instrumental support, 80
  neurobiological and psychosocial
    correlates, 79, 86
  PBL approach to, 78–81, 83–87
  process of, 78
  social support
    barriers to seeking, 80
    effects on, 80–81
    types of, 80
  sociocultural values influence, 84, 87
  spirituality influence on, 84–85, 87
  with medical adversity
    adaptive methods, 81–82

Adaptation and coping (*Cont.*)
    adaptive relational methods, 81, 83
    psychosocial interventions to facilitate,
       85–87
Adaptive
  behavior, 37
  coping, 77
  methods, 81–83
  strategies, 81
  to illness in context of family, 81–82
  See also Adaptation and coping
Adaptiveness of genotypes, with illnesses and
     other conditions, 185–187
Addictions, 82
  neurobiology of, 59
  pharmacotherapy of, 279–280
  treatment plan, 166, 283–284
Addison's disease, 311
Adherence
  in medicine, 133–138
Adjustment disorder, 48, 90, 326, 331, 404,
     424–432
  bio-psycho-social formulation, 427–428
  with depressed mood, 248
Adolescents
  cognitive and social developments, 73
  depression among, 26
  diagnoses specific to, 262
  emotional complaints, 26
  gender identity, 26
  normal development variant, 26
  parent's death impact on, 23
  physical changes, 26
  physical development, 73
Adrenal disorders, 8
Adrenocorticotropic hormone (ACTH), 144
Adults
  disorders present in childhood, 263
  psychiatric morbidity among, 23
Advice, 115
Aerobic exercise programs, 148
Affective disorders, 137
Affect–observed emotional state, 237
Age-associated forgetfulness, 367
Agency for Healthcare Research and Quality
     (AHRQ), 167
Agency for Toxic Substance and Disease
     Registry (ATSDR), 167
Aggression, 97, 256
Aggressive behaviors, 23
Agitation, 272, 274, 310, 316, 322
Agnosia, 370
Agonist, pharmacotherapy of, 279

Agoraphobia, 333
Akathisia, 299, 322
Alacrity, 129
Albers, L.J., 332
Alcohol, 8–9, 146, 269, 271, 272
  abuse, 84, 95
  death due to excessive use, 270
  dependence, 283
  induced persisting amnestic disorder, 275
  intake and sleeping, 63
  intoxication, 127
  rehabilitation program, 275
  use and sleeping problem, 53–54
  withdrawal delirium, 271–273
Alcoholics Anonymous (AA), 275, 284
Aldehyde dehydrogenase nondeficiency, 186
Aldosterone, 144
Alertness, 238
Alopecia, 321
Alpha2A agonist guanfacine, 357
Alprazolam, 279, 332
Altman, D.G., 204
Alzheimer's type dementia, 367, 372–373,
     377, 379
American Academy of Child and Adolescent
     Psychiatry (AACAP), 20, 27
American Board of Internal Medicine, 128
American College of Emergency
     Physicians, 90
American Medical Association, 220
American Psychiatric Association, 310–311,
     313, 319–320, 330, 355, 366, 374
American Society of Addiction Medicine, 284
Amitriptyline, 315
Amnestic disorders, 368–369
Amobarbital, 431
Amphetamine abuse, 297, 311, 319
Ampicillin, 311
Amyotrophic lateral sclerosis (ALS), 122
Anaclitic depression, 35, 45–46
Anal
  bleeding, 100
  stenosis, 258
Andersen, A.E., 397–399
Androgen insensitivity syndrome, 70
Anemia, 38, 311
Anger, 97, 217
  and bitterness, 23
  management issues, 293
Angina, 124
Anhedonia, 147, 272, 313, 383
Anorexia nervosa (AN), 394–396

bio-psycho-social-cultural-spiritual
    formulation, 400–401
complications from, 398
laboratory findings in, 397
signs and symptoms of, 396–397
social factors, 402
treatment, 398–400
Anoxia, 38, 48
Antabuse, 279
Antagonist, pharmacotherapy of, 279
Antecedents, 49–50
    to good or poor night of sleep, 62–63
    to tantrums, 63–64
Anterior cingulate cortex, neurons in, 41
Anthony, J.C., 314
Antiadrenergic effects, of TCAs, 315
Antiandrogen hormones, 413
Anticholinergic effects, of TCAs, 315
Anticipation, neurobiology of, 59
Anticonvulsants, 319
Anticraving agents, pharmacotherapy of, 280
Antihistaminergic effects, of TCAs, 315
Antipsychotics, 8
    due to substances and general medical
        conditions, 297
    monitoring for side effects of, 301
Antisocial disorders, 92
Antisocial personality disorder (ASPD), 137,
        355, 360
Anwar, 93
Anxiety, 23, 36, 86, 92, 178, 211, 220, 272
    disorders, 10, 137, 254, 256–257, 263,
        265–266, 315, 322, 329, 342, 402,
        403, 424, 426
        differential diagnosis, 326
        due to general medical condition,
            326, 329
        PBL approach to, 325–337
        substance-induced, 326
Anxiolytics, 330
Aphasia, 370
Apnea, 272
Apologies, in medicine, 113–114
Appearance, 129
Appetite, 172
    changes, 310, 313
Appleton, D.R., 193
Apraxia, 370
Arginine vasopressin (AVP), 144–145
Aripiprazole, 298, 300
Arnold, E., 370
Arnold, L.E., 255
Arousal system, 59

Arrhythmia, 329
Arroyo de Cabrera, E., 113
5 A's approach, to change behavior, 52
Asperger's disorder, 262
Aspirin, 220
Assess safety, in psychiatric interview and
        assessment, 234–235
Assigned gender, 70
Assignment sampling, 199
Association of State and Territorial Health
        Officials (ASTHO), 168
Asthma, 92, 145–146
Ataxia, 321–322, 332
Atherosclerotic plaques, 145
Ativan®, 332
Atopic dermatitis, 307
Attention deficit disorder, 48
Attention-deficit hyperactivity disorder
        (ADHD), 17, 254–256, 265–266,
        292–293, 318, 334, 404
Attention-deficit hyperactivity disorder, 17
Attunement, 35
Atypical antidepressants, 314
Auditory hallucinations, 305, 430
Autism, 262
Autistic disorder, 259, 263
Autonomic nervous system (ANS), 144, 148
Autonomy, loss of, 220
Autopsy, 222, 225
Aversive agents, pharmacotherapy of, 279–280
Avoidant personality disorders, 137, 364
Awakenings, and sleeping problem, 53

B
B12 deficiency, 38, 48, 311
Babinski reflex, 122
Bach, A.K., 416
Back pain, 91, 343
Baclofen, 319
Bad news communication, and physician-
        patient relationship, 114–115
Bain, D.J.G., 113
Balaban, R.B., 218, 223
Baldor, R., 156
Barbiturates, 272, 274, 319
Bargaining, 217
Barnes, T.R.E., 194
Barrows, H.S., 3
BEARS (Bedtime, Excessive daytime
        sleepiness, Awakenings, Regularity
        and duration of sleep, Snoring), 53
Beauchamp, Thomas, 123–124
Beck Depression Inventory, 314

Becoming educated strategy, 82
Bedtime, and sleeping problem, 53–54
Behavioral principles, functional analysis, 61
Behavioral strategies, 81
Behaviors, 90
    5 A's approach to change, 52
    change stages, 51–52
        action stage, 52
        contemplation stage, 52
        maintenance stage, 52
        precontemplation stage, 51
        preparation stage, 52
    coping model, 56
    extinction burst phase, 56
    functional analysis, 50–51, 55
    mastery model, 56
    principles, 49
    problems, 97
    specific self-efficacy, 138
    stages of change, 136–137
    stimulus control strategy, 53
Being female, domestic violence risk, 91
Beliefs, 86
Belmaker, R.H., 318–320, 323
Beneficence principle, 123–127
Benign parotid hyperplasia, 398
Benzodiazepines, 8, 272–274, 278–280, 283,
        299, 319, 328, 331–333, 359, 384,
        386, 431
Bereavement, 217
    in children, 22–23
Bernstein, L., 113
Bernstein, R.S., 113
Bertranpetit, J., 186
Beta blockers, 8, 74
Bicycle helmets, 137
Bilateral leg paralysis, 339, 341
Binge-eating disorder, 396, 403
Bioethics principles, 123–124
Biofeedback, 220
Biological and psychological factors,
        in psychiatric interview and
        assessment, 247–248
Bio-psycho-social-cultural formulation,
        137–138, 231, 235, 240
Bio-psycho-social-cultural-spiritual model,
        8–12, 86, 190
    biological components, 8–9, 11
        current illnesses, 8
        endocrine and hormonal, 9
        genetics, 8
        medication, 8
        pregnancy and birth, 8

    previous illnesses, 8
    substances, 9
    cultural components, 10–11
    psychological components, 9, 11
    sample formulation for, 10–12
    social components, 9, 11
    spiritual components, 10–11
Bipolar-developmental disorder, 71
Bipolar disorders, 17, 177, 180, 193, 248, 263,
        312, 318–319, 430
    medications used in, 320—323
    pathophysiology of, 320
Bipolar mania, 233
Birch, L.L., 404
Birth
    bio-psycho-social-cultural-spiritual model
        for, 8
    trauma, 8, 48
Bites, 96
Bizarre delusions, 291
Blame, 82, 85–86
Bland, J.M., 204
Bleomycin, 311
Blindness, 38
Block, S.D., 217, 219
Blood
    self-monitoring of glucose, 135
    transfusions, 126
Blunted affect, 83, 85, 86
Blurred vision, 315, 322
Bodenheimer, T.S., 154–155, 159, 163
Body dysmorphic disorder, 339
Boehmer, L.M., 389
Bolin, L., 53
Borderline disorders, 92
Borderline personality disorder, 177, 181, 249,
        360–361
Bowden, V.R., 78
Bradford, J.M., 413
Brain
    abuse and neglect effects on, 41
    damage by mercury poisoning, 38
    death, 222–224
    depression, 278
    development
        childhood sexual abuse effect on, 41
        maternal environmental conditions
            role, 36
        and mother–child attachment, 36
        verbal abuse effect on, 41
    dopamine-producing neurons, 59
    experience impact on structure and function
        of, 40–41

maturation process and gray-matter loss, 23
musical training effects on, 40–41
plasticity, 41
size, 38
tumor, 297
Brain-dead
donors, 222
Brain development
and mother–child attachment, 36
Breast cancer, 152–153, 157, 189
Breasts injuries, 91
Breath shortness, 328, 330
Bremner, J.D., 327
Brent, D., 313
Brink, T.L., 376
Briquet's syndrome, 345
Brock, C.D., 113
Brodifacoum tests, 349
Bromocriptine, 299, 319
Bronchogenic carcinoma, 311
Brown, R.H., 94, 314
Bruises, 96
Bulimia nervosa (BN), 315, 394–396, 399–402
bio-psycho-social-cultural-spiritual
formulation, 401–402
complications from, 398
laboratory findings in, 397
signs and symptoms of, 396–397
social factors, 402
treatment, 398–400
Buprenorphine, 274, 279
Bupropion, 279–280, 316, 399
Burdening others, 220
Burns, 96
Burr, W., 81, 84
Butorphanol, 283

C
Cabrera, A., 113
Caffeine, 330
induced disorder, 326
use and sleeping problem, 53
CAGE Questionnaire, 275, 282, 285–286
Calafell, F., 186
Calm, 81
Campbell, M.J., 204
Cancer, 310
cervical, 72, 189
pain management in patients, 220
Cannabis, 269
Carbamazepine, 320–321
Cardiac arrhythmias, 108, 249, 272
Cardiac disease, and coping strengths, 147–148

Cardiac event, 329
Cardiac rehabilitation program, 146
Cardiac rhythm disturbances, 298
Cardiovascular disease, 134, 189
Caregivers characteristics, 97–98
Carlson, N., 79
Case-control studies, 195–196
Case-series studies, 195–196
Cataplexy, 388, 389
Cataracts, 38
Catatonic behavior, 295
Catecholamines, 272
Cellulitis, 293
Center for Children and Families, 163
Center for Epidemiological Studies Depression
Scale, 314
Centers for Disease Control and Prevention
(CDC), 165
Centers for Disease Control and Prevention, 73
Centers for Medicare and Medicaid Services
(CMS), 157, 159–163
Cerebellum, 278
Cervical cancer
mortality from, 189
vaccine, 72
Chan, A.S., 41
Chantix, 280
Charismatic child, 36–37
Chemotherapy, 152
Chest injuries, 91
Chest pain, 328, 330
Child
abuse, 5, 9, 190, 211, 256, 266
See also Child neglect and abuse
bereavement in, 22–23
diagnoses specific to, 262
grief at parent's loss, 22–23
incest with, 97
misconceptions about care, 97
misconceptions about development, 97
resilience as basis for response rates, 36–37
response rates, 36–37
self-centered perspective, 19
sexual exploitation, 97
victimization as, 92
See also Childhood
Child Abuse Evaluation and Treatment for
Medical Providers, 101
Child Abuse Prevention and Treatment Act
(CAPTA), 96
Childhelp USA, 101
Childhood
development

Childhood (*Cont.*)
    autonomy *versus* shame and doubt
      phase, 19
    brain development, 19–20, 23, 26
    cognitive development, 19, 22
    doubt phase in, 19
    emotional development, 20
    industry and inferiority phase, 22
    learning issues, 19–20, 22–23
    motor development, 22
    neurodevelopment, 19–20
    preoperational developmental phase, 20
    skills development, 19
  disorders
    PBL approach to, 253–263, 265–267
  experience effects, 40–41
  sexual abuse and brain development, 41
Child neglect and abuse
  abusive parents and caregivers
    characteristics, 97–98
  assessments guidelines, 100–101
  brain structure and function in, 41
  categories, 96–97
  definition, 96
  exams and assessments, 99–100
  guidelines for interview and
    examination, 99
  PBL approach, 95–102
  priorities for, 102
  resources, 101
  risk factors, 97
  youth perpetrators, 102
Child Protective Services (CPS), 256
Child psychiatric evaluation
  ADHD, 254–256
  child abuse, 256
  developmental disorder, 259–263
  differential diagnosis, 254–256
  encopresis, 257–259
  PBL approach to, 253–263, 265–267
  PDD, 261
  PTSD, 256–257
Childress, James, 123–124
Child Welfare Information Gateway, 101, 411
Chiles, J., 172
Chlamydia, 73
Chochinov, H.M., 221
Cholecystitis, 108
Cholera, 186
Cholestatic jaundice, 322
Chromosomal analysis, 260
Chromosomal sex, 70
Chronic disease, 137

Chronic heart failure, 311
Chronic pain disorders, 315
Chronic physiologic changes, 146
Chronic subdural hematoma, 311
Chukwuma, C., 186
Cigarette burns, 96
Cigarette smoking, 158
Cimetidine, 283, 319
Circadian rhythm sleep disorder, 389
Citalopram, 315, 337
Civil Rights Movement, 85
Clark, C., 84
Classen, C.C., 355
Classical conditioning, 49–50
Clean Air Act, 168
Clean Water Act, 168
Clemans-Cope, L., 155
Clinical evaluation strategies, 133
Clinical reasoning
  process, 5–6
  skills of, 3
Clinical research
  analyze data, 201–202
  clean and recode data, 201
  codebook of variables, 201
  conduct of study, 201
  experimental studies, 195–198
  identify research question, 194
  instruments and diagnostic tests, 195,
    198–199
  learning issues, 194–202
  literature review, 194
  meta-analysis, 207–208
  observational studies, 195–197
  PBL approach to, 194–212
  presentation and publication of paper, 201
  protocols for study, 201
  run study on test group, 201
  sampling technique and sample size,
    199–200
  sensitivity of tests, 195, 199
  significance level and statistical errors, 200
  specificity of tests, 195, 198
  statistical test, 201–202
  study design, 194–197
  tools for measurement, 195, 198
  write paper, 201
Clinical situations, concepts, 4
Clinical trials, studies, 195–196
Clock-Drawing Test, 373
Clomipramine, 337
Clonazepam, 332
Clonidine, 257, 274, 280, 311

Closeness, 84
Clotrimazole, 311
Clotting system, 148
Clozapine, 298, 300
CNS tumors, 147, 311
Cocaine, 6, 319
    intoxication, 273–274, 276
    use, 271–272, 274–275, 278
Codeine, 220
Cognition, concept of, 367–368
Cognitive and social developments
    during adolescence, 73
Cognitive-behavioral therapy (CBT), 148, 283,
        314, 399, 412
Cognitive coping strategies, 82
Cognitive development
    in adolescence, 73
    in childhood, 19, 22
Cognitive difficulties, 77, 79, 81, 85–87
Cognitive disorders, 10
    differential diagnosis, 368
    PBL approach to, 367–379
Cognitive impairment, 321, 398
Cognitive performance, 38
Cognitive restructuring, 220
Cognitive strategies, 81–82
Cognitive system, of brain, 59
Cohen's kappa, 204–205
Cohort studies, 195–196
Collagen-vascular disease, 311
Coma, 38, 224, 272
Combat, 9
Command hallucinations, 291
Commission for the Prevention of Youth
        Violence, 102
Common illicit drugs, mechanism of action,
        5–6
Communication of bad news
    and physician-patient relationship,
        114–115
Communication skills, impact on physician-
        patient relationship, 113
Community Coalition on Family Violence
        (CCFV), 94
Community intervention trials studies,
        195–196
Community reinforcement, 284
Community surveys studies, 195–196
Comorbid mental illness, 137
Comorbid psychiatric disorder, 417–418
Complicated grief, symptoms of, 23
Compulsive masturbation, 72
Concentration, 238

Conceptual analysis, 123
Conduct disorder, 262
Conflict-escalating communication, 82
Confusion, 278
Congenital adrenal hyperplasia, 70
Conscientious, 129
Conscious
    loss of, 292
    states of, 224
Consequences, 49–50
    of action and ethical assessment, 123
Consideration, 129
Consistency and case comparison, 123
Consolidated Omnibus Budget Reconciliation
        Act, (COBRA) plan, 158, 160
Constipation, 272, 315–316, 321–322
Contact dermatitis, 307
Contemplating action, ethical assessment, 123
Contemplation stage, 137
    in behavior change, 52
Contingency management, 283
Conversion disorder, 339, 341–342, 350, 425
Cooperation with interview, 236
Cooperative learning skills, 3
Coping
    adaptive and maladaptive methods, 81
    model for behavior change, 56
    strengths and cardiac disease, 147–148
    with illness in context of family, 81–82
    with medical adversity, 81
    See also Adaptation and coping
Coprophilia, 411
Cormier, L.S., 113
Cormier, W.H., 113
Coronary artery by-pass graft surgery, 146
Coronary artery disease (CAD), 143, 145–146
    depression and, 147
    morbidity and mortality, 146, 148
    stress and, 146–148
Corpus callosum, 41
Corrigan, 177
Corruption, 96
Cortical gray-matter in brain, 22
Cortical lobes, 41
Corticosteroids, 311, 319
Corticotropin-releasing factor (CRF), 79,
        144–145
Cortisol, 37, 79, 144–145
Coumadin®, 349
Council on Ethical and Judicial Affairs, 121
Counseling, 80
Crane, 95
C-reactive protein (CRP), 145–147

Crespi, E.J., 417
Criminal Justice System, 9
Crisis counseling, 101
Crisp, 177
Cronbach's alpha, 204–205
Cross-sectional studies, 195–196
Cross-sex hormone treatment, 417
Crow, S., 398
Crystal Meth Anonymous, 293
Cultural and ethnic groups
    adaptiveness of diversity, 185–187
    basic principles and definitions, 184–185
    PBL approach to health care in, 183–190
    reducing health disparities among, 187–190
Cultural competence, 190
Cultural components, of bio-psycho-
        social-cultural-spiritual model,
        10–11
Culture, definition of, 185
Cummings, J.L., 372
Current illnesses, bio-psycho-social-cultural-
        spiritual model for, 8
Curtis, J.A., 4
Cushing's disease, 311
Cyclothymia, 321–322
Cyclothymic disorder, 312, 319, 321–322
Cyproheptadine, 328
Cystic fibrosis, 186
Cytochrome P450 2C19 ultra-metabolizer,
        186–187
Cytomegalovirus, 38

D
Dantrolene, 299
Data analysis, in clinical research, 201–202
Dauvilliers, Y., 387
Davis, M., 113
Davis, M.S., 113
DBT (dialectical behavior therapy) program,
        359, 361
Deafness, 38
Death, 38
    addressing family at time of, 215, 225
    description, 22
    diagnosing, 224
    difficulty accepting, 23
    impact on surviving spouse, 221
    PBL approach to, 215–225
    pronouncement, 225
Decision-making, aiding in, 80
Decongestants, 319
Decreased appetite, 172
De Cuypere, G., 419

Dehydration, 272
Delayed development, causes for, 37
De Leon, J., 186–187
Delirium, 6, 238, 271–272, 275, 277, 300, 322,
        367–370
    differential diagnosis, 368–371
    etiology, 374–375
Delusions, 217, 276, 291, 293–294,
        295–297, 374
    disorder, 296, 303, 307
    erotomanic, 293
    grandiose, 293
    of jealousy, 293
    somatic, 294
DeMattia, 95–97, 99
Demeanor, 129
Dementia, 79, 277, 311, 322, 367–370,
        376–379
    bio-psycho-social formulation, 378
    differential diagnosis, 368–371
    etiologies of, 371–372
    laboratory and imaging evaluation for, 373
    stages of, 377
Demerol, 271
Denavas-Wait, C., 155, 159, 161, 165
Dendrites, 20
Denial, 82, 217
Denver, R.J., 417
Denver Developmental Screening Test, 32, 36
Denys, D., 337
Depakote, 280
Department of Health and Human Services
        (DHHS), 159, 167
Dependent personality disorder, 364–365
Dependent personality traits, 249
Depersonalization disorder, 431
Depo-Provera, 412
Depressed mood, 313
Depression, 23, 25–26, 36, 48, 79, 86, 92,
        126–127, 137, 146–147, 188–189,
        211, 215–217, 220–221, 233, 244,
        247, 256, 263, 276, 310, 326,
        329–330, 367, 370, 376, 400–402
    among adolescent, 26
    diagnosis of, 313–314
    differential diagnosis, 318, 370–371
    general medical conditions associated, 311
    grief and, 217
    medications associated, 311
    medications used in, 320–323
    pathophysiology, 313, 320
    pharmacology of medications, 315–317
    pregnancy and, 317

scales, 314
symptoms, 26
treatment option, 313–314
unipolar, 311
vicious cycle of, 147
Depression disorders, 146–147, 248, 290,
        312–313
Deprivation, 90
    from institutionalization
        deficits in, 36
        effects of, 35–36
Desensitization techniques, 86
Desipramine, 315
Detachment from others, 23
Developmental and social history, in
        psychiatric interview and
        assessment, 245
Developmental coordination disorder, 262
Developmental delay, 97
Developmental retardation, 235
Diabetes insipidus, 321
Diabetes mellitus, 92, 133–136, 143, 145, 186,
        189, 311, 403
Diagnostic Interview Schedule for Children
        (DISC), 203–205
Diagnostic tests, in clinical research, 195,
        198–199
Diaphoresis, 272, 278, 330
Diarrhea, 272, 315, 321
Diazepam, 279, 332
DiClemente, C.C., 51, 135
Diencephalic glioma, 319
Diet, 137
    advice, 146
    for stress management, 148
Differential diagnosis, 7, 254–255, 259
    hypersomnias, 389
    interviewing to establish, 235
    mood disorders, 318
    process of, 231–232, 235, 240
    in psychiatric evaluation of child, 254–256
    in psychiatric interview and assessment,
        235, 248–249
    in psychotic disorders, 294
    in substance use disorders, 276–277
Diphenhydramine, 358, 384
Diplopia, 322
Direct assistance, 80
Director, T.D., 90–92
Discomfort, 137
Disinhibition, 272
Disorder of written expression, 262
Disorganized speech, 295

Disorientation, 278
Dispersed care model, 156
Disruption affects, on mother–child
        attachment, 36
Disruptive behavioral disorders, 25, 262
Dissociative amnesia, 431
Dissociative disorders, 431
Dissociative fugue, 431
Dissociative identity disorder, 431
Dissolution, 82
Distractability, 272
Distributive justice, 123–124
Disturbed appetite, 6
Disturbed sleep, 6
Disulfiram, 279, 319
Divalproate, 280
Diversion, for stress management, 148
Divorce, 82
Dizziness, 315–316, 321–322, 330, 332
Doctor-patient communication, 112
Domestic violence, 90, 245
    abuser characteristics, 92
    direct questions, 93
    emotional signs and symptoms, 92
    open-ended questions, 92
    PBL approach to, 89–95
    physical signs and symptoms, 91–92
    risk factors, 91
    screening process, 92
    steps to help victims of, 93–94
Donepezil, 377
Dopamine, 59, 147, 255, 272, 319, 356
Doubt phase, in childhood development, 19
Driving under influence (DUI) conviction, 275
Drowsiness, 322
Dry mouth, 315–316, 322
DSM-IV, 136, 205, 313, 319, 328, 330, 333,
        335, 339, 355, 364–365
DSM-IV-TR, 142, 231–232, 235, 254–255,
        257, 261, 353, 356–357, 360–362,
        370, 374, 384, 393, 410–411, 414,
        426, 427
Dubbert, Rappoport, & Martin, 134
Dulcan, M., 19, 26
Duloxetine, 316
Dwarfism, 37
Dying
    PBL approach to, 215–225
    process, 222
Dyslipidemia, 145
Dysomnias, 389
Dyspareunia, 416
Dyspepsia, 322

Dyssomnia, 382
Dysthymia, 310, 402
Dysthymic disorder, 263, 309–310, 312
Dysuria, 100

E
Early adolescence, 73
Easy going child, 37
Eating disorders, 10, 92, 310
    anorexia nervosa, 394–396
    bio-psycho-social-cultural-spiritual
        formulation, 401–402
    bulimia nervosa, 394–396, 399–402
    complications from, 398
    DSM-IV-TR recognized, 394
    genetic link in, 400
    laboratory findings in, 397
    obesity, 402–405
    PBL approach to, 393–405
    psychological factors and, 401
    signs and symptoms of, 396–397
    social factors, 402
    treatment, 398–400
Eating late and sleeping, 63
Ebert, M.H., 314, 318, 333
Ecstasy, 272, 274
Edema, 283, 301, 307
Educational neglect, 96
Edwards, H.E., 36
Effective communication, 115
    strategy, 82
Eisen, J.L., 334–335
Eisensehr, I., 385
Elder abuse, 95
Electroconvulsive therapy (ECT), 314
Electrolyte abnormalities, 311
Emanuel, E.J., 220–221
Emergency Medical Treatment and Labor
        Act, 128
Emotional
    abuse, 95–96
    complaints symptoms among adoles-
        cent, 26
    development in childhood, 20
    distancing, 82
    distress, 78
    disturbances, 97
    neglect, 96
    pain, 22
    regulation, 26, 36
    signs and symptoms of domestic
        violence, 92

    strategies, 81
    support to adaptation and coping, 80
Emotions, 84
Empathy, 115
    lack of, 95
Employer-sponsored insurance, 153, 155
Enacted-stigma, 171, 174–175, 177–178
Encephalitis, 311, 319
Encephalopathy, 38, 272
Encopresis, 258, 266
Endocarditis, 6
Endocrine and hormonal
    bio-psycho-social-cultural-spiritual model
        for, 9
Endocrine disorders, 8, 212
End-of-life, 77, 79, 81, 85, 215, 218–219
    care PBL approach to, 215–225
    diagnosing death, 224
    discussions, 218
        four-step approach to, 218–219
        goal at, 218–219
        impact on surviving spouse, 221
        issues, 218–220
        pain management, 219–220
        prognosis, 218
        spirituality and religion at, 221–222
        treatment plan, 218
        with family members, 223
Englander, 94
English National Health Service, 156
Enimatehpmahtem, 297
Environmental contaminants, 38
Environmental Protection Agency, 166
Epidemiology, 7
    of non-adherence, 133
Epilepsy, 173, 311, 319
Epinephrine (EPI), 144
Epps, H.R., 113
Erectile dysfunction (ED), 124–125, 414–416
Erikson, 19, 22, 26
Erotomanic delusions, 293, 303
Erythema, 289, 301, 307
Escitalopram, 185, 187, 315
Eszopiclone, 384
Ethical assessment
    domains of, 123
    guidelines in navigating conflicts,
        124–125, 127
    in medical practice, 123–127
Ethics and morality, 121
Ethics and professionalism
    elements of professionalism, 128–129
    learning issues, 123–127

PBL approach, 123–129
 presenting situation, 124–125, 127–128
Ethnicity and medicine, PBL approach to, 183–190
Euthanasia, 215, 220–221
Evaluation principles, PBL approach to, 233–240, 242–251
Event, sensory experience, 86
Excessive daytime sleepiness, and sleeping problem, 53
Executive functioning disturbance, 370
Exercise, 137
 late and sleeping, 63
 for stress management, 148
Exhibitionism, 411
Existential worries, 220
Experimental studies, in clinical research, 195–198
Expression of concern, impact on physician-patient relationship, 113
External validity, 204
Extinction burst phase, in behavior change, 56
Eye contact, 236

F
Factitious disorders, 137, 425
Family
 counseling, 138
 group reliance, 83
 medicine, 4
 members
  addressing at time of death, 225
  end-of-life discussions with, 223
 stressors, 425–426
 violence, 90
Fasting, 396
Fatality, 134
Fatigue, 147, 310, 383
Fear, 37
 of dying, 330
 and sadness correlates in adaptation and coping, 79–80
Feedback, 114
Feeding disorders, 97, 394
Feldhaus, Kozoi-McLain, 93
Feldman, H.H., 370
Felt-stigma, 175–176, 179
Female orgasmic disorder, 416
Female sexual arousal disorder, 74, 416
Fenfluramine, 311
Fentanyl, 220
Ferguson-Marshalleck, E., 80, 84
Fertilization, 70

Fetishism, 411
Fever, 272
Financial abuse, 95
Financial stress, 190
Fineberg, N.A., 334
Fine motor control, 36
Fiore, D.C., 52
Fisher, J.O., 404
Flat affect, 294–295, 303
Flumazenil, 274, 279
Fluoxamine, 315
Fluoxetine, 243, 315, 328, 337, 396, 399
Fluphenazine, 298
Folate deficiencies, 311
Follow rules, 129
Follow-through, 129
Follow-up appointments, 133
Folstein, M.F., 372
Food and Drug Administration (FDA), 166
Forese, L.L., 113
Fractures, 96
Fragile X testing, 260
FRAMES model, for communication of bad news, 114–115
Franko, 400
Fremon, B., 113
Frick, E., 4
Friedman, M.M., 78, 80–82, 84
Frotteurism, 411
Functional analysis
 for behavior change, 49–51, 55

G
Gabapentin, 220
Gambling, 82
Gambling behavior
 addiction, 64
 PBL approach to, 57–58, 64
 Premack principle, 58, 64
 reinforcement schedule, 58–59, 64
Gamma-hydroxy-butyrate (GHB), 272, 274
Garb, J.L., 202
Gaser, C., 41
Gastric cancer, 217
Gastroenteritis, 183
Gastrointestinal complaints, 91
Gay-lesbian-bisexual-transgender (GLBT) rights, 67
Gender, 67, 70
 identity, 67, 69, 71
  in adolescent, 26
 influence on adaptation and coping, 84
Gender identity disorders (GIDs), 71, 263, 416, 418

Gender role, 71
Generalized anxiety disorder (GAD), 326,
        329–332, 334
General lack of interest, 26
Genetics, bio-psycho-social-cultural-spiritual
        model for, 8
Genitourinary trauma, 100
George, M.S., 20
Geriatric Depression Scale, 375–376
Gervin, M., 194
GI distress, 321
Glazed eyes, 26
Glucose-6-phosphate dehydrogenase, 186
Glycogen, 144
Gochman, D.S., 134
Gonococcus, 73
Gonorrhea, 168
Good night sleep, antecedents and
        consequences of, 62–63
Grandinetti, D., 114
Grandiose delusions, 293, 303
Grant, B.F., 355
Gray, K.F., 372
Gray-matter loss, brain maturation process, 23
Greenblatt, M., 221
Grief, 22–23, 233
    depression and, 217
    stages, 215–217
Griseofulvin, 311
Gross motor control, 36
Group A beta hemolytic streptococcal
        (GABHS) complications, 334
Group model HMO, 156
Guanfacine, 257
Guerrero, A.P., 4
Guidance-cooperation model, of physician-
        patient relationship, 112
Guilleminault, C., 386
Guilt, 217
    feeling, 310
    and isolation feelings, 92

H
Hallenbeck, J., 217
Hallucinations, 6, 11, 217, 236, 238, 243, 276,
        291, 294–297, 303, 374
Hallucinogens, 272, 274, 319
Halmi, K.A., 394–400
Haloperidol, 274, 298, 300, 378
Hamilton Rating Scale for Depression, 314
Hansen's disease, 173
Harlow, Harry, 35
Harlow, N., 413

Harris, M.I., 135
Hauptman, P.J., 222
Haynes, Thomas L., 59
Headaches, 91, 283, 315–316, 322
Head size, 38
HEADSS, 133–134
Head trauma, 96, 292
Health
    care rationing, 124
    care system, 92, 157–160, 162–163
        cost of, 157–159
        dispersed model, 156
        insurance and financing in US, 154–162
        medicaid services, 152, 155,
            159–163, 165
        medicare services, 152, 155,
            159–162, 165
        nature of, 154
        PBL approach to, 151–168
        primary care, 154, 156
        public health and, 165–168
        quaternary care, 154
        regionalized model, 156
        role of, 154
        S-CHIP, 152, 155, 162–163, 165
        secondary care, 154, 156
        tertiary care, 154, 156
        uninsured population and, 164–165
        in US, 151–168
    risk behaviors, 146, 148
Health Care Financing Administration
        (HCFA), 159
Health insurance system, 152–162
    See also Health
Health maintenance organization (HMO), 152,
        156–157
Health Resources and Services Administration
        (HRSA), 167
Healthy habits, importance of, 133–134
Healthy lifestyles, promotion of, 137
Hearing
    deficit, 48
    impairment, 38
Heart
    murmur, 6
    rate, 37
Heat intolerance, 315
Heavy metal poisoning, 37
Hedley, A.A., 403
Heidenreich, T., 84
Helplessness, 217
Hematemesis, 283
Hematoma, 128

Hemodialysis, 319
Henry J.Kaiser Family Foundation (KFF),
    159–160, 162–163, 165
Hepatic disease, 311
Hepatic encephalopathy, 372
Hepatitis, 38, 189, 321–322
Hepatitis B immunizations, 73
Heroin, 271–272, 274
Herpes simplex, 38, 319
Herpes zoster, 38
Higgins, E.S., 20
Hippocampal volume, reduction in, 79
Hirschsprung disease, 258
Histrionic personality disorder, 360–362
HIV, 38, 72, 171–173, 311
HMO health insurance plan, 152
Hobbs, K.E., 404
Holmes, S.D., 146
Homeostasis, 144
Homicidal tendency, 6, 239, 311
Homosexual behaviors, 72
Homovanillic acid, 356
Honesty, 129
Hope, T., 123
Hopelessness, 173, 217, 220–221
Hospice, 215
    and palliative care, 222
House, J.S., 80
Hovering, 92
Hrabovsky, Z., 417
Hudson, P.L., 220
Hulshoff, Pol, 417
Human behavior
    change stages, 51–52
        5 A's approach to, 52
        action stage, 52
        contemplation stage, 52
        maintenance stage, 52
        precontemplation stage, 51
        preparation stage, 52
    functional analysis, 50–51
    principles, 49
    stimulus control strategy, 53
Human learning, neurobiology of, 59
Human papillomavirus vaccine, 73
Human sexual response cycle, 67, 74–75
Humor, 148
Huntington's disease, 311, 319
Huot, 36
Hutson, J.M., 417
Hydralazine, 311, 319
Hydrocodone, 220, 249
Hydroxyzine, 382, 384

Hyman, Steven E., 59
Hyperglycemia, 298
Hyperlipidemia, 158, 298, 403
Hyperprolactinemia, 300
Hyperreflexia, 122
Hypersomnias, 310, 313, 389
    differential diagnosis, 388
    epidemiology, 387
    PBL approach to, 387–388
    treatment, 388–389
Hypertension, 11, 73–74, 86, 92, 124, 143,
    145, 158, 272, 278, 282, 312, 403
Hypertensive tendency, 6
Hyperthermia, 11, 299
Hyperthyroidism, 297, 326, 329
Hypoactive sexual desire disorder, 74, 416
Hypochondriasis, 334, 339
Hypoglycemia, 329
Hypokalemia, 127, 311
Hypomania, 319
Hyponatremia, 311
Hypoparathyroidism, 311
Hypophyseal-pituitary-adrenal (HPA) axis,
    144–145
Hypophyseal-pituitary-adrenal hormonal
    system, 148
Hypopituitarianism, 311
Hypotension, 126, 298
Hypothalamic-pituitary-adrenal axis, 36–37
Hypothalamus, 59, 417
Hypothesis testing, 200
Hypothyroidism, 212, 244, 290, 309, 311, 321
Hypoxia, 38
Hysteria, 345

I
Ibuprofen, 242, 249, 311, 343
Ignorance, 96
Illegal drugs use, *see* Substance abuse
Illicit drugs, 9
Illicit substances, 8
Illness, sharing information about, 80
Imipramine, 315
Immune system, 148
    stress and, 146
Impulse control disorders, 429, 431–432
Inadequacy feelings, 92
Inappropriate sex talk, 72
Inattention, 272
Incest, with children, 97
Increased aggression, 90
Increased daily stressors, 92
Increased family cohesion, 83

Indian Health Service (IHS), 167
Individual's immediate, role in adaptation and
     coping, 80
Individual counseling, 138
Individual method, 82
Individual Practice Association (IPA), 156
Indomethacin, 311
Inductive care, 283–284
Industry and inferiority phase, in childhood
     development, 22
Infant and mother attachment, 35
Infant mortality, 189
Infectious hepatitis, 311
Infertility, 398
Inflammatory bowel disease, 145
Influenza, 311, 319
     underimmunization for, 189
Informational support, to adaptation and
     coping, 80
Inhalants, 272, 274
Injuries, 86, 134
     domestic violence signs and symptoms,
          91–92
     during pregnancy, 92
     inner thigh and arm, 91
Inner thigh and arm injuries, 91
Insight, 239
Insomnia, 243, 301, 310, 312–313, 315–316,
          322, 326, 389–390
     causes, 54, 62
     differential diagnosis, 382
     PBL approach to, 62–63, 382–384
     treatment, 384
Instable relationships, 36
Institute of Medicine (IOM), 165
Instrumental support, to adaptation and coping,
     80
Instruments and diagnostic tests, in clinical
     research, 195, 198–200
Insulin-dependent growth factor (IGDF), 145
Intelligent child, 37
Interest, loss of, 310
Interleukin-6 (IL-6), 145–147
Intermittent employment, 92
Intermittent explosive disorder, 431
Internal reliability, 204
Internal validity, 204
Interpersonal psychotherapy, 314
Inter-rater reliability, 204
Interval data, 195, 198
Interviewing
     assess safety specifically, 234–235
     components, 231–232

elicit history to establish differential
     diagnosis, 235
establish and maintain rapport, 234
PBL approach to, 231, 233–240
process of, 231
See also Psychiatric interview and
     assessment
Intimacy, 84
Intimate partner violence, 90, 97
Intimidation, 90
Intoxication
     delirium, 277
     syndrome, 271, 276
     with substance abuse treatment, 274–275
Intracranial mass, 342
Iron deficiency anemia, 38, 48
Irresponsible behavior, 26
Irritability, 26, 272, 313
Isolation, 96, 173
Isolative behavior, 25
Isoniazide, 319

J
Jacova, C., 370
Jacox, A., 220
James, S.A., 113
Jaundice, 185–186
Jealous delusions, 293, 303
Jefferson, 310, 318, 327–328, 331
Jenike, M.A., 334, 337
Job dissatisfaction, 145–146
Joint problem solving strategies, 82
Jones, E.G., 78
Judge, S., 35
Judgment, 239
Jurkovich, G.J., 225
Justice principle, 123–124
Juvenile Offenders and Victims National
     Report, 102
Juvenile victims, 102

K
Kahn, M.J., 222
Kahn, R.L., 80
Kandel, E.R., 319, 327
Kapplan, 342
Kaufman, D.M., 4
Kawas, C.H., 373
Keel, 400
Kennedy, L., 135
Kerins, D., 415
Kervasdoue, J., 154
Keshavan, M., 357
Kimberly, J., 154

Kleine–Levin syndrome, 387, 389
Kleinman, A., 185
Kleptomania, 431
Klismaphilia, 411
Klonopin®, 332
Knopman, D.S., 373, 376
Knowledge, patient-based integration, 3
Koenig H.G., 222
Koenigsberg, H.W., 355
Koerner, K., 361
Kohl, H.W., 404
Kohlenberg, B., 8
Korsch, B.M., 113
Kruijver, F.P., 417
Kubler-Ross, E., 217
Kurahara, D., 186
Kuzma, J.W., 196
Kwiatkowski, D.P., 186

L
Laboratory studies, 100
    in psychiatric interview and assess-
        ment, 247
Lactose tolerance, 186
Lamotrigine, 322
Language, 129
    delay, 259–260
    disorders, 262
    skills, 36
Laraque, 95–97, 99
Larson, D.G., 218–219, 222
Lasting cough, 26
Late adolescence, 73
Lateral nystagmus, 272
Lau, A.S., 95–97
Laughter, 148
Law and ethics, 121
Lawrence, A.A., 419
Lead poisoning, 38, 48
Learning
    affective emotional regulation, 20
    concept of lifelong interest in, 4
    disorder, 249, 254, 318
    disorder mood, 265
    issues in childhood development, 19–20,
        22–23
    lifelong interest in, 4
Lee-Chiong, T.L., 385
Left dorsal frontal and parietal lobes, thinning
        in children, 23
"Let-down" feeling, 147
Lethargy, 272
Levodopa, 319

Lewis, M., 20, 22
Lewis-Fernandez, R., 185
Lichen simplex chronicus, 307
Liebschutz, J., 93
Lifelong interest in learning, concept of, 4
Lifestyle changes, 133
Lightheadedness, 141
Limbic system, 6, 11
Linden, J.A., 90–92
Linehan, M.M., 361
Lipoproteins abnormalities, 143
Literature review, in clinical research, 194
Lithium, 320–321
Liver disease, 134
Logic, 123
Longing and searching, 23
Longstreth, W.T., 387
Long-term retention of knowledge, 4
Loosen, P.T., 314, 318
Loranger, A.W., 355
Lorazepam, 330, 332, 341
Lou Gherig's disease, 122
Low, 95–97, 99
Low birth-weight, 38
Lower educational achievement, 92
Low self-esteem, 25–26, 92, 173
Low social support, 145–146
Lung disease, 134
Luteinizing hormone releasing hormone
        (LHRH) agonists, 413
Luthar, S.S., 37
Lymphadenopathy, 310
Lymphoma, 311
Lyseng-Williamson, K., 415
Lysergic acid diethylamide (LSD), 272, 274

M
Machin, D., 204
1-2-3 Magic, 56
Magnesium sulfate, 274
Mahowald, M., 124
Maintenance stage, 138
    in behavior change, 52
Major depressive disorder, 305, 309–310, 312,
        314, 376, 383–384, 395, 404, 424
Maladaptive methods, of adapting to and
        coping with medical adversity,
        81–82
Maladaptive personality traits, 137–138
Malaria, 186
Male erectile disorder, 74, 416
Male orgasmic disorder, 416
Malignancies, 8, 309

Malingering, 136–137, 305, 424–425, 429–430
Malnutrition, 37
Malpractice risk
    and apologies in medicine, 113–114
    impact on physician-patient relation-
        ship, 112
Managed care organization (MCO), 156
Mania, 319
Manic depression, 310, 319
    See also Bipolar disorders
Manic symptoms, 243
Mann, K.V., 4
Marijuana abuse, 244, 271–272, 274, 358, 387
Marriage equality rights, 67
Martikainen, P., 221
Mastery model, for behavior change, 56
Masturbation, 72, 409
Maternal environmental conditions, role in
        brain development, 36
Mathematics disorder, 262
Mazicon, 279
McCarty, C.A., 95–97
McClure, M.M., 357
McCubbin, H.I., 81
McCubbin, M.A., 81
McDaniel, S.H., 113
McDonald, K.C., 95–97, 97
McGrew, M.C., 4
McLeer, 93
McParland, M., 4
Meagher, D.J., 374
Measurement tools, for clinical research,
        195, 198
Mechanistic case diagramming, 4
Media violence, 102
Medicaid services, 152, 155, 159–163, 165
Medical adversity, adaptively and maladap-
        tively coping with, 81
Medical fragility, 97
Medical neglect, 96
Medicare Advantage program, 160
Medicare services, 152, 155, 159–162, 165
Medication
    bio-psycho-social-cultural-spiritual model
        for, 8
    regimens, 133
    therapy, 284
    use and sleeping problem, 53
"Medigap", 160
MedlinePlus: Child Sexual Abuse, 101
Mehler, P.S., 395, 399
Meier, E.D., 222
Melham, N.M., 23

Memory, 238, 367–368
Meningioma, 372
Menopause, 9
Menses related conditions, 311, 319
Menstrual cycle, 9
Mental
    disorder, 136, 330, 430
    health services, 166
    illness, 36, 173, 177, 291, 329
    retardation, 38, 254, 259–261, 265–266
    screen for health disorders, 26
    status, 6
Mental Health Parity Act of 1996, 166
Mental status examination (MSE), 231–232,
        235–239, 372
    components of, 236–239
    in psychiatric interview and assessment,
        246–247
Menu, 115
Mepridine, 271
Mercury poisoning, brain damage by, 38
"Mesolimbic reward circuit", 59
Meta-analysis
    in clinical research, 207–208
    criteria for, 207
Methadone, 220, 271, 274, 278, 279
Methamphetamine, 6–7, 10–11, 272, 274, 358
    abuse, 187
    dependence, 294
    induced psychotic disorder, 306
    intoxication, 233
Methyldopa, 311
Methylenedioxymethamphetamine (MDMA),
        272, 274
Methylphenidate, 292–293, 319
Metronidazole, 311
Meyer, W., 418–419
Michigan Alcohol Screening Test (MAST),
        282, 286
Microcephaly, 38
Middle adolescence, 73
Migraine headaches, 311, 319, 321, 425, 428
Mild cognitive impairment, 367
Miller, W.B., 35
Miller, W.R., 135
Milliman Medical Index (MMI), 157–158
Mini Mental State Examination (MMSE),
        371–373, 375–376
Miosis, 272
Mirtazapine, 316
Miscarriages, 90, 398
Mitchell, J.E., 398
Mixed delusion, 303

Modafinil, 388–389
Modeling, 49
Molestation, 97
Moller, 419
Mongolian spots, 190
Monoamine oxidase inhibitors (MAOIs),
     314–315
Mononucleosis, 311
Mood disorders, 10, 17, 36, 254, 266, 290,
     296, 306, 311–313, 403, 426, 429
  diagnosis of, 313–314
  differential diagnosis, 318
  due to general medical condition, 309–310,
     312, 318
  PBL approach to, 309–323
  substance-induced, 312
  treatment option, 313–314
  See also Depression
Mood–expressed emotional state, 236
Mood liability, 11
Moore, 310, 318, 327–328, 331
Morbidity, 89
Morphine, 220, 224
Morrison, M.S., 222
Mortality, 89
  from breast and cervical cancer, 189
  risk factors, 134
Moscicki, E. K., 314
Mother–child attachment, 35–36
Motivation, loss of, 147
Motivational interviewing technique, 136–137
Motivations in medicine, ethical assess-
     ment, 123
Motor activity, 236
Motor cortex, 41
Motor development, in childhood, 22
Motor vehicle accidents, 311
Motor vehicle-related fatality and injury, 134
Muehlbauer, 95
Multimodal Treatment Study of ADHD
     (MTA), 255
Multiple
  infarcts, 372
  injuries, 91
  sclerosis, 145, 319, 342, 372
Multi-Society Task Force on PVS, 224
Munchausen syndrome, 350
Murphy's sign, 108
Muscle
  rigidity, 272, 299
  wasting, 398
Musical training, verbal memory and, 40–41
Musicians, gray matter volume in brain of, 41

Mutability, 37
Mutual participation model, of physician-
     patient relationship, 112
Mydriasis, 272
Myelin, 20
Myelination, process of, 26
Myocardial infarction (MI), 143, 146–147,
     205, 312
Myths, 82

N
Nalesnik, S.W., 4
Naloxone, 274, 279
Naltrexone, 279–280
Narcan, 274
Narcissistic personality disorder, 360, 362
Narcolepsy, 311, 387–389
Narcotics Anonymous, 284
National Coalition on Health Care (NCHC),
     157–158, 162
National Epidemiologic Survey on Alcohol
     and Related Conditions (NESARC),
     355–356, 360, 364
National Institutes of Health (NIH), 167
National Institute of Justice, 90
National Institute of Mental Health (NIMH),
     203–204
National Institute on Drug Abuse, 281
National Violence Against Women Survey, 90
Nausea, 141, 172, 272, 315–316, 321–322,
     330, 423
Neale, M.S., 113
Necrophilia, 411
Nefazodone, 316
Negative enacted-stigma, 174
Neglect, of child, 90
  See also Child neglect and abuse
Negrete, V.F., 113
Nelson, 19
Nemeroff, 36
Nephrotic syndrome, 321
Network model HMO, 156
Network Therapy, 284
Neural circuitry, mother–child attachment
     disruption and, 36
Neurobiological mechanisms, 7
Neurobiology
  of human learning, 59
  of psychosis, 294–301
  of reinforcement, 59
Neurodermatitis, 307
Neurodevelopment, in childhood, 19–20
Neuroimaging, 260

Neuroleptic malignant syndrome, 299
Neurological functioning, and mother–child
        attachment, 36
Neurological illnesses, 8
Neuronal circuitry, affects on global
        development, 37–38
Neuro-peptide Y, 144
Neurosyphillis, 319
New Pathways Program, 4
Nicotine, 8–9, 330
    dependence, 279–280
    use and sleeping problem, 53
Nicotine replacement therapy (NRT), 279
Nightmare disorder, 389
Nitrofurantoin, 311
N-methyl-D-aspartate (NMDA) antagonists,
        272, 278, 280, 377–379
Nocturnal bruxism, 390
Nocturnal enuresis, 390
Nocturnal myoclonus, 389
Nocturnal penile tumescence (NPT), 414
Nominal data, 195, 198
Non-abused children, brain structure and
        function in, 41
Non-adherence
    causes of, 133
    clinical attention, 136
    epidemiology of, 133
    PBL approach to, 133–138
    reasons for, 136
Non-bizarre delusions, 291, 296, 303
Noncompliance, causes for, 188–189
Noncompliant behaviors modeling, 138
Nonmaleficence principle, 123–125, 127
Non-parametric statistical tests, 195, 198
Norepinephrine (NE), 11, 144–147, 255,
        278, 327
Normal development, variant in adolescent, 26
Normalizing strategies, 82
Normal pressure hydrocephalus, 311
Norman, G.R., 3–4
Nortriptyline, 315
Nuisance, 325
Numbness, 23
Nurcombe, B., 314, 318
Nutritional deficiency, 38, 212

O
O'Connon, K.J., 222
Obesity, 133–138, 145, 173, 186, 400
    causative factors for, 404
    interventions for, 405

PBL approach to, 133–137, 403–405
psychiatric co-morbidities screened for,
        403–404
Observational studies, in clinical research,
        195–197
Obsessive-compulsive disorder (OCD), 71,
        263, 334–337, 364, 395, 402
    pathophysiology and treatment, 335–336
Obsessive-compulsive personality disorder
        (OCPD), 334, 336, 364
Obstetrics, 4
Obstructive sleep apnea, 311, 403
Occupational Safety and Health Act (OSHA),
        168
Oculogyric crisis, 299
Odds ratio, 207–208
Ohayon, M.M., 387
Olanzapine, 298, 300, 320, 322, 357, 399
Olff, 327
Olsson, 419
Operant conditioning, 49–50
Ophthalmologic studies, 100
Opioids
    abuse, 283
    use, 269, 272, 274, 278, 311, 319
    withdrawal, 273
Oppositional defiant disorder (ODD), 254,
        262, 265, 318
Oquendo, M.A., 323
Oral contraceptives, 311
Ordinal data, 195, 198
Organ donation, 215, 222–224
Organization for Economic and Co-operation
        Development (OECD), 157
Orgasmic disorder, 74
Orientation, 238
Orlistat, 405
Orthostatic hypotension, 315, 322
Osteoarthritis, 81
Ostracism, 82
Overanxious disorder, 402
Overeaters Anonymous, 399
Oversensitive norepinephrine system, 79
Oxycodone, 242

P
Pain, 272
    disorder, 339, 427–428
    management, 86
    medications, 8
    palliative care and,
        219–220
    with defecation, 100

Paliperidone, 298
Palliative care, 215
   hospice and, 222
   pain management in, 219–220
Palpitations, 141, 328, 330
Pancreatic cancer, 311
Pancreatitis, 321
Panic
   attack, 142, 329–333
      pathophysiology, 330–331
      treatment, 331–332
   disorders, 249, 315, 326, 334
Papanicolau smear, 73
Parametric statistical tests, 195, 198
Paranjape, A., 93
Paranoid delusions, 291, 305
Paranoid personality disorder, 296,
      355–356
Paraphilias
   characteristics of, 411
   treatment of, 413
Parasagittal meningioma, 319
Parasomnias, 389
   differential diagnosis, 385
   PBL approach to, 385–386
   treatment, 386
Parasuicidal behavior, 361
Parasympathetic nervous system (PNS), 144
Parent's death, preadolescent girls grief
      for, 23
Parkinson's disease, 193, 198–199, 294, 297,
      299, 311, 372
Paroxetine, 315, 328, 337
Partialism, 411
Partner problems, 136
Partner Violence Screen, 93
Passive appraisal strategies, 82
Pathological gambling, 429
Patient's support system, 221
Patient autonomy principle, 123–127
Patient barriers, in end-of-life issues, 218
Patient-based integration, of knowledge, 3
Patient-doctor relationships, 310
Pediatric autoimmune neuropsychiatric disor-
      ders associated with streptococcal
      infections (PANDAS), 334
Pediatrics, 4
Pediatric Symptom Checklist, 71
Pedophilia, 410–413
Peer identification, 284
Pelkonen, 328
Pellagra, 311
Penetration, 72

Penicillin, 168
Perceptions, 6, 238
Perinatal infectious disease, 38
Periyakoil, V.S., 217
Persecutory delusion, 303
Perseverance, 37
Personality change, 26, 290
Personality disorders, 92, 235, 263
   criteria, 355
   diagnosis, 355
   PBL approach to, 353–365
Personality traits, correlated with resilience, 37
Personal social skills, 36
Personal values, 137
Pervasive developmental disorder (PDD), 71,
      254, 259, 261, 265–266
Petronis, K.R., 314
Pharmacogenomic testing, 187
Pharmacotherapy, of addictions, 279–280
Phelan, T.W., 56
Phenacetin, 311
Phencyclidine, 272, 274, 319
Phenelzine, 315
Pheochromocytoma, 319
Phillips, D., 113
Phobias, 263, 329, 331–333–334
   diagnosis and treatment, 333
Phonological disorder, 262
Physical abuse, 90, 95–96, 243, 310, 318,
      424, 426
Physical changes, in adolescent, 26
Physical development, during adolescence, 73
Physical disabilities, 173
Physical fatigue, 26
Physical neglect, 96
Physical signs and symptoms, of domestic
      violence, 91–92, 220
Physician-assisted suicide (PAS), 215,
      220–221
Physician barriers, in end-of-life issues, 218
Physician-patient relationship
   active–passive model, 112
   apologies and, 113–114
   case tables, 116–119
   communication of bad news, 114–115
   communication skills impact, 113
   effect on outcome, 112–113
   expression of concern impact, 113
   factors affecting alliance, 113
   guidance-cooperation model, 112
   impact on malpractice risk, 112
   models, 112
   mutual participation model, 112

Physician-patient relationship (*Cont.*)
    PBL approach, 107–115
    psychological and social factors
        influence, 112
Physician-support programs, 114
Piasecki, M., 8
Pica disorder, 394
Placebo, 255
Plasticity, of child's brain, 41
Pleasure, loss of, 310
Plethysmography, 412–413
Pneumococcus, under immunization
        for, 189
Pneumomediastinum, 398
Point of Service (POS) plan, 156–157
Poor
    attention, 278
    concentration, 310
    growth inside womb, 38
    judgment, 26
    night of sleep, 62–63
Porphyria, 311
Posterior rib fractures, 96
Postpartum blues, 317
Post-partum depression, 35, 317
Postpartum period, 9
Poststroke Trauma, 319
Posttraumatic personality disorder, 355
Post-traumatic stress disorder (PTSD), 90, 92,
        212, 256–257, 325–327
    diagnostic criteria for, 328
    pathophysiology, 327
    symptoms, 327
    treatment, 328
Potter, G.G., 370, 376
Poverty, 97
Prazosin, 311, 328
Preadolescent girls, parent's death grief, 23
Precontemplation stage, 137
    in behavior change, 51
Prediction-error signal, 59
Prednisone, 311
Preferred Provider Organization (PPO) plan,
        156–157
Prefrontal cortex, 41, 59
Pregnancy, 9, 160–161, 172–173
    bio-psycho-social-cultural-spiritual model
        for, 8
    complication, 398
    injuries during, 92
    with HIV status, 171–175
Premack, David, 58
Premack principle, 58

Premarital sexual activity, 72
Premature ejaculation, 74–75, 416
Prematurity, 97
Premenstrual dysphoric disorder, 249, 317
Prenatal care, 92, 171
Preoccupation with thoughts, 23
Preoperational developmental phase, in
        childhood, 20
Preparation stage, 138
    in behavior change, 52
Prepare and repair systems, 144
Preschool-age child, sexual behavior in, 72
Primary care physician (PCP), 156, 358
Privately funded employer-sponsored health
        insurance, 153, 155
PRN analgesics, 220
Problem-based learning (PBL) approach
    adaptation and coping in medical setting,
        78–87
    analysis, 6
    anxiety disorder, 325–337
    childhood disorders, 253–263, 265–267
    child neglect and abuse, 95–102
    clinical research studies, 193–212
    cognitive disorders, 367–379
    concept of, 3–4
    culture and medicine, 183–190
    death and end-of-life care, 215–225
    domestic violence, 89–95
    eating disorders, 393–405
    ethics and professionalism, 123–129
    ethnicity and medicine, 183–190
    evaluation principles, 233–240, 242–251
    health care system, 151–168
    hypersomnia, 387–389
    insomnia, 382–384
    mood disorders, 309–323
    non-adherence, 133–138
    parasomnia, 385–386
    personality disorders, 353–365
    presenting situation, 4–6
    psychotic disorders, 289–299
    quantitative measures in healthcare,
        193–212
    sexual development, 68–75
    sexual disorders, 409–420
    sleeping problem, 53–54, 62–63
    smoking cessation, 49–53, 61–62
    somatoform disorders, 339–350
    stigma and medicine, 172–181
    stress and health, 142–148
    substance use disorders, 270–287
    suicide, 309–323

tantrums, 55–57, 63–64
   violence and abuse, 89–101
Professionalism
   elements of, 128–129
   ethics and, *see* Ethics and professionalism
   lapse in, 128
Profuse sweating, 141
Progressive exercise, 146
Promethazine, 274, 280
Propanolol, 311, 321
Propositioning strangers, 72
Prostitution, 97
Protocols, for clinical research, 201
Provigil ®, 388
Psoriasis, 321
Psychiatric disorders, 244, 403, 424
Psychiatric evaluation of child
   ADHD, 254–256
   child abuse, 256
   developmental disorder, 259–263
   differential diagnosis, 254–256
   encopresis, 257–259
   PBL approach to, 253–263, 265–267
   PDD, 261
   PTSD, 256–257
Psychiatric illness, 215
Psychiatric interview and assessment
   components of, 231–232
   developmental and social history, 235, 245
   differential diagnosis, 235, 248–249
   establish and maintain rapport, 234
   family history, 244
   formulation, 247–248
   history of present illness, 242–243
   laboratory studies, 247
   mental status examination, 246–247
   past medical history, 244
   past psychiatric history, 243–244
   PBL approach to, 233–240
   physical examination, 246
   relevant biological and psychological
      factors, 247–248
   relevant socio-cultural and spiritual
      factors, 249
   review of systems, 245–246
   specific safety assessment, 234–235
   treatment plan, 248, 250–251
Psychiatric morbidity, among adults, 23
Psychiatry, 4
Psychogenic dwarfism, 37
Psychological
   abuse, 90, 95

components bio-psycho-social-cultural-
      spiritual model, 9, 11
   distress and masturbation, 72
   and social factors influence on
      physician-patient relationship, 112
   stress, 145, 342
   unavailability, 96
Psychomotor seizure disorder, 386
Psychosis, 126, 315
   due to substances, 297
   and general medical conditions, 297, 306
   neurobiology of, 294–301
   risks associated with, 291–292
   See also Psychotic disorders
Psychosocial
   needs, 215
   stress, 143, 147
   stressors, 145, 148
Psychotic disorders, 137, 395, 404, 429
   antipsychotic agents, 297, 300–301
   differential diagnosis, 294
   due to substances, 297
   and general medical conditions, 297, 306
   mechanisms and treatments, 297, 299
   medications for, 297–298
   neurobiology of, 294–301
   pathophysiology, 294–297
   prodrome of, 290
   risks associated with, 291–292
   symptoms, 291
   treatment resistance, 303
Psychotic stress disorders, 431
   See also Psychotic disorders
Psychotic symptoms, mechanism of, 5
"Psychoto-mimetic" effect, 297
Puberty, and brain maturation, 26
Public health, 166–167
Puchalski, C.M., 222
Punishment, 49
Purposelessness and futility about future, 23
Putnam, S.M., 113
Put patient first, 129
Pyromania, 429, 430–432

Q
Q fever, 319
Quantitative measures in healthcare, PBL
      approach to, 193–212
Quetiapine, 298, 300, 301, 320, 322
Quinsey, V.L., 410

R
Radiological studies, 100
Radlow, M., 113

Rahe, R.H., 146
Ramelteon, 384
Rape, 9, 97
    misconceptions about, 94–95
Rapport, during psychiatric interview and
        assessment, 234
Rash, 322
Rasmussen, S.A., 334–335
Rasmussen Report, 166
Ratio data, 195, 198
Reading disorder, 262
Reasoning from principles, 123
Recent Life Change Questionnaire (RLCQ),
        145–146
Recovering community identification, 284
Red eyes, 26
Reflex tachycardia, 315
Refractory panic disorder, 315
Regionalized care model, 156
Regularity, and sleeping problem, 53
Reinforcement, 49–50
    for gambling behavior, 58–59
    neurobiology of, 59
    schedule for
        gambling behavior, 58–59
        tantrums, 55
Reinforcers, 50
Rejection, 96, 174, 243
Relationships
    instability in, 36
    problems, 136
Relative risk, 207
Relaxation
    for stress management, 148
    techniques, 86, 220
Reliability, 204
Religion, at end-of-life, 221–222
Religious beliefs, influence on adaptation and
        coping, 84
Renal failure, 398
Repeated health complaints, 26
Research question, identification in clinical
        research, 194
Reserpine, 311
Resilience, 36
    neural substrate and, 36
    personality traits and, 37
Respect, 129
Response inhibition, 26
Responsibility, 114, 129
Responsiveness, 129
Restless leg syndrome, 389
Retinal hemorrhages, 96

Rett's disorder, 262
Reward, 49, 59
    system of brain, 59
Reward Prediction-Error Hypothesis, 59
Rhabdomyolysis, 299
Rheumatic fever, 186, 334
Rheumatoid arthritis, 148, 311
Rheumatologic disorders, 235
Riffenburgh, R.H., 207
Right intraventricular meningioma, 319
Riluzone, 122
Risperidone, 274, 298, 300, 399
Rodriquez, F., 113
Rodwin, V.G., 154
Role flexibility, 83
Rollnick, S., 135
Ropper, A.H., 314
Rosenheck, R.A., 113
Rowley, J., 387, 389
Rubella, 38
Rumination disorder, 394
Ruth, E., 156, 160

S
Sadness, 6, 86, 217
Sadock, B.J., 312–313, 317, 332, 336–337, 342
Salinsky, J.V., 113
Sampling technique and sample size, in clinical
        research, 199–200
Samuels, J.F., 314
Satiety agents, pharmacotherapy of, 280
Scaffolding, concept of, 20
Scapegoating, 82, 85–86
Scapular, 96
Schaffer, 26
Schizoaffective disorder, 296, 321
Schizoid personality disorder, 355–357, 364
Schizophrenia, 193, 233, 237–239, 263,
        290–291, 294–296, 298–299, 303,
        305–306, 319, 321, 356–357,
        368, 372
    catatonic type, 299
    disorganized type, 299
    paranoid type, 298–299
    residual type, 299
Schizophreniform disorder, 294–295, 305–306
Schizotypal personality disorder, 294, 296,
        306, 355–357
Schlaug, G., 41
Schmidt, D., 385
Schmidt, H.G., 3–4
School-age child, sexual behavior in, 72
School performance, change in, 25

Schwartz, J.M., 337
Scratch dermatitis, 307
Screaming, 81, 83, 86–87
Seat belts, 137
Sedation, 298, 315–316, 321–322, 332
Seigel, J.M., 389
Seizures, 8, 38, 187–189, 243–244, 272, 292, 297
Self-Advocacy, 115
Self-control development, 26
Self-inflicted trauma, 98
Self-monitoring of blood glucose (SMBG), 135, 138
Self-selection sampling, 199
Self-serving behaviors, 20
Self-soothe, inability to, 36
Self-stigma, 171, 173–174
Sense
    of control and security, 23
    of failure, 383
    and reasoning integration, 26
Sensitivity of tests, in clinical research, 195, 199
Separation anxiety disorder, 424
Serious illness, 9
Serotonin, 147, 272
Serotonin-selective reuptake inhibitors (SSRIs), 8, 74–75, 314–315, 328, 412, 429
Serotonin syndrome, 315
Serotonin system, abnormal function of, 79
Sertraline, 315, 328, 337
Service, 129
Severe Stevens–Johnson syndrome, 322
Sex, 67
Sexual abuse, 90, 95–97, 243, 257, 310, 424, 426
    of adult, 90
    assessments guidelines, 100–101
    of child, 90, 318
Sexual activity, 73
Sexual acts, 72
Sexual Addiction Workbook, 412
Sexual aversion disorder, 74, 416
Sexual behavior, in preschool and school-age child, 72
Sexual brain development, 70
Sexual development
    in adolescents, 67, 72–73
    in adults, 67, 73–75
    basic definitions, 70–71
    in children, 67, 69, 71–72
    PBL approach to, 68–75

Sexual disorders
    DSM-IV-TR and, 416
    erectile dysfunction, 413–416
    PBL approach to, 409–420
    pedophilia, 410–413
    treatment of, 412–413
Sexual dysfunction, 315
Sexual exploitation, of children, 97
Sexual intercourse, 72–73
Sexuality issues, for elderly and medically –i patients, 67
Sexually transmitted disease, 134
Sexual masochism, 411
Sexual maturity rating (SMR) stage, 73
Sexual organs, development of, 70
Sexual orientation, 67, 71
Sexual sadism, 411
Shame, 175–176, 179
Sheikh, J.I., 376
Shift worker syndrome, 387
Short MAST (S-MAST), 286–287
Shulman, K.I., 373
SIADH, 322
Sibutramine, 405
Sick sinus syndrome, 321
Significance level, in clinical research, 200
Signs and symptoms, of domestic violence, 91–92
Sildenafil, 413, 415–416
Silence, 86
Simple random sampling, 199
Singhal, V., 405
Sjögren's arteritis, 311
Skaer, T.L., 414
Skills development, in childhood, 19
Sleep
    apnea, 387, 388, 389
    difficulty in, 310
    disorders
        hypersomnia, 387–389
        insomnia, 382–384
        parasomnia, 385–386
        PBL approach to, 381–388
    disturbances, 90, 217
    duration and sleeping problem, 53
    hyperhidrosis, 390
    patterns change, 25
    problem, 53–54
        causes, 54
        daily activities and, 53
        PBL approach, 53–54, 62–63
        sleep duration and, 53
        stimulus control strategy to, 54

Sleep (*Cont.*)
  stages, 386
  for stress management, 148
  walking, 389
Slurred speech, 278
Smaller hippocampus, 41
Smith, Y.L.S., 419
Smoking, 143, 146, 148, 271
  cause of premature death, 270
  cessation, 51–53, 137
    5 A's approach to, 52
    action stage, 52
    contemplation stage, 52
    education, 146
    functional analysis, 50–51
    importance of, 276
    maintenance stage, 52
    PBL approach, 49–53, 61–62
    precontemplation stage, 51
    preparation stage, 52
    stages, 51–52
    stimulus control strategy, 53
    tools, 52
Smucker, 26
Snoring, and sleeping problem, 53
Sobralske, M., 420
Social change, family role in, 81
Social components, of bio-psycho-social-
    cultural-spiritual model, 9, 11
Social isolation, 90, 97, 174
Socialization, problem with, 36
Socially adept child, 37
Social network relationship, role in adaptation
    and coping, 80
Social phobia, 263, 315, 326, 331–333,
    395, 402
Social skills, 35
Social support, 97, 145–146
  for stress management, 148
Social withdrawal, 97
Socio-cultural and spiritual factors, in
    psychiatric interview and
    assessment, 249
Sociocultural values, influence on adaptation
    and coping, 84, 87
Socio-economic status (SES), 146
Somatic delusion, 303
Somatic delusions, 294
Somatization disorder, 318, 339, 362
Somatoform disorders, 307, 339–350, 424–425
  PBL approach to, 339–350
  symptoms, 345–346, 349–350
Somatosensory cortex, 41

Somnambulism, 385–386
Somnolence, 322
Soothing support, 81
Sowell, E.R., 23, 26
Specificity of tests, in clinical research, 195,
    198–199
Specific regions thinning, in brain, 23
Speech, 6, 236
Speech slurring, 272
Spinous process, 96
Spirituality
  bio-psycho-social-cultural-spiritual model,
    10–11
  at end-of-life, 221–222
  influence on adaptation and coping,
    84–85, 87
  needs, 215
Spitzer, M., 360
Spouse
  abuse, 90, 93
  impact of death on, 221
Stable angina, 124
Stadol, 283
Staff model HMO, 156
Stages of Change model, 136
State Children's Health Insurance Plan
    (S-CHIP), 152, 155, 162–163, 164
Statistical errors, in clinical research, 200
Statistical power, 200
Statistical test, in clinical research, 201–202
Statistics, 193
"StaT" Screening Tool, 93
Staying in bed and worrying, effects on
    sleeping, 63
Steffens, D.C., 370
12-Step facilitation, 283
Sternal fractures, 96
Steroids, 8
Stigma, 82–83, 86
  effects on seeking and receiving health
    care, 171–176
  enacted, 171, 174–175, 177–178
  faulty assessment and treatment due to,
    171, 173–174
  felt, 175–176, 179
  PBL approach in health care, 172–181
  physician role to reduce effects of, 171,
    175–176, 180–181
  positive and cooperative responses,
    176, 180
  of pregnancy with HIV status, 171–176
  self, 171, 173–174
  of suicidal ideation, 177–181

Stiles, W.B., 113
Stimulants, 269
Stimulus control strategy, 49
   for change in human behavior, 53
   for smoking cessation, 53
Stoic disposition, 77, 79, 85–86
Stop Child Molestation Book, 413
Strains, 81
Stratified sampling, 199
Streptococcal pharyngitis, 187
Streptomycin, 311
Stress, 37, 310
   management techniques, 148
   PBL approach, 142–148
   psychological, 145
   psychosocial, 143, 147
   reducing communication, 81
Stressors, 81, 144, 235
   family, 423–424
   psychosocial, 145, 148
Stroke, 311–312
Strosahl, K., 172
Structured Clinical Interview for DSM-IV TR
      (SCID), 282, 286
Student health plan, 166
Study design, for clinical research, 194–197
Subacute bacterial endocarditis, 311
Sub-clinical depression, 147
Subdural hematoma, 372
Submersion burns, 96
Substance abuse, 92, 95, 97–98, 137, 148, 167,
      173, 189–190, 244, 249, 277, 310,
      329, 400
   mechanism of action, 5
   program, 11
   treatment of intoxication with and
      withdrawal from, 274–275
   See also Substance use
Substance Abuse and Mental Health Services
      Administration (SAMHSA),
      162, 167
Substance dependence, 290, 305
   disorders, 277
Substance-induced disorder, 326
Substance-induced mood disorder, 249,
      309–310, 318
Substance-induced persisting amnestic
      disorders, 277
Substance intoxication, 329
Substance use, 25–26
   and addiction, 270
   bio-psycho-social-cultural-spiritual model
      for, 9

disorders, 10, 82, 235, 431
   assessment, 282–284
   categories of, 276–277
   clinical manifestations, 271–275
   cost of, 270–271
   differential diagnosis, 276–277
   epidemiology, 270–271
   management, 277–281
   mechanisms, 271–275, 278
   morbidity and mortality, 270–271
   PBL approach to, 270–287
   prevention, 281
   treatment, 271–275, 279–280, 283–284
   See also Substance abuse
   induced psychotic disorder, 306
   symptoms of, 26
Substance withdrawal disorders, 277
Sudden mood changes, 26
Suicide, 239, 296, 311–314, 317, 326
   attempts, 8, 82, 92, 310
   ideations, 147, 217
   PBL approach, 309–323
   physician-assisted, 220–221
   thoughts, 310
Sulfamethoxazole, 311
Supplementary Medical Insurance Trust
      Fund, 159
Support, 129
Sympathetic nervous system (SNS), 144–145
Symptoms, 349–350
Synapse, 20
Syncope, 347
Syphilis, 38, 73, 189, 311, 372
Systematic sampling, 199
Systemic lupus erythematosus, 311, 319, 372
Systems barriers, in end-of-life issues, 218

T
Tachycardia, 11, 126, 272, 278, 293, 315, 328,
      330, 374
Tachycardic tendency, 6
Tachypnea, 329
Tadalafil, 415
Tagamet, 283
Tangentiality, 11
Tantrums
   antecedents and consequences to,
      63–64
   coping model, 56
   extinction burst phase, 56
   extinguishing phase, 57
   functional analysis, 55
   mastery model, 56

Tantrums (*Cont.*)
    PBL approach to, 55–57, 63–64
    reinforcement schedule, 55, 63–64
Tardive dyskinesia, 299
Taylor, D.J., 381
Tearfulness, 83, 85
Teicher, M.H., 41
Telephone scatologia, 411
Temporal lobe epilepsy, 311, 386
Tennyson Center for Children, 101
Terminally –i patient, 217, 222
Terrorism, 96
Testosterone, 73, 412
Tetracycline, 311
Thalassemia, 186
Thiamine, 274–275
    deficiencies, 311
Thorazine, 298
Thought content, 237
Thought process, 6, 237
Threatened physical abuse, 90
Threats, 82
Thrombocytopenia, 321–322, 398
Thyroid disorders, 8, 249, 310, 319, 329
Thyromegaly, 310
Tibial edema, 310
Tic symptoms, 334
Time for self-care, 84
Time management, for stress management,
    129, 148
Tissue necrosis factor alpha (TNF-a), 145, 147
Tobacco use, 269, 277
Tobin, D.R., 217
Toga, A.W., 23, 26
Tongue, J.R., 113
TORCH infection, 38, 48
Tourette's disorder, 262
Tourette's syndrome, 334
Toxoplasmosis, 38
Tramadol, 282
Transient global amnesia, 431
Transitions, 81
Transsexualism, 417
Trans-theoretic Model of Change, 94
Transvestic fetishism, 411
Tranyl-cypromine, 315
Trauma, 243–244, 311
    developmental stage and, 84
    effects, 36, 84–85
    history of, 9
Traumatic stress, 327–328
Trazodone, 274, 280, 382

Treatment plan, in psychiatric interview and
    assessment, 248, 250–251
Treatment planning, bio-psycho-social-cultural
    formulation process of, 231,
    235, 240
Trembling, 330
Tremors, 272, 278, 316, 321–322, 329
Triamcinolone, 311
Triangling, 82
Trichotillomania, 429
Tricyclic antidepressants (TCAs), 220,
    314–315, 319
Troubled relationship, 85–86
Trzepacz, P.T., 375
Tuberculosis, 189, 311
Tuomilehto, J., 186

U
Unhealthy diets, 146
Uninsured US population, health care for,
    164–165
Unintentional injury, 311
Unipolar depression, 319
United States
    health care
        cost, 157–159
        expenditure on, 157–160, 162–163
        per capita spending on, 157–158
        system, 157–168
        uninsured population and, 164–165
        See also Health
    health insurance and financing in, 154–157
Up to date, 129
Uremia, 311
Urinary retention, 315
Urophilia, 411
Urticaria, 322
US Census Bureau, 163
US Public Health Service (USPHS), 167, 277
US Public Health Service Commissioned
    Corps, 167
Uvulopalatopharyngoplasty (UPPP), 389

V
Vaginal
    bleeding, 100, 172
    discharge, 100, 172
    infections, 91
Vaginismus, 416
Valeri, S.M., 95–97
Validity, 204
Valium®, 332
Valkonen, T., 221
Valproate, 320

Valproic acid, 321, 430
Van der Heide, A., 220
Vardenafil, 415
Varenicline, 279–280
Vasospasm, 272
Vegetative state, 224
Venlafaxine, 316
Ventral tegmentum, 59
Verbal abuse, 92
    effect on brain development, 41
Veteran's Administration, 9
Veterans Affairs (VA) system, 152–153, 155
Vetulani, Jerzy, 59
Viagra ®, 413, 415
Vinblastine, 311
Vincristine, 311
Vineland Adaptive Scales, 260
Violence, 82, 239
    cycle of, 94
    exposure to, 36
    PBL approach to, 89–101
Vision deficit, 48
Visual Diagnosis of Child Abuse, 101
Visual disturbances, 329
Visual hallucinations, 293
Vivitrol, 280
Vomiting, 172, 272, 315,
            321–322
Voyeurism, 411

W
Wagstaff, A.J., 415–416
Waitzkin, H., 113
Walsh, F., 80
Warfarin, 349
Washington, E.T., 4
Watching television in bed and sleeping, 63
Waxy flexibility, 299
Weight
    changes, 310

gain, 313, 315–316, 321–322
    loss, 217, 316, 383
Weisser, R.J., 113
Weissman, D.E., 223
Weisz, J.R., 95–97
Wernicke's encephalopathy, 275
Weschler Intelligence Scale for Children
            (WISC), 254, 266
Wiener, J., 19, 26
Williams, G., 94, 225
Williams, S.K., 263
Wilson's disease, 311, 319
Wise, M.G., 375
Withdrawal
    from substance abuse treatment, 274–275
    syndrome, 271, 276
Wolf, M.H., 113
Women, infants, and children (WIC)
            program, 168
Wood's Lamp of Skin, 260
World Health Organization, 220
Worthlessness feeling, 217, 247, 310

X
Xanax®, 332
Xerosis, 301, 307, 398

Y
Yager, J., 397–399, 402
Yelling, 82
Yesavage, J.A., 376
Yohimbine, 319
Young adults, health habits importance for, 134

Z
Zhou, J.N., 417
Ziprasidone, 298, 300
Zisook, S., 4
Zolpidem, 282, 382
Zoophilia, 411